ANAESTHETIC
EQUIPMENT

Second Edition

ANAESTHETIC EQUIPMENT

PHYSICAL PRINCIPLES AND MAINTENANCE

C. S. Ward MB, BS, FFARCS

Consultant Anaesthetist
The Royal Infirmary
Huddersfield, England

Baillière Tindall   London   Philadelphia   Toronto
Sydney   Tokyo

Baillière Tindall
W.B. Saunders

24–28 Oval Road
London NW1 7DX

The Curtis Center,
Independence Square West, Philadelphia,
PA 19106–3399, USA.

1 Goldthorne Avenue
Toronto, Ontario M8Z 5T9, Canada

Harcourt Brace Jovanovich Group (Australia) Pty Ltd
32-52 Smidmore Street, Marrickville,
NSW 2204, Australia

Harcourt Brace Jovanovich Japan Inc.
Ichibancho Central Building, 22–1 Ichibancho
Chiyoda-ku, Tokyo 102, Japan

© 1985 Baillière Tindall

First published 1975
Second edition 1985
Reprinted 1987 and 1989

Typeset by Inforum Ltd, Portsmouth
Printed and bound in Great Britain by Mackays of Chatham PLC, Letchworth

British Library Cataloguing in Publication Data
Ward, C.S.
  Anaesthetic equipment.—2nd ed.
  1. Anesthesiology—Apparatus and instruments
  I. Title
  617′.96′028   RD78.8

  ISBN 0–7020–1008–1

Contents

Preface

The first edition of this book was written primarily for the anaesthetist, though it was also intended to help the theatre technician, the anaesthetic nurse and the staff of the intensive care ward. However, it also proved to be of value to the manufacturer, his service engineer and his technical representative. Anaesthetic apparatus is described in many of the larger textbooks of anaesthesia, but these may not be read by some of the above or by the trainee anaesthetist during the earlier part of his career. Nor do all these books give the more practical details of the day-to-day management of anaesthetic equipment.

Those in charge of anaesthetic departments need more than a general understanding of anaesthetic apparatus. A knowledge of the mode of operation of the equipment and the maintenance required, as well as of some of the commoner causes of mechanical failure, is important. It is the intention of this book to provide this information, as well as to suggest a 'cockpit drill' for the regular checking of equipment. Accidents, both trivial and serious, have occurred only too often as a result of damage to, or misuse of, anaesthetic apparatus. These accidents might often have been prevented by a better understanding of the mechanical principles involved and more efficient maintenance. It is not, however, intended that this book should act as a passport to anyone to interfere with anaesthetic apparatus in any manner beyond his capabilities.

The instruction of trainee anaesthetists includes so many complicated aspects of anaesthesia and para-anaesthetic subjects that the practical use of the anaesthetic machine is often left to be 'picked up as they go along'. They become familiar only with the type of apparatus and the methods used in the particular hospital where they train. Many of these anaesthetists will eventually work in remote parts of the world, where the apparatus available may be quite different, being limited by lack of funds, manpower and long lines of communication. It is for this reason that some types of equipment that will be regarded by many readers as primitive and old-fashioned are described. Indeed, some items, particularly in the chapters on ventilators and dental anaesthesia, are no longer manufactured. However, they are still in use in large numbers, and they have been included also because they demonstrate principles that are important to the practice of anaesthesia. In any case, some items seem to get regularly reinvented from time to time, apparently without the innovator knowing of their prior existence!

In many countries the anaesthetist does not have the assistance of the operating department assistant (theatre technician), which he has come to expect in Great Britain. He will need to supervise the checking and maintenance of apparatus himself.

The chapter on dental anaesthesia may seem unusual, if not extraordinary, to those who work in countries where this is not carried out. However, it is (still) a reality in others and must therefore be included. In contrast, those working in the more developed countries will be surprised to learn how much reliance is placed on systems such as the EMO and OMV elsewhere.

The list of ventilators described in Chapter 11 may disappoint some readers until they realize that this is not a catalogue of the most recently developed models. Such a catalogue would soon become out of date. Instead, the chapter describes a number of ventilators which exemplify the principles involved, so as to equip the anaesthetist with enough knowledge and experience to understand the newer developments as they occur.

Paediatric anaesthesia has a chapter to itself, and a new chapter has been devoted to the control of atmospheric pollution.

The chapter on sterilization does not describe all methods, but rather a few that are considered adequate and yet relatively easy to institute in any hospital that may not possess facilities for more sophisticated methods.

It has been difficult to decide which units of measurement should be given in the text. There are many instances where the older units have been employed, and equivalents given, because of their popularity or the fact that much equipment is still calibrated in these rather than SI units.

There are instances where the terms used are not those that are listed in British Standard 6015 (ISO 4135), 'Terms Used in Anaesthesiology'. This is because many of the older terms will remain in common parlence for a long time to come.

The book has been enlarged, with the addition of new chapters. Therefore, some material, such as the monitoring of functions other than those directly concerned with the anaesthetic machine, have had to be deleted.

Exhaustive lists of references have not been given, since it is unlikely that the reader for whom this book is intended will need them! However, under 'Further Reading' there are references to some of the 'classic' texts and to important information that the reader might otherwise find difficult to trace.

C. S. Ward

Acknowledgements

In the preparation of this book I have received help from so many people that I beg forgiveness from any whom I might inadvertently fail to mention here.

I have received much assistance from many manufacturers and their representatives, both in the provision of photographs, drawings and samples of their equipment for evaluation, and in the courtesy extended to me when I visited their factories to see in detail how the equipment was manufactured, assembled and serviced. Rather than mention them here, I have given a list of the names and addresses of these companies at the end of the book.

Many figures were prepared by the Department of Medical Illustration at Huddersfield Royal Infirmary, under the supervision of Mr M. E. Morris. Much of the artwork was drawn, as for the first edition, by Mrs C. Barrett (formerly Miss C. Morten). I am indebted to them for the great care and attention to detail that they have so willingly shown. The members of the Reprographics Department have assisted considerably by special techniques which have helped in the creation of many of the diagrams.

Various pieces of information have been provided by Mr L. Small of the DHSS and his colleagues, and several illustrations have been provided by Professor S. Jorgensen of Odense, Denmark and Dr J. A. Lack of Salisbury, England. The original of the cartoon used for Figure 21.1 was provided by Miss P. Moody.

I am grateful to Professor P.A. Foster of Stellenbosch, South Africa, for details of (and also the gift of) the equipment shown in Figure 12.1; and to Dr H.H. Samson, formerly of Johannesburg, South Africa, for drawings and samples of his 'valveless' breathing system, shown in Fig. 7.3.

The library staff of the Postgraduate Medical Centre, Huddersfield Royal Infirmary, provided much reference material and I appreciate all their hard work.

The heavy burden of secretarial work in preparing and revising manuscripts, as well as making enquiries from other quarters, has fallen upon the secretaries of the Department of Anaesthetics and of the Operating Theatres at Huddersfield Royal Infirmary, under the supervision of Miss I. M. Kennedy.

Dr Nicholas Ball, resident anaesthetist, and Mr Stephen Lunn, operating department assistant (theatre technician), have undertaken the most tedious task of proof reading.

Baillière Tindall, and in particular their senior medical editor, Mr P. Gill, have been most helpful, encouraging and patient in putting the book together.

It is probably that only those involved in the preparation of a textbook appreciate how much the author depends on the help and forbearance of friends, colleagues and, in particular, his family.

Terminology

The interpretation of the various terms employed in anaesthetic practice tend to vary from one anaesthetist to another. Some terms that were incorrectly derived have become so common in usage that they are likely to remain. To prevent confusion a few definitions are given below:

1. *Pulmonary ventilation* (breathing) may be spontaneous or passive and is also known as respiration. Passive ventilation may be achieved by rhythmically inflating the lungs by applying gases at fluctuating pressure to the patient's airway. This is usually abbreviated to *IPPV* (intermittent positive pressure ventilation).
2. *Breathing.* This is divided into three phases:
   (a) *Inspiration* or inhalation;
   (b) *Expiration* or exhalation;
   (c) A period after the end of expiration and before the next inspiration, when no movement takes place, known as the *expiratory pause*. During IPPV there may be a pause after inspiration, before expiration commences, known as plateauing (the airway pressure curve shows a plateau).
   The following terms are also employed:
   (d) *Tidal volume* — the volume of a single breath.
   (e) *Stroke volume* — the volume delivered by a ventilator during the inspiratory phase of IPPV. Part of this volume may fail to enter the patient.
   (f) *Minute volume* — the sum of the tidal volumes of all the breaths in one minute.
   (g) *PEEP* (positive end-expiratory pressure) — which implies that a positive pressure is maintained in the breathing system during the expiratory pause.
   (h) *NEEP* (negative end-expiratory pressure) — which implies that a negative pressure is maintained in the breathing system during the expiratory pause.
3. *Respiratory exchange* is the process in which oxygen in the alveolar air passes into the plasma and carbon dioxide is given up by the plasma to the alveolar air.
4. *Rebreathing* is the reinhalation of any gas that has previously entered the patient's respiratory tract. The rebreathed gases may have previously occupied only the patient's dead space, and therefore this does not constitute functional rebreathing, which is the rebreathing of gases that have already taken part in respiratory exchange.
5. Pressure. *Positive pressure* indicates a pressure above the ambient, and *negative pressure* one below it.
6. *Upstream* is the direction from which gases are flowing. *Downstream* is the direction to which gases are flowing.
7. The *back bar* is that part of a continuous flow anaesthetic machine which dispenses gases and vapours. It includes flowmeters, vaporizers and an outlet.
8. The *breathing system* is that part of the anaesthetic apparatus downstream from the back bar, in which gases are at, or not far from, atmospheric pressure, and from which, and into which, the patient breathes. (For classification, see p. 122.)
9. Gas. Whereas oxygen is a true *gas* (see p. 1), nitrous oxide, carbon dioxide and cyclopropane are strictly speaking *vapours*. They are, however, frequently termed gases, as in (10) and (11) below.
10. *Mixed gas flow* is the mixture of gases (and vapours) that have been metered through the flowmeters.
11. *Fresh gas flow* (*FGF*) consists of the mixed gas flow and vapours of the volatile agents from the vaporizers, which are supplied from the back bar to the breathing system.
12. *Back pressure* is the pressure that has to be overcome by the mixed gas flow as a result of it having to do work, for example by driving a minute volume divider ventilator or passing through a constriction. The term does not imply that the gases flow in a reverse direction to normal.
13. *Dead space.* (See pp. 136–138.)
14. *Rotameter* is a commonly used name for a flowmeter with a rotating bobbin. In fact, 'Rotameter' is the trade name for one particular manufacturer.
15. *Expiratory valve* is a valve through which all expired gases pass, or should pass, either to the external atmosphere or to part of the breathing system.
16. *APL valve.* The adjustable pressure limiting valve allows the escape of excess gases from the breathing system.
17. *Overpressure valve* is a valve which will open under fault conditions to allow the escape of gases if the pressure in it exceeds a preset limit.
18. *Dumping valve* is a valve which allows the ingress of atmospheric air to the breathing system if the pressure in it falls below a preset limit.
19. *Scavenging* is the collection and removal of waste anaesthetic gases from the operating theatre or recovery room. This is usually achieved by attaching hoses and other components to the breathing system.

Abbreviations

AE	Anaesthetic Equipment Ltd (once part of Cyprane)
APL	Adjustable pressure limiting (valve)
atm	Atmosphere (unit of pressure)
BOC	British Oxygen Company (now Ohmeda)
BS	British Standard
BSP	British Standard Pipe (screw thread)
CA	Compressed air
cmH_2O	Centimetres of water (unit of pressure)
COELCB	Current-operated earth-leakage circuit breaker
CSSD	Central Sterile Supply Department
DHSS	Department of Health and Social Security
DISS	Diameter indexed safety system
EBME	Electronic and Biomedical Engineering (Department)
EXH	Exhaust
EXP	Expiratory (valve)
FGF	Fresh gas flow
HEI	Health Equipment Information (issued by the DHSS)
HFPPV	High frequency positive pressure ventilation
HME	Heat and moisture exchanger
HTM	Hospital Technical Memorandum (issued by HM Stationery Office)
ID	Internal diameter
IPPR	Intermittent positive pressure respiration (IPPV is the preferred term)
IPPV	Intermittent positive pressure ventilation
ISO	International Organization for Standardization
INSP	Inspiratory (valve)
lb/in^2	Pounds per square inch (unit of pressure)
MDM	Monitored dial mixer
MGI	Medical Gas Installations Ltd
MIE	Medical and Industrial Equipment Ltd
mmHg	Millimetres of mercury (unit of pressure)
MOH	Ministry of Health (now superseded by the DHSS)
MV	Minute volume

NEEP	Negative end-expiratory pressure
NIOSH	National Institute for Occupational Safety and Health (USA)
NIST	Non-interchangeable screw thread
OD	Outside diameter
OMV	Oxford Miniature vaporizer
Pa	Pascal (unit of pressure)
PEEP	Positive end-expiratory pressure
PI	Pin index
PMGV	Piped medical gas and vacuum (system)
PTFE	Polytetrafluoroethylene (= Teflon; = Fluon)
ppm	Parts per million
PPM	Planned preventative maintenance
psi	Pounds per square inch (unit of pressure)
SDU	Sterilizing and Disinfecting Unit
SI (units)	Système International d'Unités (International System of Units)
SVP	Saturated vapour pressure
TILC	Temperature indicated, level compensated (vaporizer)
TV	Tidal volume
VAM	Vinesthene/aether mixture
VIBS	Vaporizer in breathing system
VIC	Vaporizer in circle
VIE	Vacuum insulated evaporator
VOC	Vaporizer out of circle

1
Physical Principles

The art of anaesthesia is essentially practical. For this reason the anaesthetist must be able to master the physical and mechanical aspects of the apparatus and techniques which he employs. Many unnecessary accidents have occurred as a result of a simple mechanical fault which the anaesthetist had failed to observe, or were caused by the misuse of equipment, the physical principles of which he did not appreciate. The anaesthetist should have the practical manipulations at his fingertips in order that he might devote the necessary proportion of his attention to clinical considerations. The first two chapters of this book are therefore devoted to the physical and mechanical principles of anaesthetic apparatus and the practice of anaesthesia.

In these chapters only the information required to give a simple working knowledge of the apparatus is included. Mechanical details have been given only when they are important for its routine use and maintenance and no mention is made of the more complicated principles that are often involved in its design.

One of the problems besetting the medical profession today is the clinician's inability to discuss his requirements with the engineer in terms that they can both understand. It is to be hoped that the expansion of EBME (Electronic and Biomedical Engineering) Departments will improve this. To this end we should start with the basic concepts of the nature of matter.

Solids, Liquids, Vapours and Gases

In order to understand the functioning of an anaesthetic machine it is necessary to appreciate the difference between the three states of matter.

A *solid* is compact and relatively dense. It maintains its shape unless subjected to quite large forces and is not easily compressed. Its molecules, although in a state of constant agitation, do not change their position relative to each other; hence a solid tends to maintain its shape. Different solids, in contact with each other, do not normally mix.

A *liquid* is also compact. Its molecules are constantly moving relative to each other and, owing to their being densely packed, there are frequent collisions between them. Because its molecules move freely, a liquid takes the shape of the container in which it is confined and moves to one part of it under the influence of gravity. Its shape may be distorted by small forces. Different liquids, in contact with each other, may or may not mix.

A *vapour* or *gas* expands to evenly fill the space within which it is confined. Different vapours or gases in contact with each other normally mix. They are easily compressible. In general, vapours have the same properties as gases and obey the same laws (see pp. 4–5) In everyday terms a vapour is a substance in a gaseous state and at a temperature below or not very much above its boiling point.

The correct distinction between a gas and a vapour is as follows. For any substance there is a maximum temperature at which it can be compressed so as to convert it from a gas to a liquid. Above that temperature, known as the *critical temperature,* no amount of compression will liquefy it. Under these conditions the substance is defined as a *gas.* Below the critical temperature it is termed a *vapour.* For example, the critical temperature of carbon dioxide is 30.9°C. Therefore, unless it is being used at a temperature above 30.9°C (which is unlikely to be the case in anaesthetic practice), it is, correctly speaking, a vapour and not a gas. The *critical pressure* is that which is required to liquefy a gas at its critical temperature. The critical temperatures and pressures of various gases are shown in Table 3.2.

Behaviour of molecules of solids and liquids

The molecules of a solid or liquid attract each other. They may also be attracted by the molecules of another substance. The mutual attraction between the molecules of a substance is termed *cohesion,* and their attraction to those of another substance is called *adhesion.* Let us suppose that there are three

1

molecules of mercury placed in a straight row. Each molecule would attract its neighbour, but the first would also attract the third, so that they would at once move to take up a more compact form (Fig. 1.1).

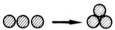

Figure 1.1   The cohesion between three molecules arranged in a straight row causes them to take up a more compact form.

If we now consider a much larger number of molecules of mercury, each one attracting the others, they would tend to take up the shape of a sphere. The force that preserves the periphery of the sphere is called *surface tension*. With a still larger quantity of mercury the sphere would be so large that it would be distorted by the force of gravity (G) and the pressure exerted by the surface on which it rests (Fig. 1.2).

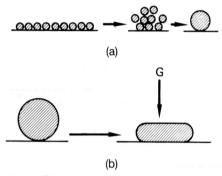

Figure 1.2   (a) The cohesion between a number of molecules causes them to group together in the most compact form, a sphere. (b) The sphere is distorted by the effect of gravity.

Note that the edges of the blob are still circular. This may be observed when a quantity of mercury is spilled and blobs of various sizes are formed. The small ones are nearly spherical, while the larger ones are flattened.

The molecules of other substances may exert less mutual attraction and the force of adhesion to another substance may be greater than the force of cohesion. Thus if there are a number of, for example, water molecules on a glass slide, the outer molecules have a greater attraction for the glass than for the inner ones, so they 'wet' the glass (Fig. 1.3). However, water will not wet a greasy surface, on which it takes up a globular form.

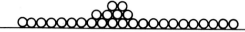

Figure 1.3   The molecules of a substance for which the force of adhesion is greater than the force of cohesion spread out as they wet the surface on which they rest.

If a vertical tube of about 1 cm diameter is dipped in a vessel of water, the top surface of water within the tube forms a *meniscus* with an upturned edge because the water wets the walls of the tube (Fig. 1.4a). Water is drawn a little way up the tube by molecular attraction, against the force of gravity. However, if the water is replaced by mercury, which does not wet the glass, the shape of the meniscus is reversed and the edges are depressed (Fig. 1.4b) since the edge of the meniscus is pulled inwards by cohesion and it resembles the blob of mercury described above (Fig. 1.2).

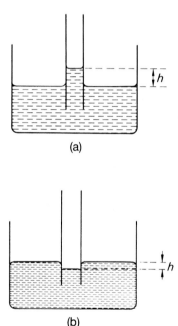

Figure 1.4   (a) If a narrow tube is dipped into a vessel of water, the wetting effect causes the water to rise up the tube and the edge of the meniscus is turned up. The height of the water column *h* depends, apart from other factors, on the diameter of the tube. (b) If the same tube is dipped into a vessel of mercury, the level of mercury within the tube is depressed and the edge of the meniscus is turned down.

Returning to the case of the tube filled with water, if it is an extremely narrow one, known as a capillary tube, a high column of water may be drawn up by the wetting effect of the water on the tube. The force of attraction of the wall of the tube on the column determines the height of the column of water which will be raised. This phenomenon is known as capillary action or *capillarity*. It may also occur, for example, when two closely fitting smooth surfaces of any shape are separated by a thin film of water. Considerable force may be needed to prise them apart.

Use is made of capillarity when a wick is employed in a vaporizer. Since it dips into the liquid agent, the latter rises up it and so presents a larger surface area from which vaporization occurs.

Heat and Temperature

Temperature

Temperature means relative hotness or coldness and is measured in degrees. At normal atmospheric pressure water freezes at a temperature of 0°C (degrees Celsius, formerly Centigrade) and boils at 100°C. Other scales of temperature in common use are the Kelvin (formerly Absolute) and Fahrenheit (0°C = 32°F; 100°C = 212°F) scales.

Kelvin (Absolute) scale. As will be seen on p. 5, the volume of a gas is directly proportional to its temperature. From this it would seem that if it were cooled indefinitely, it would eventually disappear, the temperature at which this would happen being − 273°C or 0K (Kelvin). Of course this does not actually happen because the gas liquefies before that stage is reached, and the gas laws (*see* p. 5) no longer apply. The Kelvin temperature scale starts at this point and the freezing and boiling points of water are 273K and 373K, respectively. Temperature conversion tables are given in Appendix 1, on p. 360.

Heat

In order to raise the temperature of an object it must be made to acquire an additional quantity of energy in the form of heat. Although this should correctly be measured in joules, it is more commonly the practice to express it in calories: 1 calorie equals 4.2 joules. One calorie (cal) raises the temperature of 1 g of water from 14.5°C to 15.5°C (i.e. by 1°C). Other units of heat used are the kcal (kilocalorie or Calorie, which is used in physiological measurements; 1 kcal equals 1000 calories), and the British thermal unit (BTU) which raises the temperature of 1 lb of water by 1°F. 1 BTU is equivalent to 0.252 Calories or 252 calories.

Heat may be transferred by one of the following means:

Conduction. In conduction, heat simply travels along a substance from molecule to molecule. Metals such as copper are good conductors of heat, while, for example, glass and expanded polystyrene are bad conductors. The latter are termed thermal insulators.

Convection. If part of a fluid is heated, it expands and becomes lighter than the fluid around it. Being free to move, it rises, and as it travels upwards its place is taken by the cooler, denser fluid from around it, which in turn is heated and rises. There is, therefore, a constant rising stream above a source of heat, the latter being carried by 'convection'.

Radiation. The amount of heat radiated from a surface depends not only on its temperature, but also on its nature. A matt black surface radiates far more than a smooth shiny one. Heat 'rays' can be focused and directed, as is seen in the electric radiant heater with a reflector.

Specific heat

The quantity of heat required to raise the temperature of a given mass of a substance by a specified amount varies from one substance to another. This is termed *specific heat*, which is defined for a particular substance as the quantity of heat required to raise the temperature of unit mass of that substance by unit temperature. Specific heat may be expressed either in absolute terms or relative to water, 1 cal being required to raise the temperature of 1 g of water by 1°C. For example, as 0.095 cal are required to raise the temperature of 1 g of copper by 1°C, the specific heat of copper is 0.095 cal/g per °C or 0.095 (relative to water).

Latent heat

Considerably more heat is required to vaporize a

liquid than to raise its temperature from room temperature to its boiling point. The heat required to vaporize a liquid is called its *latent heat of vaporization*. For water, this is 539 cal/g at 100°C and normal atmospheric pressure.

The heat required to melt a solid is known as its *latent heat of fusion*. For ice, this is 80 cal/g at 0°C and normal atmospheric pressure.

It is evident that since energy is needed to raise the temperature of a substance, that substance must store energy as *potential energy*. This is achieved by the fact that the molecular agitation and movement become faster and more violent. In the case of a gas, this leads to a greater force of bombardment of the walls within which it is confined and, therefore, to a rise in pressure.

Vaporization

As stated above, the molecules of a liquid are in constant motion, but they also have a mutual attraction for each other.

If the liquid has a surface exposed to air or other gases, or to a vacuum, some molecules will escape from the surface when the force with which they move exceeds that of their mutual attraction to other molecules at the surface. This is the process of *evaporation*. It is increased if the temperature of the liquid is raised, since the molecules move faster and possess more energy. If the atmosphere is enclosed, some of the molecules that have escaped, while moving freely in a gaseous state, impinge on the surface of the liquid and re-enter it. The vapour formed by the molecules exerts a pressure — the *vapour pressure*. Within a confined space there may occur an equilibrium in which the number of molecules re-entering the liquid equals the number leaving it. At this stage the vapour pressure is at a maximum for the temperature and is called the *saturated vapour pressure* (SVP).

If the liquid is heated progressively, a point is reached at which the SVP becomes equal to the ambient atmospheric pressure. Vaporization now occurs not only at the surface of the liquid, but also in the bubbles that develop within its substance. The liquid is boiling and this temperature is its *boiling point*.

From the above it is evident that the boiling point of a liquid depends on the ambient pressure. At high altitudes there is a significant depression of the boiling point. This may render the use of agents such as ethyl chloride, divinyl ether and diethyl ether difficult.

A test for an efficient suction pump is that it can lower the pressure within the receiver to such a point that water within it, at a temperature which can be tolerated by the hand, will boil.

Expansion of solids

As any substance is heated it expands and different metals expand to a different extent. There is a considerable difference between the coefficients of expansion (an index of the amount of expansion per unit of temperature rise) of various metals. If strips of two dissimilar metals are joined tightly together, side by side, and heated, one expands more than the other, causing a deflection of the 'bimetallic strip' that they form (Fig. 1.5). This principle is used in thermostats, some dial thermometers and the temperature-compensating mechanisms of vaporizers.

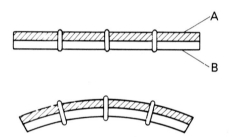

Figure 1.5   A bimetallic strip. Two tightly joined strips of dissimilar metal A and B are initially the same length, but when heated A expands more than B, causing the deflection shown.

Expansion of gases

The molecules of a gas are far more widely separated than those of a solid. This results in two phenomena that do not occur in the case of solids or liquids:
1. A gas expands to evenly fill the space within which it is confined.
2. Gases expand to a greater extent when heated than do solids or liquids.

Properties of Gases

As is the case with all substances, the smallest

particle of a gas that can exist separately is a molecule. Gas molecules are in constant motion, moving about in all directions and occasionally bombarding the walls of the space in which they are confined. It is this bombardment of the walls that exerts the pressure due to the gas.

A vessel may be occupied by more than one gas, in which case the total pressure within it is the sum of the pressures exerted independently by each of the gases. Each gas is said to exert a *partial pressure*.

If a gas is heated, the movement of its molecules becomes more intense and this leads to a rise in pressure. If the volume in which it is confined is constant, its pressure varies directly with temperature. These facts are expressed in Dalton's, Boyle's and Charles's laws as follows:

Dalton's laws relating to vapours

1. The maximum pressure exerted by a particular vapour, in a closed space, at a given temperature, depends only on that temperature, and is independent of the pressure of other vapours or gases (provided they have no chemical action upon it).
2. When several vapours or gases, having no chemical action upon each other, are present in the same space, the pressure exerted by the mixture is the sum of the pressures that would be exerted by each of its constituents if separately confined in the same space.

Boyle's law

Boyle's law states that at a constant temperature, the volume of a mass of gas is inversely proportional to the pressure.

Charles's law

Charles's law states that the coefficient of expansion of any gas at a constant pressure is 1/273. This means that when the pressure is kept constant, the volume of a gas is directly proportional to its absolute (kelvin) temperature.

From the last two laws we may derive the equation

$$\frac{P_1 V_1}{T_1} = \frac{P_2 V_2}{T_2}$$

where P_1, V_1 and T_1 are the pressure, volume and temperature of one case, and P_2, V_2 and T_2 are the corresponding quantities of a second case. T must be expressed in absolute units (kelvin).

The above formula may be used to calculate the results of a change of pressure, temperature or volume of a gas.

The Poynting effect (overpressure effect)

The critical temperature and critical pressure of one gas may be affected by its admixture with another.

If a cylinder is partially filled with liquid nitrous oxide, inverted and then further filled from a high-pressure source of oxygen, an unexpected phenomenon occurs. This may be viewed through the glass observation window of a high-pressure rig. The bubbles of oxygen diminish in size as the gas is partially dissolved in the liquid nitrous oxide through which they pass. Simultaneously, the volume of liquid nitrous oxide diminishes as it evaporates and mixes with the oxygen. Eventually the cylinder, filled to a pressure of nearly 2000 lb/in² (psi) (~ 140 bar), contains mixed nitrous oxide and oxygen, both in the gaseous state. A 50:50 mixture of these two gases is marketed under the name Entonox. Further details of the use of this and the correct handling of the cylinders are given on pp. 32–37. The precautions concerning the cooling of cylinders are necessary because the new critical temperature (known as the pseudocritical temperature) of the nitrous oxide is −6 °C.

Temperature Changes in Anaesthetic Apparatus

The performance of some items of anaesthetic equipment is affected by changes in temperature. A rise in temperature:
(a) increases the vaporization rate of a volatile agent;
(b) causes a fall in density of fluids due to expansion;
(c) reduces the viscosity of liquids;
(d) increases the viscosity of gases owing to increased molecular activity.

As vaporization proceeds there is a fall in the temperature of the liquid, and the vaporizer in which it is contained, owing to the latent heat required, so that unless there is some form of compensation the vapour concentration falls.

Three different measures may be taken to counteract this effect:

1. The temperature of the vaporizer may be indicated on a thermometer so that the anaesthetist can make the appropriate adjustments in order to maintain the desired concentration. Very accurate vaporizers such as the 'Vapor' are temperature indicated, level compensated (TILC) and the calibration takes account of temperature. There is a built-in thermometer.

2. Automatic compensation for temperature changes may be made within the vaporizer, as in the case of the 'Fluotec' halothane vaporizer.

3. A supply of heat may be made available to satisfy the needs of latent heat of vaporization, as a rule by either physically attaching a large mass of metal such as copper, or by immersing the vaporizing chamber in a large mass of water which may be warmed. Again, heat may be obtained by attaching fins, which present a greater surface area in contact with the air and so assist in heat transfer by conduction and convection. Some vaporizers are electrically heated.

Force and Pressure

It is important to understand the terms force and pressure. *Force* causes an object to move in a certain direction. The amount of force does not vary with the area over which it is exerted. The unit of force is the newton. One newton causes a mass of 1 kg to accelerate by one metre per second per second (1 m/s^2). Other units are the kgf and the lbf which exert a thrust of 1 kg and 1 lb, respectively.

Pressure is exerted in all directions and is a measure of force per unit area, i.e.

$$P = \frac{F}{A}$$

Let us consider the intravenous syringe. The user exerts a force on the plunger in one particular direction. The pressure in the fluid in the syringe is exerted in all directions, and if there were a leak in

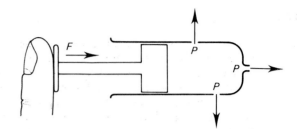

Figure 1.6   When the user exerts a force, F, to the plunger of an intravenous syringe, it is applied in one direction only, while the resulting pressure, P, in the fluid is exerted in all directions.

the barrel of the syringe, the liquid would squirt out sideways (Fig. 1.6).

If a wide-bore syringe is used, the force exerted by the thumb acts over a large area and so the pressure in the syringe is lower than it would be if the same force were exerted on the plunger of a narrower bore syringe.

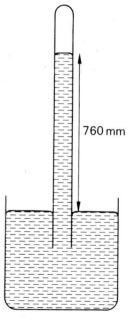

760 mm

Figure 1.7   A simple barometer. The long tube is closed at the top, and although it was filled with mercury before being inverted and placed in the mercury reservoir, the mercury level in the tube has fallen, leaving a virtual vacuum at the top of the tube. The height of the column of mercury indicates the atmospheric pressure.

Pressure and partial pressure

The air in which we live exerts a pressure. At the surface of the Earth this atmospheric pressure is due to the influence of gravity on the mass of air supported, as may be demonstrated as follows:

A long tube, closed at one end, is filled with mercury and then inverted so that its open end rests in a reservoir of mercury (Fig. 1.7). The column of mercury falls until its meniscus is about 760 mm above the level in the reservoir. Above the column there is a vacuum (or near vacuum). The atmospheric pressure acting on the reservoir supports a column of mercury 760 mm high, and is said to be 760 mmHg or 760 Torr. If the column had a cross-sectional area of 1 cm^2, it would weigh 1033 g and the pressure would then be said to be 1.033 kg per square centimetre (kg/cm^2). The average atmospheric (i.e. barometric) pressure at sea level is therefore 1.033 kg/cm$^2 \approx 15$ lb/in$^2 \approx 1.01 \times 10^5$ newtons/m^2 (pascals). However, in many instances it is more convenient to use the units mmHg.

As seen on p. 5, the pressure (or partial pressure) of a gas is the result of the energy expended by its molecules impinging on its confines, and if two or more gases are mixed, the total pressure is the sum of all the partial pressures measured as if they were acting independently of each other. Within a gas or liquid, pressure is exerted equally in all directions.

PARTIAL PRESSURE

If the pressure of a mixture of two gases is 760 mmHg, the partial pressures of each gas added together equals 760 mmHg. If, for the sake of argument, we consider that air contains approximately 20% oxygen and 80% nitrogen, then the partial pressures of these two gases at sea level are:

Oxygen: 20% of 760 = 152 mmHg
Nitrogen: 80% of 760 = 608 mmHg (disregarding other gases and water vapour)

and the barometric pressure equals 760 mmHg (152 mmHg + 608 mmHg).

As the altitude above sea level increases, the barometric pressure decreases, because for each unit of area a shorter column of air is being supported. The relationship between altitude and average barometric pressure is shown in Fig. 1.8.

When treating patients at high altitudes, a larger percentage of oxygen in a gaseous mixture is required to maintain the same partial pressure, and it is the partial pressure rather than the oxygen percentage that is important. It is also necessary to remember that most oxygen analysers measure the partial pressure and not the percentage of oxygen. Therefore, the barometric pressure should be taken into account when oxygen analysis is performed.

Direct methods of measuring pressure

SIMPLE MANOMETER

Figure 1.9 shows the principle of a simple manometer, which is a U-tube partially filled with water. A gas with pressure P has been applied to end A of the tube and end B is open. The pressure P causes the water to be pushed across to the opposite limb of the tube. At a the water level has been depressed by 5 cm from its former position and at b it has been raised by 5 cm. The pressure P is therefore 10 cm of water. If the U-tube were filled with mercury, the pressure would be expressed in millimetres of mercury (Torr). Figure 1.10 shows the basic principle of the mercurial sphygmomanometer, in which the two limbs are of different diameter. The pressure reading is still taken as the difference between the levels of the two columns of mercury, but the reser-

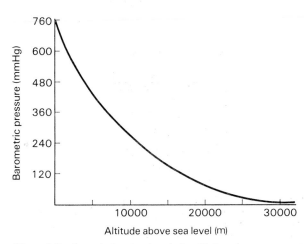

Figure 1.8 A graph showing the relationship between barometric pressure and altitude above sea level.

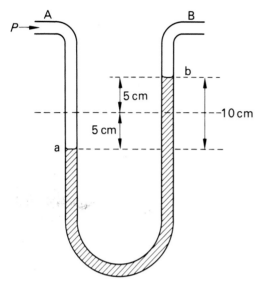

Figure 1.9   A simple manometer. A pressure *P* is applied at A. This causes a depression of the fluid level at a and a corresponding rise of the fluid level at b. In this case the tube is filled with water and the pressure *P* is 10 cm of water.

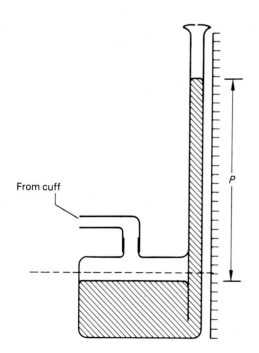

Figure 1.10   The principle of the mercurial sphygmomanometer.

voir limb, being so very much wider than the other, exhibits a very much smaller change in level.

PRESSURE GAUGES

A simple type of *diaphragm* gauge is shown in Fig. 1.11. The gas enters at C and the diaphragm D is distended against the force of the spring S. The rod attaching the diaphragm to the spring has a rack, R, which turns a pinion on which is mounted the pointer. In practice the rack and pinion is replaced by a sophisticated train of gear wheels, and the spring is not needed if the elastic recoil of the diaphragm itself is sufficient. There may, however, be a hair spring to steady and improve the performance of the pointer. The larger and more compliant the diaphragm, the lower are the pressures that can be measured.

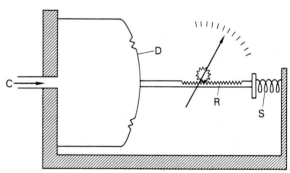

Figure 1.11   A diaphragm pressure gauge. Pressure exerted at C causes deflection of the diaphragm D. This pushes the rack R against the pressure of the spring S, thereby turning the cogwheel so that the pressure is indicated on the scale by the pointer.

The Bourdon tube is a development of the diaphragm pressure gauge. It is normally used for much higher pressures, such as those in a full oxygen cylinder, and may be calibrated up to 30 000 kPa($\sim$ 2000 lb/in^2) or even higher. As will be seen in Fig. 1.12, the chamber with the diaphragm has been replaced by a curved and flattened tube. When the pressure is applied to it, the tube expands and the curvature is straightened out, thus moving the rack and the pinion. Again the rack and pinion is usually replaced by a compound train of gear wheels and there is a hair spring. The inlet to the gauge is fitted with a constriction to prevent sudden surges of pressure damaging the mechanism.

Another type of pressure gauge for both high and

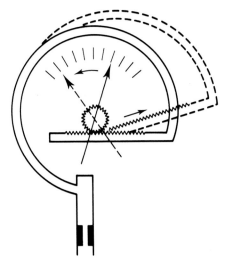

Figure 1.12 The principle of the Bourdon tube pressure gauge. Note the constriction at the inlet.

low pressure is the aneroid gauge. This is frequently used in barometers. Figure 1.13 shows a typical low-pressure aneroid gauge, and Fig 1.14 a typical arrangement for a barometer. Note that in the latter case the capsule is completely sealed; it expands and contracts as pressure changes are applied to its exterior. Changes in atmospheric pressure compress it or allow it to expand, thereby causing movements of the pointer.

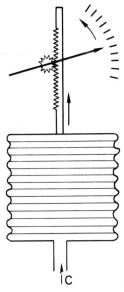

Figure 1.13 A low-pressure aneroid gauge.

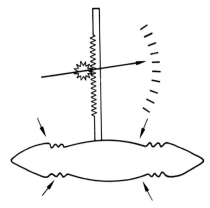

Figure 1.14 A typical arrangement for a barometer. Note that the capsule is closed and the atmospheric pressure acts on its exterior.

Gauges for very low pressure have diaphragms made of neoprene or rubber; these may perish. In some low- and all high-pressure gauges the diaphragm, tubes or capsules are made of various types of metallic alloy.

PRESSURE TRANSDUCERS

Electronic devices may measure pressure, or changes in pressure, by means of a transducer, which converts the pressure into electrical units. Usually action of the pressure on a compressible part of the capsule causes changes in its electrical conductivity or capacitance (see Fig. 1.15).

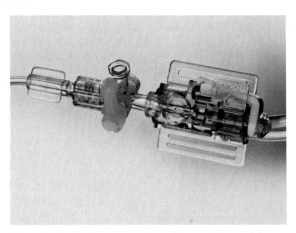

Figure 1.15 A minature transducer for measuring arterial pressure.

Indirect methods of measuring pressure

In some instances it is not practicable to connect a pressure gauge directly to a system in which it is desired to measure the pressure. For example, the routine estimation of arterial blood pressure is made by measuring the equal and opposite pressure that is just sufficient to occlude the artery. A cuff is wrapped around the upper part of the arm and the pressure of air within it is steadily increased by a small hard pump or other device until the pulse in the lower part of the arm is no longer perceptible. At this point the pressure in the cuff, which can be measured using a manometer, is equal to the systolic blood pressure.

Calibration of pressure gauges

A British Standard specification for oxygen cylinder contents gauges recommends that they be marked with calibrations ¼, ½, ¾ and Full, the lowest segment between 0 and ¼ being marked in red in order to urge the anaesthetist to change to a new cylinder in good time. Contents gauges for nitrous oxide cylinders may have a wide segment marked 'Full at varying temperature', below which the only calibration is a small red segment marked 'change' just above zero (Fig. 1.16).

Pressure gauges for high pressures are usually calibrated in lb/in², kg/cm², atmospheres (1 atm ≈ 15 lb/in² ≈ 1.03 kg/cm²), kPa or bars. They are normally calibrated in *gauge pressure*, i.e. the pressure above atmospheric pressure. In this case 'g' may be written after the pressure.

In some circumstances gauges are calibrated in *absolute pressure* (P_{abs}). In such a case a pressure gauge open to the air would indicate a pressure of 15 lb/in² or 1 atm. Examples are the barometer and gauges used in connection with hyperbaric oxygen therapy. Where it is not stated which of these units is used, it is usually understood that *gauge* pressures are being described. It is important to make this distinction in apparatus such as hyperbaric oxygen equipment, where a gauge pressure of, say, 2 atm may be used, which equals an absolute pressure of 3 atm.

For lower pressures, gauges are often calibrated in millimetres of mercury (mmHg) or centimetres of water (cmH₂O). The term 'Torr' is now commonly used in place of millimetres of mercury (normal

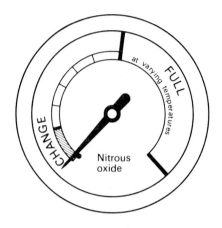

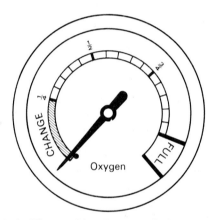

Figure 1.16   Nitrous oxide and oxygen cylinder contents gauges.

atmospheric pressure = 760 Torr).

Conversion tables for the different units of pressure are given on pp. 356–8.

The pressure within a bubble or a balloon

A bubble or droplet is maintained intact by the effect of *surface tension* (T) acting on its surface as if it were enclosing it in a capsule. Since the sphere is the shape that has the smallest surface area per unit volume, a bubble or droplet will tend to take this form. In the case of a bubble, the wall may have two surfaces, an inner and an outer one, as for example when it is floating free in air.

Now if we consider a soap bubble bisected by an

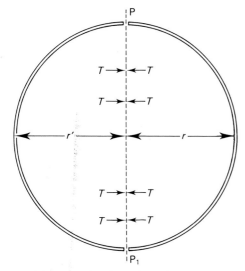

Figure 1.17 A soap bubble bisected by an imaginary plane PP₁. r = internal radius; r' = external radius; T = the surface tension holding the two halves together round the cut circumference.

imaginary plane PP₁ (Fig 1.17), the force preventing the separation of the two halves is the surface tension (T), which acts over the whole of the circumference, i.e. over a length of $2\pi r$ for the inner surface and $2\pi r'$ for the outer. It is usually measured in dynes/cm. In practice r and r' are so nearly equal that they may be taken as identical, so the total force preventing the separation of the two halves of the bubble, $2\pi rT$ plus $2\pi r'T$, may be written as $4\pi rT$.

Now pressure may be expressed as force/area,

i.e.
$$P = \frac{F}{A}$$

A, the area of the cut face of the bubble, is πr^2

So,
$$P = \frac{4\pi rT}{\pi r^2} = \frac{4T}{r}$$

In other words, the pressure in a bubble is inversely proportional to its radius. This was first demonstrated by Laplace and is of particular importance in pulmonary physiology and open chest anaesthesia.

Note that when the anaesthetist inflates the patient's lungs by squeezing the breathing or reservoir bag, if the bag is nearly empty, a greater pressure is exerted on the patient by the same manual effort than when the bag is relatively full.

There is a difference between a gas bubble within a liquid and a balloon constructed of a material such as rubber. In the former, the wall is fluid and the surface tension remains the same however much the bubble is increased in size. In the case of the balloon (i.e. a reservoir bag), as it is distended there is a preliminary stage when the wall assumes a progressively more spherical shape but is not under appreciable tension. Then there comes a time when the material of the wall becomes stretched against its own elastic recoil. Hooke's Law (see pp. 21–22) now begins to apply, and the pressure within the balloon becomes related to the elastic recoil of its walls and therefore to its diameter. This occurs when ventilators such as the East–Freeman Automatic Vent are used, but on the Mapleson A system the expiratory valve usually opens first. Eventually either the elastic limit of the rubber is reached or there is rupture. In this respect the nature of the material from which the bag is constructed is of importance, since some types of rubber are easily stretched, and in the case of accidental closure of the expiratory valve, the reservoir bag becomes distended to an alarming degree, yet the pressure within it does not rise sufficiently (in the short term) to injure the patient. On the other hand, there have been disposable reservoir bags, constructed of other materials, which were by no means so distensible, and within which dangerously high pressures could develop very quickly. Some reservoir bags — such as that in the Flomasta ventilator — are surrounded by a net or similar device to limit distension, since in these cases it is the intention to develop sufficient pressure to inflate the patient's lungs.

The Flow of Fluids Through Tubes and Orifices

By definition a tube has a length considerably greater than its diameter, whereas an orifice has a diameter greater than its length.

Three factors affecting the rate of flow of a fluid through a tube or orifice are its density, its viscosity and the pressure difference across the tube or orifice. The resistance to flow also depends on the diameter and length of the tube, or the diameter of the orifice.

The *viscosity* of a fluid is a measure of its resistance to flow. If we consider a fluid passing along a tube,

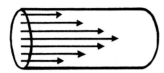

Figure 1.18 The viscosity of moving fluid may be considered to be the resistance between layers within that fluid slipping over one another.

the fluid in the centre of the tube flows more rapidly than that at the periphery, which tends to adhere to the walls of the tube. We can imagine that there are layers of fluid slipping over each other (Fig. 1.18). It is the friction between these layers that causes viscosity. Viscosity is measured in poises (1 poise = 0.1 Pa·s), named after the French physiologist Poiseuille, but a more useful measure for both liquids and gases is the coefficient of viscosity as compared with water.

Both the viscosity and density of a fluid are affected by changes in temperature. In the case of an orifice it is the density that has the most effect, and in the case of a tube, the viscosity.

The flow of fluids through a tube

The relationships between the factors relating to a fluid (which may be a liquid or gas) flowing with laminar flow (see below) through a tube are set out below:

Flow rate $\propto \dfrac{1}{L}$ where L = length of tube,

Flow rate $\propto P$ where P = the pressure difference between the two ends of the tube,

Flow rate $\propto \dfrac{1}{V}$ where V = the viscosity of the fluid,

Flow rate $\propto r^4$ where r = the radius of the tube.

Thus Flow rate $\propto \dfrac{P \times r^4}{L \times V}$

Laminar and turbulent flow
The above formulae refer to fluids, the entire stream of which flows in a straight line. This is known as *laminar flow*. However, under certain circumstances, although the general flow is in a straight

line, eddy currents occur. This is known as turbulence. These eddy currents cause resistance to flow. For any system there is a *critical velocity*, above which the flow becomes turbulent and below which it remains laminar.

Turbulence may also be caused by the flow being deflected by rough areas, passing through a tube of irregular diameter, or passing around sharp bends (Fig. 1.19).

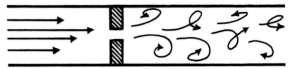

Figure 1.19 Laminar flow becoming turbulent as its smooth pathway is obstructed by an obstacle.

As examples, the design of the inlet to flowmeter tube is important, since turbulence would render the reading inaccurate, and in breathing systems, especially those of the circle type, it increases the resistance and therefore increases the work done in spontaneous breathing. Where there is turbulence a greater pressure is required to maintain the same rate of flow.

The wider the tube, the lower the flow velocity for the same flow rate (volume per unit time) and therefore the less the likelihood of turbulence.

The flow of fluids through an orifice

When a fluid passes through an orifice there is usually turbulence. The flow rate is determined by the pressure difference across the orifice, the density of the fluid and the area of the orifice.

Thus Flow rate $\propto \sqrt{P}$ where P = the pressure difference across the orifice,

Flow rate $\propto \dfrac{1}{D}$ where D = the density of fluid

and Flow rate $\propto r^2$ where r = the radius of the orifice.

Thus Flow rate $\propto \dfrac{\sqrt{P}(r^2)}{\sqrt{D}}$

The effect of changing the bore of a tube

Where the bore of a tube is diminished, the flow velocity is increased, since the flow rate (volume per unit time) must remain the same. The change in diameter acts to some extent as an orifice, and because of this, and the fact that turbulence may occur, the density of the fluid becomes significant. The kinetic energy required to accelerate the fluid through the narrower part of the tube can be calculated and may be expressed as resistance or the pressure difference required to overcome it.

It will be seen, therefore, that for any system through which fluids flow there are three elements of resistance to overcome: (a) those due to the dimensions of the tube, (b) those of an orifice, and (c) those associated with initiating the flow and changing its velocity. A combination of all three is always present, but one or other tends to dominate under different circumstances.

The fact remains that the passages in anaesthetic equipment should be as wide, short, smooth, straight and uniform as possible.

The Bernoulli effect and the venturi

Let us consider a tube which has, along part of its course, a constriction. When a gas passes through the tube it will accelerate when it encounters the constriction.

If pressure gauges are attached at various parts of the tube it is found that as the gas accelerates, the pressure falls (Fig. 1.20a). This is known as the Bernoulli effect. When the gas emerges from the constriction into the wider tube the linear velocity of flow decreases and the pressure increases again. The pressure may rise to a level almost as high as that before the constriction, the extent of this rise being dependent on the design of the tube and the constriction

Advantage of this phenomenon was taken by Venturi, who found that if the shape of this constriction was suitably designed, and there was a side branch to the tube in a suitable position, fluid from the branch would be entrained by the main stream (Fig. 1.20b). In order to achieve this, not only must the constriction be of suitable shape, but also the distal limb of the tube needs to be of gradually increasing diameter.

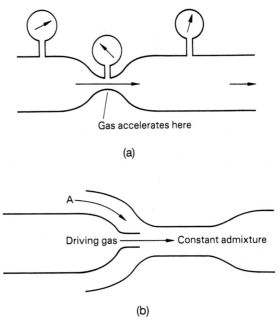

Figure 1.20   (a) The Bernoulli effect. (b) The venturi.

The rate of flow of fluid per unit time is a function of the cross-sectional area of the tube and the flow velocity. Energy is expended in accelerating the flow of fluid to increase its velocity as it passes into the constriction. When it leaves the constriction it will tend to continue to flow at the same velocity, but since the cross-sectional area of the tube is gradually increasing, either it will be slowed down or further fluid may be entrained through the side branch mentioned above or the fluid close to the walls of the tube of expanding diameter will stagnate.

It is one of the features of a venturi that provided the velocity of the driving gas is adequate and there is no change in the configuration of the orifice from which it emerges or of the side branch, the volume of gas entrained will bear a constant proportion to the driving gas. It may, therefore, be used for the mixture of nitrous oxide and oxygen in an anaesthetic machine or in mixing valves such as some oxygen/air blenders.

Apart from their use in mixing gases, venturis may also be used to provide a medical vacuum. Very often the extra cost of using oxygen to drive the venturi is considerably less than the capital expense of installing a separate vacuum line.

Venturis have also been used for assisting the circulation of gases in a breathing system (see p. 166).

The Joule–Kelvin Principle
(Joule–Thompson Effect)

Work has to be done to compress a gas and the energy expended is converted into heat. In some circumstances, such as the compression ignition (diesel) engine, the compression is sufficiently rapid to cause a considerable rise in temperature, resulting in ignition of the fuel vapour. In the same way, if a part of an anaesthetic apparatus contained oil, grease or some other inflammable material and was subjected to a sudden rise of pressure in the presence of oxygen, as when a cylinder is turned on suddenly,

an explosion could occur. For this reason all apparatus using high-pressure oxygen must be free of oil, grease or other inflammable material. Pressure gauges are fitted with a constriction in the inlet to reduce the shock wave that occurs when a cylinder is turned on. Conversely, when a gas expands it does work and the temperature drops. Under normal circumstances in anaesthetic practice, the expansion of a gas leaving the cylinder is not sufficiently rapid to cause a great fall in temperature. The fall in temperature is, for example, much less than the latent heat of vaporization, which is the main cause of cooling of cylinders of nitrous oxide when in use.

Methods of Joining Tubes and Pipes

Metal tubing

Permanent joints are usually brazed or hard soldered. After making such a joint it is important that all traces of flux are removed. More recently a system of brazing copper pipes and brass fittings without flux has been evolved. This is used particularly for medical gas pipeline installations. In the case where provision has to be made for the subsequent disconnection and reconnection of a joint, a *union* is used. This consists of two parts which are held together in a gas-tight manner, usually by a nut or *cap*, which screws onto a parallel male thread. Figure 2.1 shows a *ball-and-cone* or *cone-seated* union, in which the seating is by direct metal-to-metal contact. A *flange* or *flat-seated* union (Fig. 2.2) requires a washer to complete the seal. With pipes carrying oxygen this washer should be of non-flammable material.

Figure 2.3 shows a screwed high-pressure joint such as that where a pressure gauge is fitted to a regulator. It will be noticed that a parallel thread is used and the actual seal is made by a non-flammable washer. For some other purposes tapered threads (Fig. 2.4) may be used and the seal made either by screwing them down extremely tightly or interposing a sealing compound such as PTFE (polytetrafluoroethylene or Teflon), which is supplied as a tape. The joint between the valve block and the body of the cylinder is sealed by a metal foil between two tapered threads. Liquid jointing compounds

such as Locktite may also be used where a screw connection is to be permanent. A joint between a tapered thread and a parallel one (Fig. 2.5) cannot be either pneumatically or mechanically sound.

For low-pressure tubing, compression fittings are commonly used. Figure 2.6 shows a compression fitting, known as the 'Simplifix connection', which is used by several manufacturers. Other types of low-pressure fittings are shown in Fig. 2.7. Compression joints are made by squeezing a soft ring, known as an 'olive', of metal or a suitable plastic between the pipe and the parts of the union, thus making a mechanically strong, gas-tight joint.

2
Mechanical Principles, Pneumatics and Fluidics

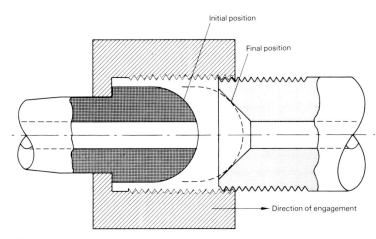

Initial position

Final position

Direction of engagement

Figure 2.1   A cone-seated union.

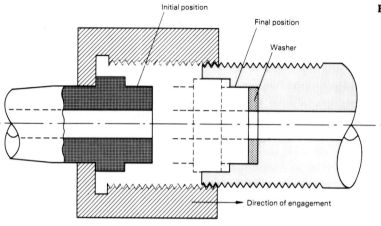

Figure 2.2   A flange- (or flat-) seated union.

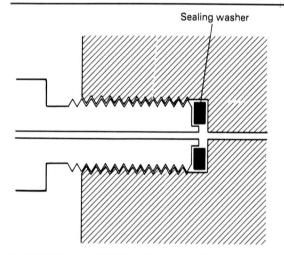

Figure 2.3   The joint such as that between an oxygen regulator and a pressure gauge. Note that the threads are parallel and that a sealing washer is required.

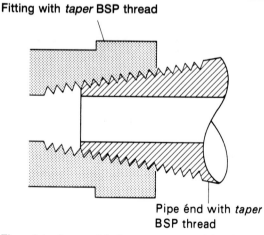

Figure 2.4   A correct joint between two tapered threads.

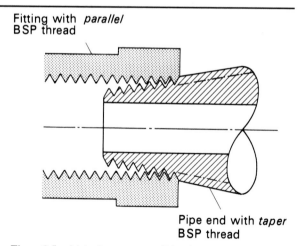

Figure 2.5   A joint between a parallel and a tapered thread. This is both mechanically and pneumatically unsound.

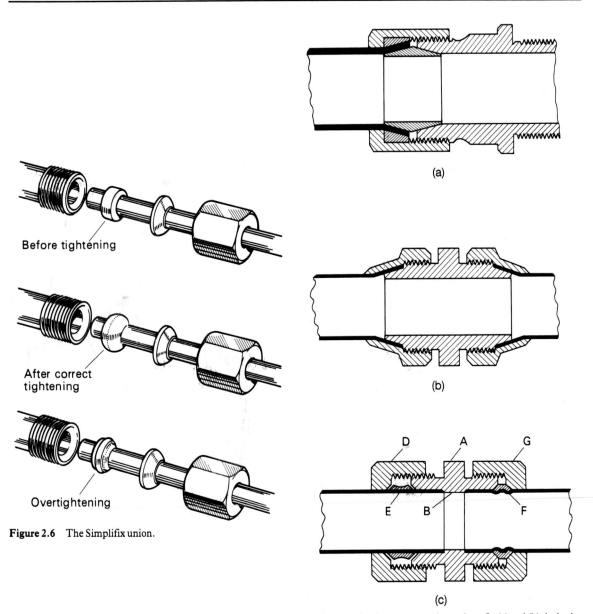

Before tightening

After correct
tightening

Overtightening

Figure 2.6   The Simplifix union.

(a)

(b)

(c)

Figure 2.7   Various compression unions. In (a) and (b) the body
of the tube has been flared. In (c), A is the body of the joint; B, the
shoulder against which the end of the tube abuts; E, the olive
before tightening; F, the olive when tightened; D and G, the nuts
(G has been tightened).

Rubber tubing

Joints in rubber tubing may simply be a push fit over a plain piece of metal tubing (Fig. 2.8). The metal tubing may terminate in a bulbous tip or have a serrated shank (Fig. 2.9). The joint may be made stronger and more permanent by adding a ferrule fixed on by a special crimping tool or pliers (Fig. 2.10). In the case of larger sizes of tubing a 'Jubilee' clip (Fig. 2.11) or O-clip (Fig. 2.12) may be used to secure the joint. Unlike ferrules, Jubilee clips may be released and retightened.

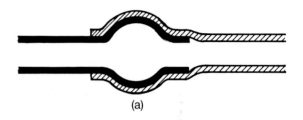

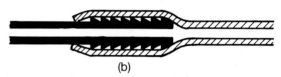

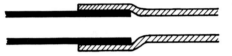

Figure 2.8 A joint made between metal and rubber tubing by a simple push fit.

Figure 2.9 The end of the metal tube has been shaped so as to improve the strength of the joint. (a) The metal tube has a bulbous tip. (b) The metal tube has a serrated edge.

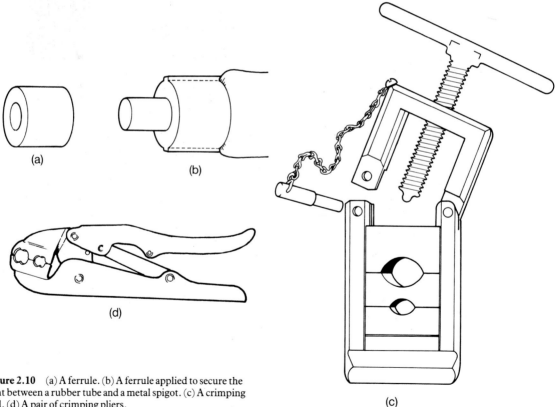

Figure 2.10   (a) A ferrule. (b) A ferrule applied to secure the joint between a rubber tube and a metal spigot. (c) A crimping tool. (d) A pair of crimping pliers.

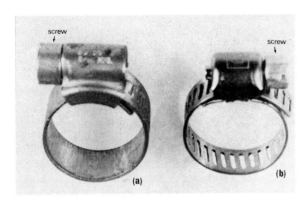

Figure 2.11 (a) A Jubilee clip. Note that these clips can be released and retightened many times. They make a secure joint, but should not be used for joining medical piped gas hoses, where there could be a danger of misconnection; for such connections only permanent joints should be made. (b) A Parker clamp. This is similar to the Jubilee clip, but if applied to soft rubber tubing, the latter may be damaged by the serrations.

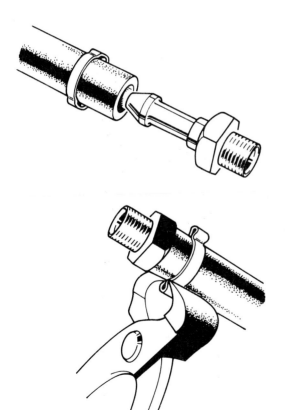

Figure 2.12 The O-clip. This should be used once only and is not suitable for repeated applications.

In so many accidents — including fatal ones — it has been the willing but ill-informed action taken by people not trained in the care of anaesthetic equipment that has led to the accidental cross-connection of pipeline hoses, made possible by this type of fixing.

For the nylon tubes of small diameter used in the interconnection of pneumatic components, joints such as those shown in Fig. 2.13 may be employed. The tube is simply pushed into the orifice, where it is gripped by serrations or some other locking device. Pressure of gas in the tube acts in such a way as to cause slight expansion, which can only tighten the grip.

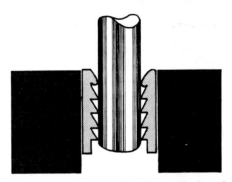

Figure 2.13 A barbed push-in fitting for a rigid nylon tube. A special pair of tube holding pliers may be used for both the insertion and the removal of the tubing: if the tube is reinserted after removal, the end should be trimmed off.

Whenever there is a possibility of mistake, such as the crossover of nitrous oxide and oxygen hoses, permanent connections should be used. In this respect the ferrules now available are far more robust, that of one manufacturer being applied by a 30 ton press! (Fig. 2.14). Where a rubber tube is stretched over a joint it is advisable to protect it from the light to prevent perishing. Rubber tubing supplying compressed gases should be colour coded throughout its length or at least close to a joint, to prevent connections being made to a circuit carrying the wrong gas. Self-coloured hoses are now available.

Screw threads

That screws and nuts have threads of varying diameters and pitches requires no further comment. The threads used for jointing metal tubes and their fittings however, do require further explanation.

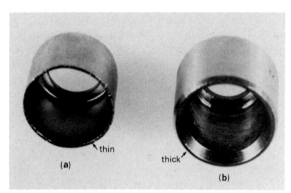

Figure 2.14 Ferrules. (a) An old type by BOC, of thin metal which may be crimped by hand. (b) A more recent type by MIE, constructed of stainless steel and of much greater thickness. A 30 ton press is required for its application.

Traditionally the two threads commonly used in Great Britain were the British Standard Pipe (BSP) thread and Brass thread, which is considerably finer. However, there being a need for non-interchangeable unions, as, for instance, on the inlet to a four-gas flowmeter block, a variety of sizes and types of thread have been employed. Special couplings such as NIST and DISS may be used. On cylinders for certain gases, a left-hand rather than the usual right-hand thread is used.

A further type of connection, which may be dismantled using a spanner, is a banjo union (Fig. 2.15). The name 'banjo' is used since in former types of this connection one part of the union was shaped very similar to the musical instrument. One part of the union consists of a threaded orifice, into which may be screwed a hollow member which passes through the body of the second part of the union. Two washers ensure a good seal when the union is tightened. The advantage of this type of union is that the body of the banjo may be swivelled to any desired angle before the union is tightened. The banjo union is used for both gases and liquids.

Some Mechanical Points

Glands (stuffing boxes)

Where a valve spindle passes from an area of high pressure to one of low pressure, as in a cylinder valve, provision must be made to prevent the leak of gases along the line of the spindle. This is achieved by means of a *gland* or, as it is colloquially known, a 'stuffing box' (Fig. 2.16). In Fig. 2.17 the contents of the cylinder flow through the valve in the valve block and out through the outlet. If the spindle is turned fully clockwise (down), the valve is closed. If it is turned counter-clockwise, to open the valve, the gas is permitted to escape from the cylinder and could do so by one of two routes — either through the outlet as intended or along the line of the spindle and past the nut N (Fig. 2.16). However, the latter course is prevented by the packing, or stuffing, P in the stuffing box. The nut N is screwed down so tightly that the packing is applied so closely to the spindle (S) that no gas can escape by this route. There is provision for the nut to be tightened down further as the packing wears.

This principle can be used for a high-pressure gland such as that of an oxygen cylinder (as shown in Fig. 2.17) or in a low-pressure gland such as that in a flow-control (fine-adjustment) valve (see Fig. 6.6). In the case of high-pressure valves, a special type of

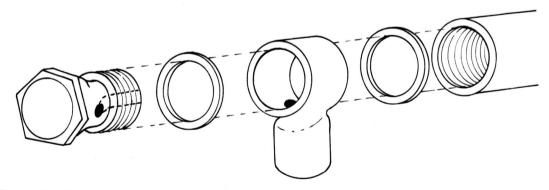

Figure 2.15   The Banjo union. Note that two washers are required to make a satisfactory seal.

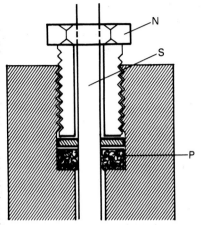

Figure 2.16   A gland (stuffing box). The packing P is compressed by screwing down the nut N until it is applied sufficiently tightly round the spindle S to prevent the gas from leaking.

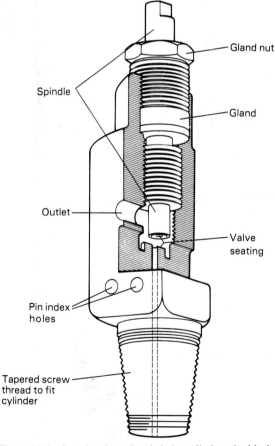

Figure 2.17   A section through a pin index cylinder valve block.

leather or long-fibre asbestos was at one time used for the packing, but modern stuffing boxes are sometimes filled with specially shaped nylon. Stuffing boxes in low-pressure flow control valves may be filled with rubber, nylon, neoprene or cotton.

O-rings

In certain circumstances the packing of a stuffing box may be replaced by an O-ring (Fig. 2.18). This consists of a simple ring made to a fine tolerance out of a material such as neoprene. If the spindle S and casing C are suitably designed, an O-ring is all that is needed to prevent leakage at this point. O-rings can withstand remarkably high pressures and yet cause very little friction between the spindle and the casing. One recent innovation is the use of an O-ring in the bull-nose oxygen cylinder coupling. Whereas a spanner was previously required to tighten the union sufficiently to prevent leaks, the O-ring now makes such an efficient joint that the nut needs to be turned down only hand-tight to prevent a leak.

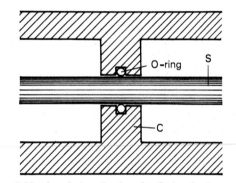

Figure 2.18   A typical application of an O-ring. Leakage between the spindle S and the block C is completely prevented.

Springs

There are two types of coil spring: tension springs, which are normally closely wound and are extended when force is exerted upon them, and compression springs, which are shortened by an applied force. There are also leaf springs, which are deflected by an applied force, and hair springs, as are seen on the balance wheel of a clock and on the mechanism of a pressure gauge.

Provided that there is neither fracture nor fatigue, the extent to which a spring is distorted is governed by Hooke's law, which states that the length of extension (or compression) is proportional to the tension or force producing it.

When considering the operating characteristics of adjustable pressure limiting or relief valves, it is important to realize that whereas much the same pressure is required to lift a gravity valve, however wide it is opened, the degree of opening of a spring-loaded valve varies with the pressure applied. The spring can be set at a tension to prevent opening before a predetermined pressure is reached.

Bistable Mechanism

A bistable arrangement is one that will rest in either of two modes, but is unstable and refuses to remain in an intermediate position. It may apply in mechanical, electric or fluid systems, and is particularly indicated where a change of function needs to be complete, rapid and decisive.

Perhaps the most familiar example of a bistable mechanism is the 'good quality' electric light switch, which will rest in the 'on' or 'off' position, but will not stay in between unless forced to do so. The

bell-push is a monostable device, which rests in the 'off' position and can remain 'on' only as long as the operator's finger is applied.

Let us consider the cycling mechanism of the Manley ventilator. The change over between the inspiratory and expiratory phases is actuated by a lever which is required to pass from one end of its traverse to the other. The locus of the free end of the lever is described by the arc $L_1 L_2 L_3$ of a circle with centre O (Fig. 2.19). Attached to the free end of the lever is a spring, the other end of which is fixed at a point S, more distant than O. From the diagram it will be seen that $L_1S = L_3S$ but L_2S is longer than either of these. If the lever is held in the position L_2 and then released, it will move to L_1 or L_3 owing to the tension on the spring being greater at L_2 than at L_1 or L_3. If the lever is at L_1 and is pushed towards L_3, there will come a time when it is 'over the top' and the spring will accelerate rather than oppose the movement of the lever.

Another example of mechanical bistable mechanism is found in ventilators such as the Bird Mk 7 (p. 228), where metal masses move between magnets. They fly towards the nearest magnet since the attraction exerted by the magnet increases as the distance between it and the metal is reduced. The

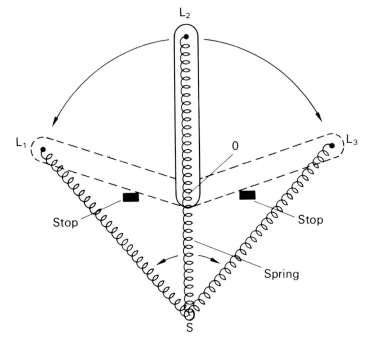

Figure 2.19 A bistable mechanism. Notice that the distance between L_1 and S, and L_3 and S are shorter than the distance between L_2 and S. The lever will therefore pass to position L_1 or L_3, rather than remain in an intermediate position between them. O is the centre around which the lever pivots.

operation is similar to the spring loaded bistable mechanism described above.

In Fig. 2.32a the 'flip-flop' fluidic logic is also a bistable element. The 'and', 'or' and 'not' elements are examples of monostable systems since in the absence of a signal the output is always on one particular side.

Pneumatics and Fluidics

Pneumatics and fluidics are concerned with the behaviour of fluids as they flow through chosen pathways and orifices. As applied to anaesthesia, they are concerned with air and/or other gases, in the manner by which they may control or actuate equipment such as anaesthetic machines or lung ventilators. In other applications fluidic devices may be used to handle liquids rather than gases, but they function in the same manner.

Pneumatic and fluidic equipment may perform functions somewhat analogous to those of electric and electronic devices, but as will be seen below the analogy often breaks down when details are considered.

Pneumatics

The principal components in pneumatic equipment are spool valves which perform switching functions and activators such as cylinders with pistons. Both of these contain moving parts in which wear and damage may occur, requiring service maintenance and replacement. The pressure of the driving gas is between 30 lb/in² (~ 2 bar) and 150 lb/in² (~ 10 bar). In all the earlier equipment the compressed air which operated it contained a specially added oil mist to lubricate the components — but more modern developments have obviated the need for this lubrication in many instances and 'dry' devices, more appropriate to medical applications, have been developed. High-pressure equipment using oxygen rather than air should not be lubricated with inflammable materials. If lubrication is required, a non-flammable grease such as Fomblin should be used. This substance is similar to a hydrocarbon, except that the hydrogen atoms have been replaced by those of fluorine.

In the industrial field, where large-diameter cylinder activators are employed, heavy-duty tasks may be performed. For instance, if a cylinder of 200 mm bore is operated at a pressure of 150 lb/in² (~ 10 bar), there is a thrust of over 30 kN. In anaesthetic equipment, much smaller cylinders are employed and the activating pressure is between 30 lb/in² (~ 2 bar) and 60 lb/in² (~ 4 bar).

The spool valve operates by means of a shuttle, usually in the shape of a cylinder of varying diameter, which moves from one end to the other in a passageway divided by seals into a number of chambers, the sides of which are pierced by inlet and outlet ports. By means of the recesses and seals, the gases passing through the valve are directed in one direction or the other. By virtue of there being multiple sections with inlets and outlets, these valves may control several operations simultaneously. Figure 2.20 shows a three-port spool valve, which is analogous to a two-way electric switch. In the 'on' position, gases pass from port 1 to port 2, while in the 'off' position they pass from port 1 to port 3. Here lies the essence of the difference between electric and pneumatic functions. In the for-

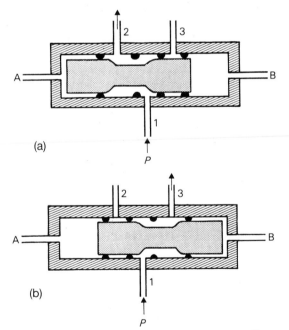

Figure 2.20   A three-port spool valve. (a) When the spool is to the left-hand side the driving gas passes from port 1 to port 2. A pneumatic or mechanical force applied at A will cause the spool to travel to the right, as seen in (b), so that the driving gas now emerges from port 3. *P*, driving gas supply.

mer, when the signal ceases, the effect becomes zero; whereas in the latter, when the signal ceases, it may still be stored in the position of the activator (as a 'trapped signal') until it is exhausted to atmosphere.

Spool valves with three, five or more ports are commonly employed, as will be seen in Fig. 2.21. The importance of the five-port valve will be seen when the activator cylinders are considered.

Spool valves may be operated by:
(a)   a pilot air pressure (between 2 and 10 bar);
(b)   a low-pressure air signal acting on a diaphragm;
(c)   a toggle or push rod; or
(d)   an electric solenoid.

The driving gas passes from the spool valve to an activator which is usually a double-acting cylinder (Fig. 2.22). The fact that the cylinder can be driven from either end permits it to be used in a reciprocating manner, with the strokes in each direction doing work.

Advances in technology have led to the development of pneumatic logic components (also known as 'moving part logics'), which may be used without lubrication. It should be pointed out, however, that before these are employed in conjunction with high-pressure oxygen they should be degreased. There are now logics with many functions, and these with their fluidic and electrical equivalents are described on p. 29.

Fig. 2.23 shows the type of pneumatic logic circuit that might be used to control a lung ventilator.

The actual work of driving the bellows in the breathing system may be done by a reciprocating cylinder. The driving gas is applied alternately to its two ends via a spool valve, the action of which is controlled by two other valves, which are in turn activated, via levers, by the movement of the piston rod of the cylinder. The timers determine the interval between the end of one stroke and the start of the return stroke, i.e. length of inspiratory and expiratory pauses, while the restrictors regulate the speed at which the piston travels, i.e. the inspiratory and expiratory flow rates. Note that the restrictors control the gas flow in the exhaust direction only, since they are connected in parallel with low-resistance diodes, which present little resistance to the flow of gas in the reverse direction.

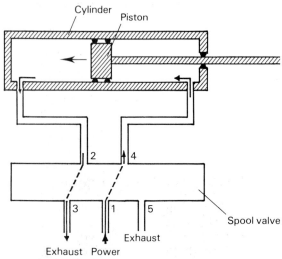

Figure 2.21   The pneumatic power is applied to port 1 of the spool valve. With the spool valve in one position the power passes through port 4 to the right-hand side of the cylinder, thus causing the piston to move to the left. At the same time the gas from the left-hand end of the cylinder escapes to the atmosphere via ports 2 and 3 of the spool valve. When the spool valve moves so as to alter the direction, the power passes to the left-hand side of the cylinder via ports 1 and 2 and the gases from the right hand end of the cylinder are exhausted through ports 4 and 5.

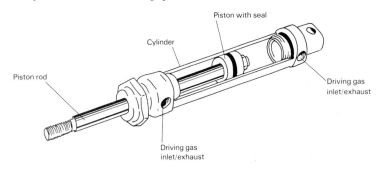

Figure 2.22   A pneumatic cylinder. Note that there are ports at either end which, according to the direction of movement of the piston, act as the inlet or exhaust for the driving gas.

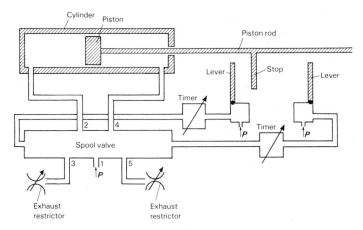

Figure 2.23 A pneumatic logic ventilator cycling system. The output of the spool valve drives the piston in the cylinder. The piston rod may have a stop which operates triggers on the actuators for inspiration and expiration. The output of these actuators may pass through timers that can delay the onset of inspiration or expiration. The exhaust from each end of the cylinder may be controlled by flow restrictors which may be used to slow down the movement of the piston during either the inspiratory or the expiratory phase. The piston rod might be used to operate a bellows that is part of the breathing system. *P*, driving gas supply.

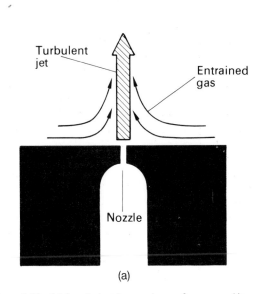

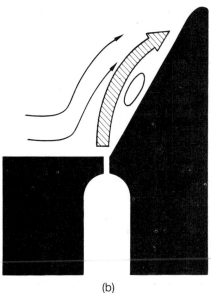

Figure 2.24 (a) A turbulent jet entrains gas from around it.

(b) If the supply of gas to be entrained is limited, a 'bubble' of reduced pressure is produced.

Fluidics

Pneumatic equipment has been used for many years, but the scope of fluid engineering was greatly enhanced by the exploitation, during the development of space rockets, of the discovery published in 1932 by Henri Coanda of the phenomenon of wall attachment. Coanda described the behaviour of a jet of fluid emerging from a nozzle. For present purposes a jet of gas is considered, but the same phenomenon occurs with liquids. Being turbulent, the jet entrains with it molecules of the surrounding gas

(Fig. 2.24a). The presence of a wall on one side of the jet, thus limiting the availability of molecules of gas to be entrained, causes a 'bubble of reduced pressure' to develop. This results in the jet being diverted towards the wall and under favourable conditions becoming attached to it (Fig. 2.24b).

If there is a choice of walls to which it might become attached, the entire jet goes either one way or the other; it does not split (Fig. 2.25). These devices may, therefore, be described as digital logics, having two possible outlets only, 'on' and

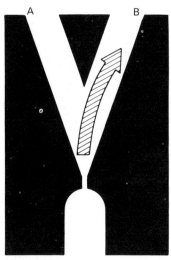

Figure 2.25   If there is a choice of two walls, the entire jet will attach itself to one of them.

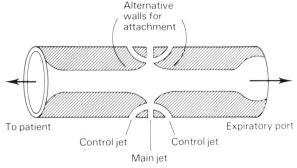

Figure 2.26   The principle of a simple fluidic ventilator. Although the control jet (see below) may be used to switch between inspiration and expiration, back pressure towards the end of the inspiratory phase will cause the main jet to return to the expiratory end.

'off'. (Splitting logics operating on an analogue rather than digital basis also exist and are described below.) Referring again to Fig. 2.25, when the jet is flowing through the right-hand limb B it may, by the Venturi effect, entrain gas from the left-hand limb A. Obstruction of the jet as it passes to one outlet may, by back pressure, cause it to transfer to the other. This is seen in the simple fluidic respirator shown in Fig. 2.26. More important, however, is the fact that a small puff of gas injected at the site of the bubble will deflect the main jet to the opposite wall (Fig. 2.27).

The signal required to deflect the jet is very much smaller than the main jet itself, so this device may be regarded as not only a switch but also an amplifier. Switching frequency of up to 100 kHz may be obtained. The dimensions of such a fluidic device may vary enormously from control units with very fine passages, measuring 2.5 cm in their largest dimension, to large pipes conducting liquids such as corrosive chemicals.

Anaesthetists were interested originally in designing single fluidic elements through which the actual patient gases pass. An example of this is shown in Fig. 2.28. This simple device, constructed of clear plastic, is driven by oxygen or other gas at a pressure of 52 ± 3 lb/in^2 (3.6 ± 0.2 bar.) It is monostable, the preferred direction for the jet being towards the port attached to the facepiece. When the lungs are inflated the back pressure increases to a point where it

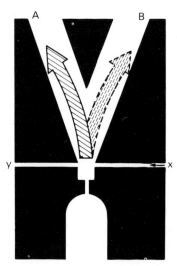

Figure 2.27   A small control port has been drilled at each side. A signal at x will cause the jet to be deflected to the left-hand limb A.

causes the jet to switch to the other limb. Both the driving gas and the expired air escape via the expiratory port. At the end of expiration the jet switches back to the original direction and the cycle starts again. This type of system is not very satisfactory in anaesthetic practice owing to its lack of fine control and its dependence on driving gas at a precise pressure. It is more appropriate to employ fluidic logic systems to control ventilators, usually using gas that is not destined to be breathed by the patient.

By changing the design of the passages through which the jet passes, 'gates' or switching devices with various functions have been elaborated. For

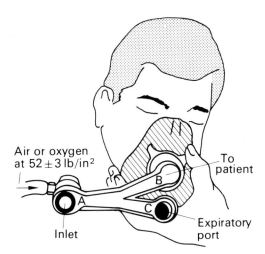

Figure 2.28   Another fluidic ventilator, consisting of one large fluidic element. The gas enters at A and, this being a monostable element, passes via B to the patient. When, however, the airway pressure rises sufficiently, the jet from A changes over to C, allowing expiration to occur. When the pressure in B falls sufficiently the jet returns to that side. Note that the input pressure must be within narrow limits.

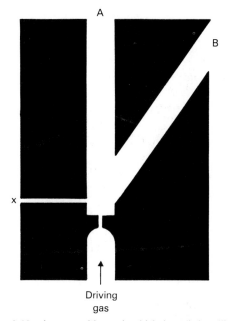

Figure 2.29   A monostable gate in which the main jet will emerge at A, except when a control signal is applied at x, when it will transfer to B. When the signal x ceases the jet will return to A.

instance, in Fig. 2.29 the jet will normally pass to output A, but when a signal is applied at x it will be deflected to B and remain there only as long as the signal at x is operating. In Fig. 2.30 a logic is shown with two signal inputs either of which will cause the jet to switch to output B.

In Fig. 2.31 the main gate is a flip-flop, but the signal ports on the two sides are different. A signal at x *or* y on its own will have no effect since it exhausts via y or x. The operation of x *and* y together will switch the output to B. On the other hand a signal at r *or* s, or at both, will result in an output at A.

The input signal may be derived from various devices including a push button with a small balloon, a plunger, a proximity sensor (Fig. 2.32g) or the output from another element.

Terminology of logics

As stated above there is now a wide diversity of logics available in pneumatics, fluidics and electronics. The analogy between these three breaks down at times and the several manufacturers have tended to use their own classifications, terms and symbols, which has added to the confusion. Figure 2.32 shows a variety of logics and some of the symbols

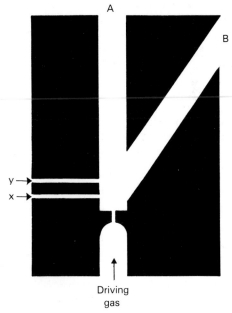

Figure 2.30   A monostable gate in which the main jet will switch from A to B only as long as a signal is applied at x or y or both. An OR gate.

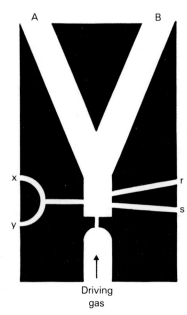

Figure 2.31   AND/OR flip-flop gate. Signals at x *and* y will cause the jet to pass to output B, whereas signals at r *or* s will cause it to return to A.

commonly employed. Note that in the case of the fluidic and pneumatic logics the terminology indicates the mode of action when the signal is applied.

An example of a fluidic system that may be used to control a variety of ventilators is shown in Fig. 2.33. A somewhat similar device is employed in the Campbell ventilator (Fig 2.34). Although reliable, this device is somewhat noisy and does require a high flow rate of driving gas (average 11 *l*/min), but it is most flexible in use and requires no other power source than the driving gas, which may be oxygen from a cylinder.

There are applications of fluid control other than those depending on wall attachment. For instance 'gates' may be constructed to perform various functions. Figure 2.35 shows a passive AND gate in which each of the jets a and b blowing on its own is voided through its own separate output, A and B, respectively, but if they operate together they together pass to a third output AB. No power supply is required. This is therefore an economical application and, indeed, in some circumstances an AND gate can replace up to three active NOR logics.

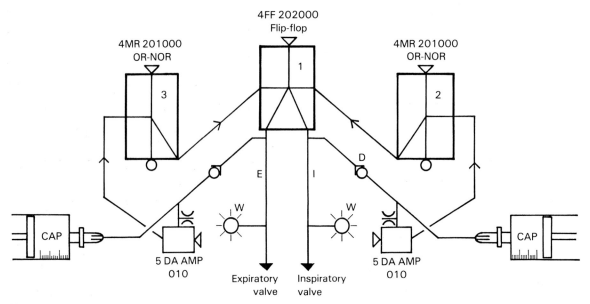

Figure 2.33   A fluidic control 'circuit' for a lung ventilator. Let us suppose that the output from a flip-flop fluidic element 1 is going via I to the inspiratory valve and also the inspiratory indicator. Gas passes via the diode/restrictor D to the variable capacitor CAP and the diaphragm amplifier. The length of time taken for the diaphragm amplifier to act depends on the volume of the capacitor. Eventually a signal is passed to the monostable gate 2 and from there to the flip-flop logic 1. This then switches to the expiratory mode via E and the train of events is then repeated on the opposite side via gate 3. The duration of inspiration and expiration is controlled by the capacitors CAP.

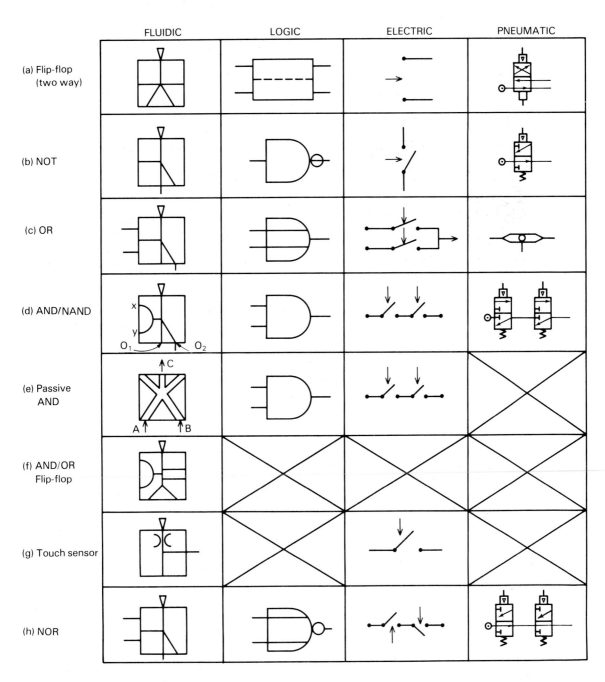

Figure 2.32   Conventional signs for various logics.

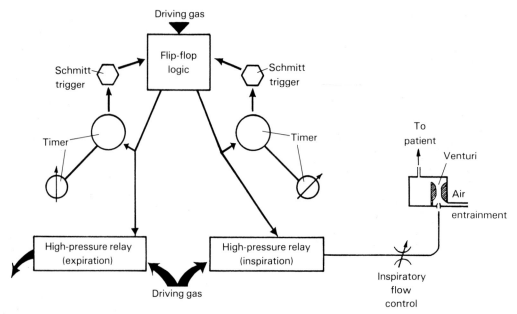

Figure 2.34   The working principles of the cycling control system of the Campbell ventilator. Note that the outputs from the bistable (flip-flop) logic control the expiratory and inspiratory high-pressure relays. The outlet from the inspiratory relay may be restricted by the inspiratory flow control. This operates a venturi through which the air may be entrained. The patient system may include a 'bag in a bottle'.

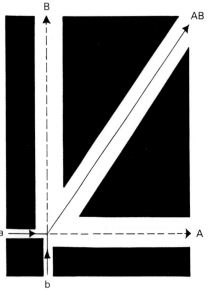

Figure 2.35   A passive AND gate.

Proportional (analogue) logics

Not all fluidic devices are digital, i.e. 'on/off'. The splitter (mentioned above) operates proportionally. Figure 2.36 at first resembles a flip-flop, but on closer inspection it will be seen that the power jet passes through a chamber so shaped as to prevent wall attachment. In the absence of any control signal the jet is divided into two equal parts by the splitter. A control jet from one side deflects the power jet towards the opposite side to an extent proportional to its power. The flow from each output is therefore proportional to the power of the control signal applied to the opposite side.

Turbulence amplifiers

Turbulence amplifiers are not currently in favour and are mentioned only for the sake of completeness. They operate on the principle of a low-pressure *laminar* jet (15–25 mbar $\approx$ 15–25 cmH$_2$O) passing across a chamber with side ports (Fig. 2.37a). In the absence of a side signal the jet passes into a chosen

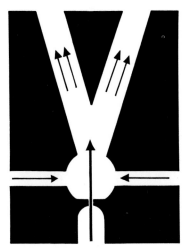

Figure 2.36   The proportional splitter.

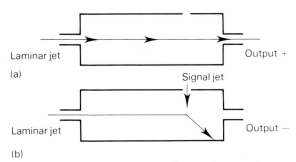

Laminar jet

(a)

Signal jet

Output +

Laminar jet

Output −

(b)

Figure 2.37   The turbulence amplifier. (a) With no signal. (b) With a signal.

orifice and an output signal is registered. A side signal (Fig. 2.37b) interferes with the signal and interrupts the output. The advantage that these devices operate on so low a pressure is offset by the fact that on this account they are liable to interference by stray air currents and are therefore unreliable.

Terminology of logic units

The logic units employed in anaesthesia are virtually all binary, i.e. they are either 'off' or 'on'. In the terms of Boolean algebra or truth tables they may be described as '0' and '1' or − and +. Space does not permit a discussion of Boolean algebra or truth tables in this volume, but the reader is strongly advised to consult a work such as *Introduction to Boolean Algebra and Logic Design*, mentioned in the Further Reading references at the end of the book, if he has not yet studied this fascinating subject.

Each unit is named according to the function that it performs while the control signal is applied. Thus a logic that permits the supply air to pass to the designated output during the absence of a signal, but prevents it while the signal is operating, is termed a NOT logic. The reverse of this is referred to as YES logic.

Figure 2.32 shows a number of logics, with the symbols, as appropriate, for their pneumatic, fluidic and electrical equivalents. The terminology employed by the various manufacturers does not strictly follow that laid down in the terms of Boolean algebra. Thus a logic such as that shown in Fig. 2.32d may be termed an AND/NAND, in that in the absence of a signal at both x and y the output is sustained at O_1, whereas when a signal is entered at *both* x and y the output is at O_2. If the output at O_1 is considered normal, the logic is a NAND; if the output at O_2 is considered normal, it is an AND.

The flip-flop logic (Fig. 2.32a) is bistable and sometimes referred to as 'memory', since provided that the driving air supply is uninterrupted, the last instruction continues, even after it has ceased, to be reflected in the mode of the output.

In the NOT logic (Fig. 2.32b), also known as an inverter, a signal causes the output to be diverted away from the designated port.

In the OR logic (Fig. 2.32c) a signal at any one of two or more inputs will cause the output to come from the designated port, while in the AND logic (Fig. 2.32d) *both* of two signals are required.

In the passive AND logic (Fig. 2.32e) no power is required. If, and *only if*, signals are applied at A and B is there an output at C.

Thus compound logics may be built up, such as the AND/OR flip-flop (Fig. 2.32f) and many others, performing multiple functions.

3

The Supply of Anaesthetic Gases*

Cylinders

The anaesthetic gases are usually supplied in cylinders, though oxygen is supplied to some of the larger consumers in liquid form (p. 54). Modern cylinders are made from molybdenum steel and because of the greater strength of this alloy, they have thinner walls than their heavier and larger carbon steel predecessors and are known as 'light-weight' cylinders. Alu-

minium cylinders are not, as yet, widely used in the medical field in Great Britain.

Oxygen, nitrogen, air and helium are stored in cylinders as a compressed gas (Table 3.1). Nitrous oxide, carbon dioxide and cyclopropane, being strictly speaking vapours and not true gases, liquefy at the pressures to which the cylinders are filled. Indeed, the greater part of the contents of cylinders of these 'gases' are in the liquid form. The cylinder is not completely filled with liquid, since if this were the case, a comparatively moderate rise in temperature would lead to a very great increase in pressure, which would result in rupture. It is filled to a 'filling ratio' which may be taken as the weight of the substance with which it is actually filled, divided by the weight of water that it could hold. In Great Britain, which has a temperate climate, nitrous oxide and carbon dioxide cylinders are filled to a ratio of 0.75; in tropical climates this is reduced to 0.67. For cyclopropane the figures are 0.51 and 0.48 respectively. Since they contain liquid, it is important that cylinders of nitrous oxide, carbon dioxide and cyclopropane are mounted in the vertical position when in use. The temperature of the cylinder and its contents drops during vaporization, and

Table 3.1 Cylinder sizes equivalents

Size	C	D	E	F	G	J
Maximum dimensions						
mm	406 × 89	559 × 102	864 × 102	914 × 140	1372 × 178	1435 × 229
in.	16 × 3½	22 × 4	34 × 4	36 × 5½	54 × 7	56½ × 9
Weight of empty cylinder						
maximum (kg)	4.5	7.3	11.3	23.6	56.2	73.5
(lb)	10	16	25	52	124	162
minimum (kg)	2	3.2	5.2	13.6	31.8	65
(lb)	4½	7	11½	30	70	141
Oxygen						
litres	170	340	680	1360	3400	6800
cubic feet	6	12	24	48	120	240
gallons	36	72	150	300	750	1495
Nitrous oxide						
litres	450	900	1800	3600	9000	—
gallons	100	200	400	800	2000	4000
Entonox (litres)	—	500	—	2000	5000	—
Carbon dioxide (lb)	2	4	7	—	—	—
Air (medical)						
litres	—	—	—	—	3200	6400
cubic feet	—	—	—	—	110	220

Cyclopropane is supled in smaller cylinders containing 36, 90 or 180 litres (8, 20 or 40 gallons).

* Including nitrous oxide, carbon dioxide and cyclopropane, which are, strictly speaking, vapours.

where high-flow rates of nitrous oxide are taken from a small cylinder, the fall of temperature, and consequently pressure, may be marked. Water vapour from the surrounding air condenses on the exterior of the cylinder as it cools and if the temperature falls still further this may freeze. In a 'dental gas session' the pressure in a 3600 *l* cylinder may fall from 750 to 500 lb/in² (~ 50 to 35 bar) before the liquid nitrous oxide is exhausted.

In the case of oxygen and other gases that do not normally liquefy, the contents of the cylinder may be estimated with a pressure gauge, since the amount of gas is proportional to the pressure. Fluctuations of pressure due to changes of ambient temperature are not usually of a significant order in clinical practice. However, in the case of nitrous oxide, carbon dioxide and cyclopropane, it is not until all the liquid content has evaporated that the pressure within the cylinder falls appreciably, provided that there has not been significant cooling. Therefore, in this case the contents gauge falls rapidly only when the contents are nearly exhausted. Some contents gauges for these gases are therefore calibrated with a wide segment marked 'Full at varying temperatures'. The pressure of gases in full cylinders is shown in Table 3.2.

The contents of nitrous oxide, carbon dioxide and cyclopropane cylinders are more accurately determined, if required, by weighing the cylinders. As shown in Fig. 3.1a, the weight of the empty cylinder (Tare) is stamped on the side of the valve block. The weight of the gas in terms of its density in ounces per gallon or grams per litre is shown on the label on the neck of the cylinder, and by weighing the cylinder and subtracting its weight empty, the weight of the contents of the cylinder can be estimated at any time. The densities of various gases are shown in Table 3.2.

The cylinder for each gas is painted in a distinctive colour, as shown in Table 3.3. They are also marked with the chemical symbol for the gas they contain.

Medical gas cylinders are hydraulically tested every five years and the test recorded by a mark which is stamped on the neck of the cylinder. Other marks on the neck and the valve block (Fig. 3.1) relate to the name of the owner, the serial number of the cylinder and the pressures to which the cylinder has been tested and may safely be filled.

A simple test as to whether a cylinder is empty or at least partially full is to hold it by the valve and to gently bump the bottom on a concrete or other hard

Table 3.2 Physical properties of compressed vapours and gases

	Oxygen	Nitrous oxide	Entonox	Carbon dioxide	Cyclo-propane
Symbol	O_2	N_2O	$O_2 + N_2O$	CO_2	C_3H_6
Physical state in cylinder	Gas	Liquid	Gas	Liquid	Liquid
Pressure when full (15°C)					
lb/in²	1980	639.5	1980	723	64
kg/cm²	139.2	44.9	139.2	50.8	4.5
atm	134.7	43.5	134.7	49.2	4.3
Type of cylinder valve*	PI BN HW	PI HW	PI	PI	PI
Critical temperature (°C)	−118.4	36.5	(Gases separate at −7°C)	31	125
Critical pressure (atm)	50.14	71.7		72.85	54
Boiling point (1 atm)	−183	−89	—	−78.5	−33
Flammability	Supports combustion	No	Supports combustion	No	Yes
Approximate weight (for calculation of cylinder contents)					
g/l	—	1.87.	—	1.87	1.8
gal/oz	—	3.3	—	3.3	3.5

* PI, pin index; BN, bull nose; HW, hand wheel.

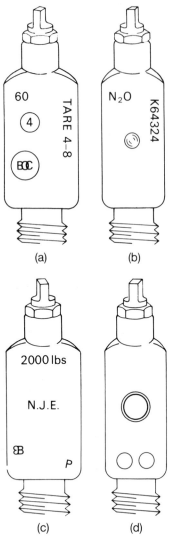

Figure 3.1 The four faces of a pin index cylinder valve block. Note on (a) the weight of the empty cylinder, 'Tare' (in pounds and ounces), on (b) the symbol for nitrous oxide, on (c) the pressure of the hydraulic test, and on (d) the outlet and pin index holes.

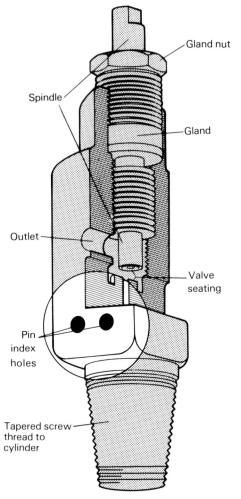

Figure 3.2 A section through a pin index cylinder valve block, showing the position of the pin index holes.

floor. A dull thud indicates that it is empty, whilst a cylinder containing gases under pressure gives a ringing noise.

Pin-index system (International Standard)

This system has been devised in order to prevent the accidental fitting of a cylinder of the wrong gas to a yoke, thus making interchangeability of cylinders of different gases impossible. One or more pins project from the yoke, and these locate in holes bored in the valve block of the cylinder (Fig. 3.2). The configuration of the pins varies for each gas, as illustrated in Fig. 3.3. If the wrong cylinder is accidentally offered up to a yoke it is impossible to fit it. When piped medical gas systems were first employed, the supply hose to the anaesthetic machine often terminated in a block similar to the valve block of a cylinder and drilled for the appropriate pin index. Full details of the pin index system are given in British Standard 1319 of 1955.

The Department of Health and Social Security

Table 3.3 Colour codes for cylinders and flow control knobs

Gas	Symbol	International Standard			USA	West Germany
		Valve end (shoulder)	Cylinder body	Control knob		
Oxygen	O_2	White	Black	White	Green	Blue
Nitrous oxide	N_2O	Blue	Blue	Blue	Blue	Grey
Carbon dioxide	CO_2	Grey	Grey	Grey	Grey	—
Cyclopropane	C_3H_6	Orange	Orange	Orange	Orange	—
Air (medical)	AIR	White and Black	Grey	White and Black	Yellow	Yellow
Entonox 50/50 N_2O/O_2	$N_2O + O_2$	Blue and White	Blue	Blue and White		
Vacuum		—	—	Yellow		

advised in 1973 that pipeline hoses should be connected permanently to anaesthetic machines using a union such as a cap and liner. Although this is now the common practice, many of the earlier types still exist, though they may have been modified by the removal of the tommy bar and its replacement by an Allen (hexagon wrench) screw.

Medical gases are also supplied in cylinders other than those with pin index outlets, and those still available in Great Britain are shown in Fig. 3.4. Note that the 'handwheel' type cylinders (Fig. 3.4b) of nitrous oxide and oxygen, used commonly in dental practice, have different sizes of thread on the outlet and are therefore non-interchangeable. The British Oxygen Company (BOC) has now replaced handwheel cylinders for oxygen by 'bull-nosed' cylinders, but other companies such as Kingston Medical Gases have retained the handwheel type for both nitrous oxide and oxygen.

Full cylinders are usually supplied with plastic dust-covers over the outlet in order to prevent contamination by dirt or grit; this should be removed immediately before fitting the cylinder. When a cylinder is fitted, care should be taken to see that the sealing washer is present and in good order. If it is not so, it should be replaced by a new one, and this must be of non-combustible material. ('Bodok' seals supplied by BOC have a metal periphery, which keeps them in good order for a long period (Fig. 3.5).) The screw or clamp securing the cylinder in the yoke should not be tightened excessively, or damage to the washer or even the cylinder may occur. Immediately before fitting it is advisable to open the valve gently and to allow some gas to

escape, in order to blow from the outlet any dirt or grit which might cause damage to the pressure regulator or could even lead to an explosion. The cylinder valve should be opened slowly so as to prevent a sudden surge of pressure (shock wave) on the contents gauge and regulator. It should be closed with no more force than is sufficient, or damage to the seating of the valve may result. If, after a cylinder has been turned on, there appears to be a leak, this may be tested for with water or a soapy solution. Occasionally there is a leak of gas around the spindle of the valve; this can be prevented by gently screwing down the gland nut (see Fig. 3.2). If high pressure oxygen is allowed to come into contact with combustible materials, especially oil or grease, fire or an explosion is liable to occur.

In the USA cylinders are fitted with a Wood's metal fusible plug in the valve block which melts at low temperature. This is to prevent the risk of explosion if the cylinders are exposed to very high temperatures, such as in a fire. (In Great Britain the sealing material between the valve and the neck of the cylinder is often made of a fusible material which in the event of involvement in a fire would melt and allow the contents of the cylinder to escape around the threads of this joint.)

Cylinders should be stored in a clean place in order to prevent the admission of dirt and possible infection to the operating theatre. They should be kept in a rack in such a manner that they are used in rotation, to prevent any being stored for a long period and thereby reducing the possibility of their being empty when brought into use. Cylinders of Entonox (50% nitrous oxide plus 50% oxygen)

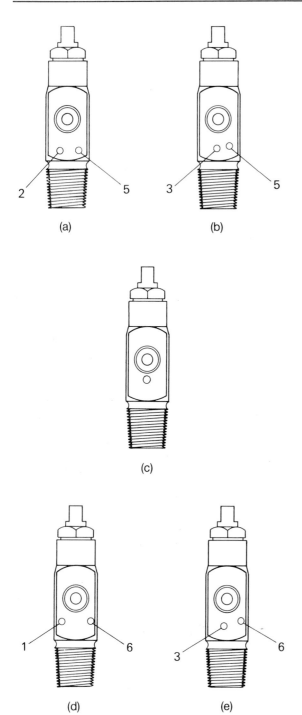

Figure 3.3   Pin index configuration. (a) Oxygen (O_2);
(b) nitrous oxide (N_2O); (c) Entonox (50% N_2O + 50% O_2);
(d) carbon dioxide (CO_2); (e) cyclopropane (C_3H_6).

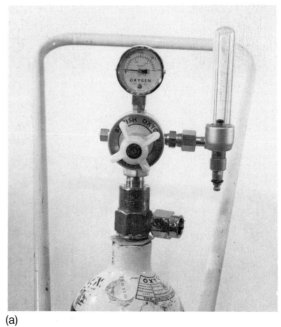

(a)

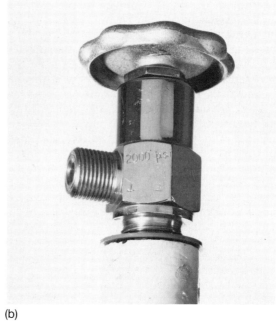

(b)

Figure 3.4   (a) A bull-nosed cylinder valve. (b) A handwheel
cylinder valve. These are for larger cylinders.

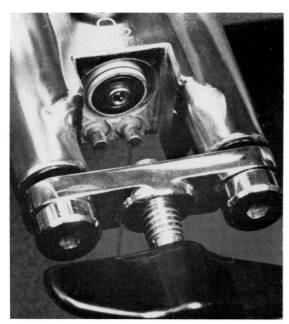

Figure 3.5   A Bodok seal, shown in position on a pin-index yoke.

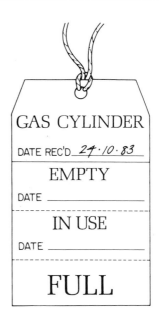

GAS CYLINDER

DATE REC'D _24·10·83_

EMPTY

DATE _____

IN USE

DATE _____

FULL

Figure 3.6   A cylinder label.

should never be stored under conditions in which the temperature might fall below 0°C, since if the temperature falls below the pseudocritical (condensation) temperature for this mixture, the nitrous oxide and oxygen could laminate (separate). If this does happen, the instructions for remixing the contents printed on the neck of the cylinder should be followed. This involves gentle rewarming and repeated inversion of the cylinder.

Empty cylinders should be stored separately from full ones and marked accordingly with chalk. It is customary to use the letters 'MT' for empty. In some instances labels such as that in Fig. 3.6 are employed, but the danger of these becoming detached and lost probably renders them less reliable than chalk marks. Faulty cylinders should be appropriately marked and returned to the supplier. Cylinders should not be stored under conditions where very high temperatures may occur.

Further information on medical gas cylinders may be found in British Standard 1319, 1955, and for aluminium cylinders in Health and Safety Executive Specifications HOAL 3 and HOAL 4 as revised in June 1980, *Seamless Aluminium Alloy Containers for the Conveyance of Compressed and Liquefied Gases.*

Pressure Regulators (Reducing Valves)

Pressure regulators are used on anaesthetic and oxygen therapy apparatus for three main reasons:
1. The pressure delivered from a cylinder is far too high to be used with safety in apparatus where a sudden surge of pressure might accidentally be delivered to the patient.
2. If the pressure were not reduced, flow-control (fine-adjustment) valves, tubing and various other parts of the apparatus would have to be very much more robust, and a fine and accurate control of gas flow would be difficult to achieve. There would also be a danger of pressure building up and damaging other components of the apparatus.
3. As the contents of a cylinder are used, the pressure within the cylinder falls. If there were no regulating mechanism to maintain a constant reduced pressure, continual adjustment would have to be made of the flow-control valve in order to maintain a constant flow rate.

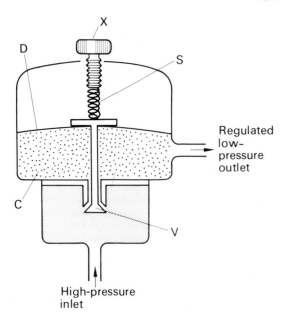

Figure 3.7   A simple pressure regulator. D, diaphragm; S, spring; C, low-pressure chamber; V, valve seating; X, adjustment screw.

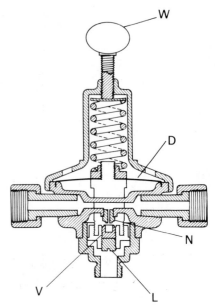

Figure 3.8   A McKesson regulator. W, wing screw; N, nozzle; V, valve seat; L, lock screw; D, diaphragm.

Not only is the pressure reduced, but it is also kept constant, and for this reason the correct term for this type of valve is a *pressure regulator*. The working principle of a pressure regulator is shown in Fig. 3.7. The chamber C is enclosed on one side by the diaphragm D. As gas enters the chamber through the valve V, the pressure is increased and the diaphragm distended against its own elastic recoil plus the tension in the spring S. Eventually the pressure rises so much and the diaphragm moves so far that valve V is closed. The pressure at which this occurs may be varied by adjusting the screw X so as to alter the tension in the spring. If gas is allowed to escape from the outlet of the chamber, the pressure falls and valve V reopens. When the regulator is in use a steady pressure is maintained in the chamber by the partial opening of valve V.

There are several types of pressure regulator available, the choice being dependent on the maximum flow rate required, the regulated pressure to which it is to be set and the maximum input pressure that it is to handle. For low-pressure regulators, the diaphragms are frequently made of rubber or neoprene, whereas in those for higher pressures, such as the McKesson regulator shown in Fig. 3.8, the diaphragm is made of metal. Where there is to be a considerable pressure reduction and at the same time a high flow rate is required, it is common practice to use a two-stage regulator, as shown in Fig. 3.9. Adjustments to alter the regulated pressure should normally be made only by service engineers, except in the case of the McKesson regulator, which is provided with means for easy adjustment to equalize the pressures of nitrous oxide and oxygen. Adjustments should be made with the gas flowing.

On some anaesthetic machines 'universal' regulators are used (see also p. 40). These operate equally well from an input of 60 lb/in² (~ 4 bar) from the pipeline, as from a maximum of 2000 lb/in² (~ 140 bar) from cylinders. They are of the Adams type (see Fig. 3.10).

The Accuracy of regulators

If we consider Fig. 3.11, the push-rod is pushed downward by two forces, the tension in the spring and the elastic recoil of the diaphragm. Let these be added together and represented by S. The force that opposes S consists of two parts: the high-pressure (P) of the gas pushing on the valve V over an area of a; and the low pressure (p) acting on the diaphragm over an area A, so:

$$S = Pa + pA$$

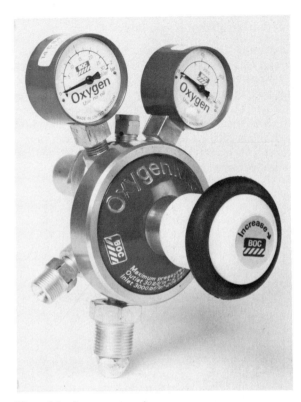

Figure 3.9   A two-stage regulator.

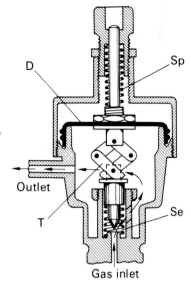

Figure 3.10   The Adams regulator. D, diaphragm; Sp, spring; Se, seat; T, toggle levers.

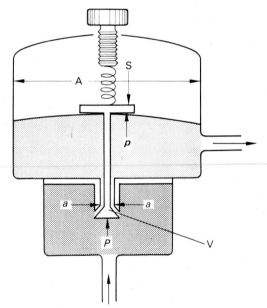

Figure 3.11   Forces acting in a simple regulator.

Thus if S remains constant, as P falls, p rises. So that as the cylinder empties, the regulated pressure increases. In fact, as P falls, the valve V will have to open further to permit the same flow rate. The spring expands and therefore the tension in it is reduced, and in the same way the tension in the diaphragm is reduced. Therefore as P falls, there is a small reduction in S, which partially reverses the effect shown here.

In the case of the Adams valve, however, the formula is different, since the push-rod is replaced by a 'lazy tongs' toggle arrangement, which reverses the direction of the thrust transmitted from the diaphragm.

In Fig. 3.12 it will be seen that the pressure P exerted by the high-pressure gas on the valve V to open it is assisted by the spring and the recoil of the diaphragm S. These forces jointly oppose the force exerted by the low-pressure gas on the diaphragm, so:

$$Pa + S = pA$$

Now as P falls, so does p; therefore the regulated pressure falls slightly as the cylinder pressure drops. At the same time the valve V opens slightly and this, by allowing the spring to *expand*, reduces S, which slightly accentuates the fall in p. The fall of p can be minimized by making S great compared with Pa.

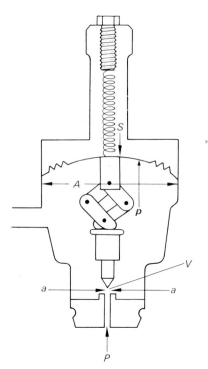

Figure 3.12   Forces acting in an Adams regulator.

A more accurate regulated pressure may be more easily produced by using a two-stage regulator. The pressure is considerably reduced in the first stage. In the second stage there is little variation in the input pressure and therefore the final regulated pressure is relatively constant.

Effect of flow rate on the performance of regulators

The above description of a regulator shows what happens in static conditions or when there is a low flow rate. However, when there is a high flow rate the input to the valve may not be able to keep pace with the output, in which case the regulated pressure will fall. For this reason a sufficiently heavy duty regulator for the flow rate required must be used. For high gas flows, two-stage regulators are usually employed; these are sometimes referred to as 'endurance' regulators. Examples of the performance of an oxygen therapy regulator are shown in Fig. 3.13.

Interchangeability of regulators

Regulators for different gases may have individual design features and should be used only for the gas for which they are intended. One make of regulator is called 'universal' in that the same body is used for all gases, but different seatings and springs are fitted for each particular gas. This should not be confused with the regulators for universal use at input pressures of 60 or 2000 lb/in² (~ 4 or ~ 140 bar), as described on p. 38.

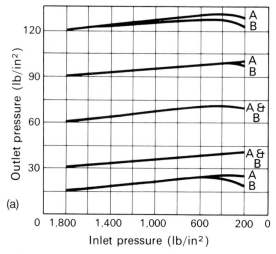

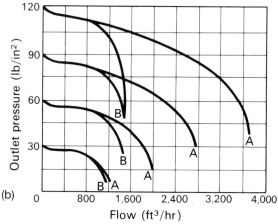

Figure 3.13   Graphs showing the performance of an oxygen therapy regulator. (a) Note that as the cylinder (inlet) pressure falls, the regulated pressure rises. A, 50 ft³/hr flow; B, 500 ft³/hr flow. (b) The outlet pressure falls as the flow rate increases. A, 1800 lb/in² inlet (when the cylinder is full); B, 200 lb/in² inlet (when the cylinder is empty).

Common faults in regulators

1. Damage to the soft seating of valves may occur as a result of the presence of grit or dust, usually from a dirty cylinder. This may cause a steady build up of pressure in the apparatus when the cylinder is left turned on but with no gas flowing.
2. A hissing noise may indicate a leaking or burst diaphragm. The regulator will need replacing or repairing by the manufacturer or service engineer.
3. Adams valves (Fig. 3.10) sometimes develop a fault that causes continual 'jumping' of the flowmeter bobbin — indicating an intermittent change of pressure and flow rate. This is usually due to the 'lazy tongs' sticking as a result of wear, but it may also be caused by small particles of grit or metal in the lazy tongs or the valve seating.

   On older patterns of the Adams valve there were fins on the nitrous oxide regulator to conduct heat from the surrounding air to prevent excessive cooling of the valve. It was not uncommon for the nitrous oxide to contain a significant quantity of water vapour as an impurity, and this condensed upon the valve seating and then froze, jamming the valve. The extra heat conducted by the fins was sufficient to prevent this freezing. Another method of preventing freezing was to install a small heater adjacent to the regulator. This was more commonly used in dental anaesthetic apparatus where high gas flows were usual. Water vapour is no longer a problem, but the fins remain as a relic.

Maintenance of regulators

Regulators should be checked during each routine service of the apparatus. Where apparatus is commonly out of use but kept available for emergencies it is wise to have rubber diaphragms renewed or a service exchange every five years.

Master and slave regulators

In some circumstances it is desirable to link two or more regulators together so that they give the same output pressure for their respective gases under any circumstances. Should the output pressure of one regulator fall, the others would follow suit. This is achieved by a principle using master and slave regulators. The output pressure of the master regulator is applied above the diaphragm of the slave regulators, thus replacing the screw and spring of an ordinary regulator. Such an arrangement is shown in Fig 3.14, where the principle is used to regulate the pressure of nitrous oxide relative to that of oxygen. Oxygen at between 40 and 100 lb/in^2 ($\sim$ 3 and 7 bar) is supplied to the input of the master regulator and the output of this master regulator is applied above the diaphragms of the slave regulators. A very small leak is allowed from the master output so that in the case of failure of the gas supply, the pressure on the secondary side of the master regulator would fall. If the oxygen supply fails, the pressure above the diaphragms of the slave regulators drops and these regulators close, preventing further flow of nitrous oxide.

Another example of master and slave regulators is seen in the Walton Five anaesthetic machine (see p. 177).

Flow restrictors

Where anaesthetic machines are supplied from the pipeline at a pressure of 60 lb/in^2 ($\sim$ 4 bar), it has become a common practice to omit regulators. Sudden pressure surges at the patient end of the anaesthetic machine are prevented by flow restrictors. These consist of constrictions in the regulated pressure pipework upstream of the flowmeters (Fig. 3.15). The disadvantage of using flow restrictors without regulators is that changes of pipeline pressure are reflected in changes of flow rate, which makes readjustment of the flow control valves necessary. Also there is a danger that if there is an obstruction at the outlet from the anaesthetic machine, pressure could build up in the vaporizers and cause damage. This is normally prevented by the inclusion of a 'blow-off' safety valve (as shown in Fig. 6.17). Flow restrictors do not normally require any maintenance. A different form of flow restrictor may be fitted in the downstream end of the vaporizers to maintain them under some pressure and so reduce the effect of back pressure when controlled ventilation or minute volume divider ventilators are used (see Fig. 5.19).

Relief valves on regulators

Safety blow-off valves are often fitted on the

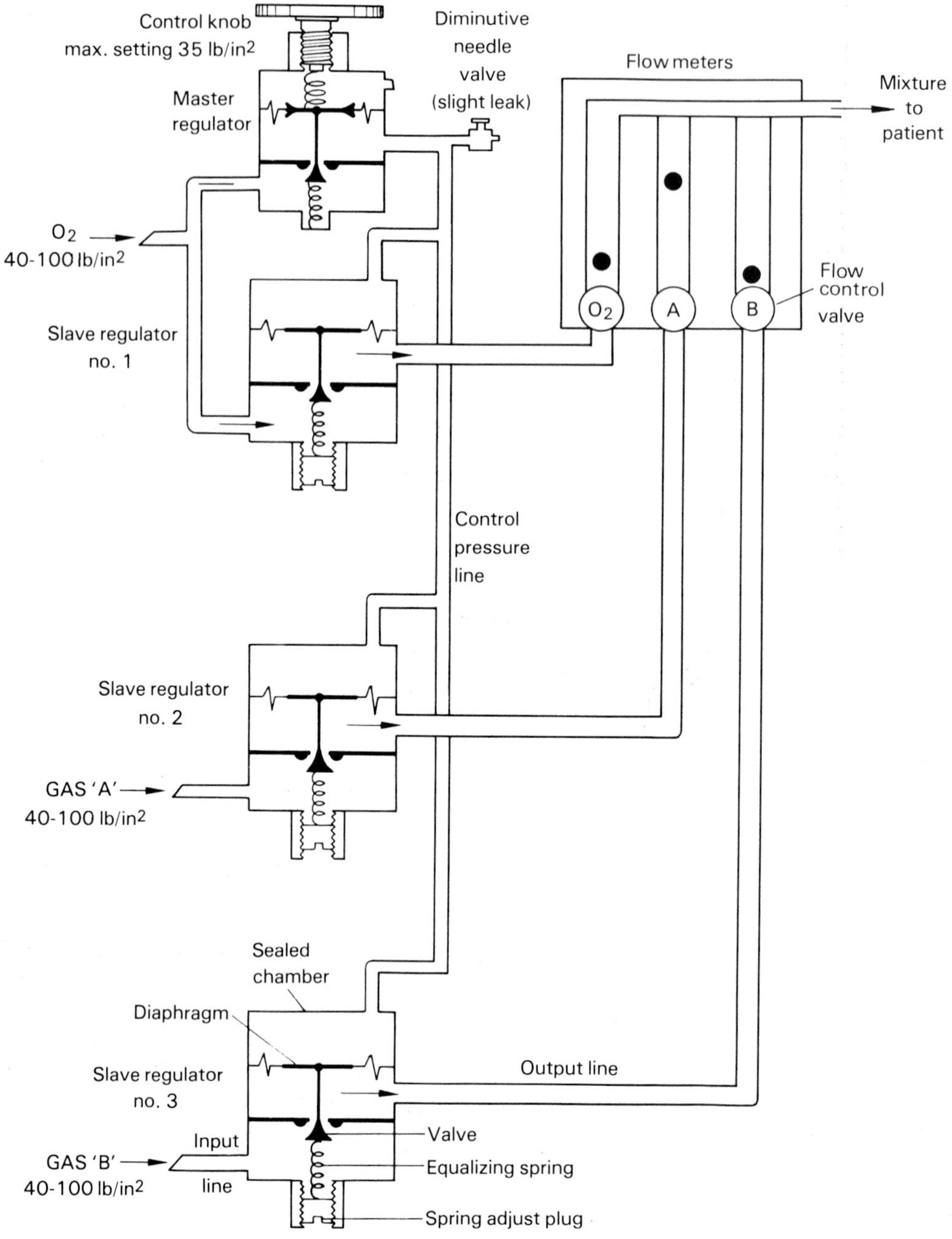

Figure 3.14 Master and slave regulators. The output of the master regulator, which can be adjusted by the control knob, is relayed through the control pressure line to the space above the diaphragm of each slave regulator. It acts on the diaphragm of the slave regulator in the same way as the spring shown in Fig. 3.10. If the oxygen supply fails, the pressure in the control pressure line falls due to the small leak from the needle valve. This, by virtue of reducing the pressure above the diaphragm of the slave regulators, leads to their closure and interruption of the output of the slave regulators. Thus if the main oxygen supply pressure begins to fall, the nitrous oxide and carbon dioxide pressures also fall. Should the oxygen supply fail altogether, they are completely cut off.

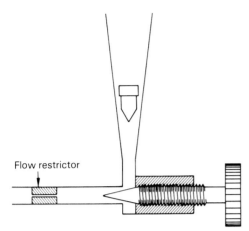

Figure 3.15 A flow restrictor. The narrow orifice causes a considerable pressure drop when there is a high flow rate, thus protecting the patient from sudden surges at the supply pressure of 60 lb/in^2 ($\sim$ 4 bar).

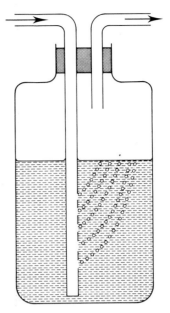

Figure 3.16 A water sight flowmeter.

down-stream side of regulators to allow the escape of gas if by accident the regulators were to fail and allow a high-output pressure. With a regulator designed to give a pressure of 60 lb/in^2 ($\sim$ 4 bar), the relief valve may be set at 100 lb/in^2 ($\sim$ 7 bar). These valves may be spring loaded, in which case they close when the pressure falls again, or they may operate by rupture, in which case they remain open until repaired.

Flow Rate of Gases

Although present day apparatus almost exclusively uses either the rotameter or the ball-and-tube type of flowmeter, it is necessary to mention the more primitive types of flowmeter so that the basic principles involved may be understood.

The earliest Boyle's machine, and some oxygen therapy equipment, employed the 'water sight' flowmeter (Fig. 3.16). The end of the tube through which the gas is supplied is immersed in water, and in this portion of the tube are drilled a number of holes. If there is a very low flow rate, the gas emerges through only the first hole, giving rise to a single stream of bubbles passing through the water. If, on the other hand, there is a very high flow rate, the bubbles stream from all the holes. Thus by observing the number of bubbles and the number of holes through which they emerge, a rough estimation of

flow rate can be made. This type of flowmeter is now obsolete. However, when one such oxygen therapy flowmeter/humidifier was taken from the museum and tested, the flow rates from the six holes marked 2, 4, 6, 8, 10 and 12 l/min were remarkably accurate.

Modern flowmeters depend on the fact that when a gas passes through an orifice there is a difference of pressure between the two sides. The fall in pressure is proportional to the flow rate of the gas and inversely proportional to the diameter of the orifice. If the orifice is of a fixed size, the pressure difference across it will be proportional to the gas flow through it. Conversely, if the pressure difference is kept constant, i.e. that required to lift a bobbin, the gas flow rate will vary with the diameter of the orifice. The resistance to flow of an orifice also varies with the density of the gas concerned, so that a flowmeter calibrated for one gas will not be accurate for another. Also, if a gas is at a different pressure than that for which the flowmeter is calibrated, its density will be altered and the calibration will be inaccurate.

Figure 3.17 represents a situation where gas is flowing along a tube in which there is a constriction with an orifice O. The flow rate is proportional to the difference between the pressures at P_1 and P_2. This principle is still used in some oxygen therapy

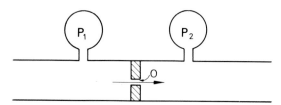

Figure 3.17 A constant orifice flowmeter. The diameter of O is constant. The difference between the pressures at P_1 and P_2 is proportional to the flow rate.

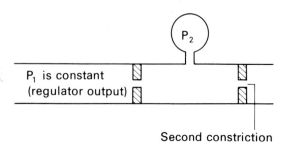

Figure 3.18 A variation of the above. The gauge at P_1 has been omitted since the pressure is constant, being the output of a regulator. A second constriction downstream from P_2 minimizes the effect of the output resistance on the pressure at P_2.

equipment. It has the great disadvantage that it depends on the accuracy of the pressure gauges, which, being delicate, may be damaged and become inaccurate. Its advantage is that it may be used in any position and does not have to be kept upright. In practice only one pressure gauge is needed, since the regulated pressure (at P_1) is constant. A false reading of flow rate may be produced by changes in the outlet resistance of the system. Thus if there is a resistance in the delivery tube, a high reading will be obtained. A second constriction downstream from P_2 may be used to produce a permanent output resistance for which the meter is calibrated and this minimizes the effect of resistance in the delivery tubing (see Fig. 3.18).

Variable area flowmeters

The flowmeter described above measures the pressure difference across a fixed construction, i.e. an orifice of constant area.

Most modern flowmeters depend on the principle of maintaining constant pressure but with an orifice of variable area. Examples of these are the 'dry bobbin' flowmeter, the 'Rotameter' and ball float meters (see p. 49), which are described below.

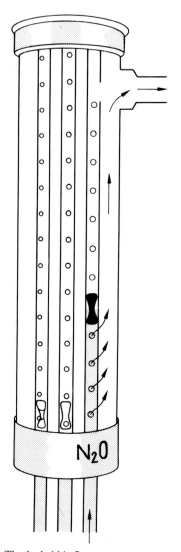

Figure 3.19   The dry bobbin flowmeter.

THE DRY BOBBIN FLOWMETER (Fig. 3.19)

Here a tube of uniform diameter has a series of holes bored in one side of it at intervals along its length. Running freely, but as a close fit in this tube, is a bobbin. The weight of the bobbin, which is analogous to the difference between the pressures at P_1 and P_2 in Fig. 3.17, is constant. The flow rate of the gas is proportional to the number of holes below the point to which the bobbin is lifted, i.e. the effective total diameter of these orifices. The higher the flow

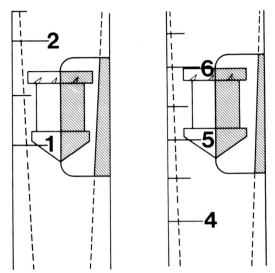

Figure 3.20   The Rotameter. In each case a portion of the tube has been cut away to show that the gap, or annulus, varies with the flow rate. The calibration should be read from the top of the float, (e.g. in the right-hand diagram the flow rate is 6 *l*/min).

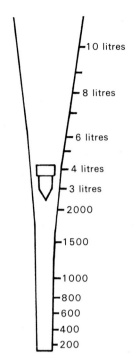

Figure 3.21   A flowmeter tube with varying taper to give an elongated scale at lower flow rates but allowing calibration for high flow rates also.

rate, the higher the bobbin is pushed up the tube. The disadvantage of this type of flowmeter is that it is rather inaccurate, partly because the bobbin tends to stick on the walls of the tube.

THE ROTAMETER* (Fig. 3.20)

This has now replaced the dry bobbin flowmeter. The tube has no holes drilled in it, but the bore is tapered so that the higher the bobbin is lifted, the wider is the gap between it and the wall of the tube. This variable gap or 'annulus' is the orifice. The bobbin is replaced by a 'float' of special shape which, having oblique notches cut in the rim, rotates freely in the middle of the gas stream and does not normally touch the walls of the tube. There is, therefore, no tendency for it to stick to the wall of the tube unless the rotameter is out of the vertical plane. The taper of the bore of the rotameter tube may be constructed so that it varies in order to elongate part of the scale, as shown in Fig. 3.21. This has the advantage that, even with a short tube, low flow rates may be measured accurately, while high flow rates are also indicated. The rotameter is capable of great accuracy.

---

* 'Rotameter' is strictly speaking the trade name used by one particular manufacturer, but in practice it has become synonymous with flowmeter.

Causes of inaccuracy in flowmeters

Tube not vertical
The orifice between the float and the tube is an annulus of a complicated shape (see Fig. 3.22). The resistance (across which there is a pressure difference) is caused by: (a) the effect of the density of the gas passing through the orifice (of diameter D), plus (b) the element caused by the viscosity of the gases passing through the tubular element (of length L) of the annulus.

If the tube is not vertical, the shape of the annulus becomes asymmetrical and at certain flow rates there is a significant variation in the proportions of the orifice and tube elements of the resistance, and therefore inaccuracies occur. If the flowmeter tube is further tilted, the float may actually touch the tube and the resulting friction may cause an even more inaccurate reading.

Static electricity
The float may also stick to the side of the tube as a result of static electricity, particularly in very dry

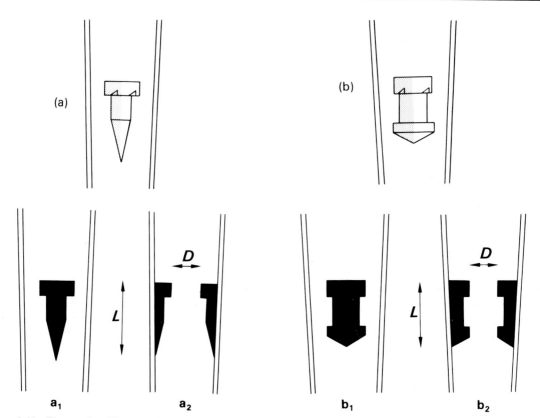

Figure 3.22   The annulus of flowmeter bobbins. (a) and (b) are two different types of bobbin. a₁ and b₁ show the space around them. a₂ and b₂ show how the effective tubular and orificial elements of these annuli differ. Note that this is a two-dimensional representation of a three-dimensional situation.

atmospheres. Moist air can leach away static from the outside of the tube. The effects of static may be reduced by spraying the outside of the tube with an antistatic agent such as Croxtine (BOC), which is supplied in an aerosol can. Improvements can be made by coating the inside of the tube with a material such as gold, in a film so thin as to be transparent, yet sufficient to be conductive of static electricity.

Dirt
Dirt on the tube or float may also cause sticking, especially in the case of nitrous oxide. Even if it does not cause sticking, particles of dirt either on the float or on the inner wall of the tube can change the effective diameter of the annulus and therefore cause an inaccurate reading.

In some of the older rotameters the wire stop at the upper end of the tube is shaped in such a way that the float can become impaled upon it. When the gas supply is turned off or fails, the float may remain at the top of the tube and give the impression that there is still a high flow rate. Some flowmeters are so constructed that the top of the tube is hidden by a bezel. This has resulted in patients being given a gross overdose, for instance of carbon dioxide, when the float, being at the top of the tube, was hidden by the bezel and not observed. This has also occurred in the case of cyclopropane, where the float is usually very small, and not readily observed.

Calibration of flowmeters

Flowmeter tubes are individually calibrated with their floats, at a specific temperature and pressure. Should there be any back pressure, for example when a minute volume divider ventilator is used, the density of the gas is increased and therefore the

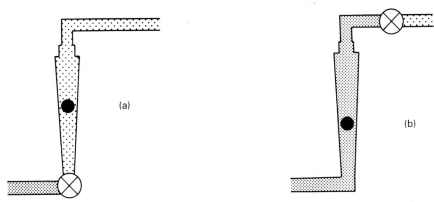

Figure 3.23 A pressure-compensated flowmeter. In (a) the flow control valve is upstream from the flowmeter tube. Any output resisance, as for example when minute volume divider ventilators are being used, will result in compression of the gas, leading to a false reading. In (b) the flow control valve is downstream from the flowmeter tube. The flowmeter tube is therefore constatntly pressurized (pressure compensated) at the supply pressure, at which the tube must be calibrated.

calibrations are inaccurate. In some anaesthetic machines, particularly in the USA, the flow control valves are fitted on the downstream side of the flowmeter tube. This results in the flowmeters being pressurized at the regulated pressure, and they need to be appropriately calibrated for these conditions. It prevents variations due to back pressure, and would seem to be a logical development. Figure 3.23 shows a pressure-compensated oxygen therapy flowmeter, and is included to demonstrate this principle.

Changes of temperature, except when extreme, produce insignificant inaccuracies. Flowmeters should be read from the top of the float. They are not calibrated from zero to the top of the scale, but from the lowest accurate point, and this is the first mark on the scale. Readings by extrapolation below this mark should not be attempted. A typical tube may be calibrated from 100 to 5000 cm^3/min, with the lower part of the scale elongated by a more gradual taper.

Causes of failure of flowmeters

On a number of occasions patients have suffered from oxygen deprivation due to leakage from a

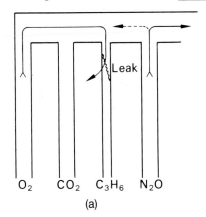

(a)

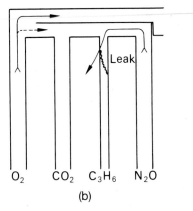

(b)

Figure 3.24 Diagram to show the effect of a leak from one of the rotameter tubes. (a) A leak from the cyclopropane tube in the traditional form of flowmeter block would result in back pressure from the nitrous oxide, causing oxygen to escape through the leak. The patient would therefore receive an anoxic mixture.

(b) A rearrangement whereby the oxygen is the last gas to enter the mixed gas flow and nitrous oxide rather than oxygen would be expelled through a leak. This would not lead to the patient receiving an anoxic mixture.

broken flowmeter tube in a flowmeter block arranged so that the oxygen is at the upstream end. If, for example, the carbon dioxide tube is broken, the force of the nitrous oxide flow will tend to cause a much higher proportion of oxygen than nitrous oxide to leak out of the fractured tube. This could be prevented by better design of the block so that oxygen is the last gas to enter the mixed gas flow (Fig. 3.24) In fact, ISO 5358 now requires that '. . . the oxygen shall be delivered downstream of all other gases. . .'.

Sequence of Gases in the Flowmeter Block

It is most unfortunate that although ISO 5358 requires that '. . . the oxygen shall be delivered downstream of all other gases. . .', there is no international agreement for the sequence of gases in the flowmeter block. It is even possible to find, in one hospital, anaesthetic machines, some of which have the control and flowmeter for oxygen on the left-hand side of the block and others on the right. To date the only other matter on which there is international agreement in this respect is that the oxygen flow control valve should have a knob of distinctive size and shape (Fig. 3.25).

Although the standardization of the sequence of gases in the flowmeter block is obviously desirable, there is still the possibility of the accidental production of an anoxic mixture owing to a mistake made by the anaesthetist using a machine in which the sequence is different from that to which he is accustomed. Here, again, there is no *international* standard for the colour coding of the cylinders, tubing, control valves, etc. for the gases, and this, too, can lead to dangers of confusion.

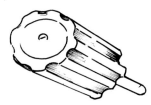

Figure 3.25 Specially profiled knob to identify the flow control valve for oxygen.

Routine Maintenance of Flowmeters

The tube and float should be regularly dismantled and cleaned. This is best done by a trained service engineer, who will often clean the tubes in rotation, one during each routine maintenance visit. It is essential that each float is replaced in its original tube.

Other Examples of Flowmeters

THE HEIDBRINK FLOWMETER (Fig. 3.26)

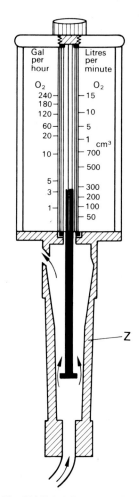

Figure 3.26 The Heidbrink flowmeter. Z, conical tube.

The Heidbrink flowmeter has a metal tube, the inside of which is tapered in the same way as a rotameter tube. The bobbin is replaced by a rod, the top of which may be seen through a glass tube which is an extension of the metal one. On either side of the glass tube is a scale, which is calibrated on one side in litres per minute and on the other side in gallons per hour. The tube has a varying taper (Z) which makes accurate measurements of small flow rates relatively easy and yet can measure flow rates of up to 15 litres/min. In Great Britain this meter is mostly used in oxygen therapy apparatus.

BALL FLOAT FLOWMETERS

Ball float flowmeters, like rotameters, have a tapering bore and are therefore variable orifice meters. The bobbin is replaced by a special ball of stainless steel or sapphire. If the tube is mounted on an inclined plane, one ball is sufficient, but if it is vertical, there may be an oscillation of a single ball which can be prevented by using two ball floats. The reading is taken from the point of contact between the two. The Connell flowmeter is set on an inclined plane and also has two ball floats in contact.

A single ball may also be used if the bore of the tube is not only tapered but also trefoil or triangular in section (Fig. 3.27). The ball is prevented from oscillating by its closeness to the ridges of the bore, and it is the depth of the grooves that varies along the length of the tube. Where there is one ball only, the reading is taken from its centre.

With inclined plane meters it is important that they are set at the correct angle, otherwise inaccuracies will occur.

THE FOREGGER FLOWMETER (Fig. 3.28)

This is a differential pressure, fixed area meter, and instead of the Bourdon pressure gauge (see p. 8), a water manometer is used. Gases pass through an orifice, the pressure across which is measured by the water manometer whose two limbs are of different diameter. The narrower limb is visible from the

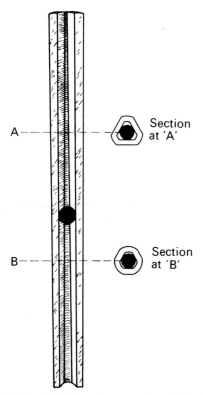

Figure 3.27   Trefoil ball float flowmeter. Note that the ball is prevented from oscillating by the shape of the bore of the tube. This type of meter is capable of greater accuracy than a ball float meter with circular bore.

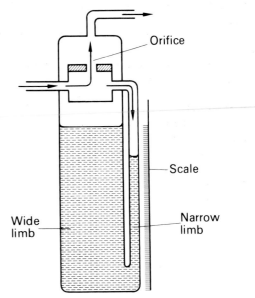

Figure 3.28   The Foregger water manometer flowmeter. The visible limb of the manometer is of relatively narrow bore compared with the hidden limb, which acts as a reservoir. The orifice is large, and therefore inaccuracies due to dirt are minimized.

front of the meter and the degree of depression of the water level indicates the flow rate of gas. Provided that the water level is properly maintained, this is an accurate flowmeter and there are no working parts to go out of adjustment and upset the calibration. Since the gas passages and orifice are relatively large, there is less chance of inaccuracy caused by dirt.

A Possible Danger with Flowmeters

One particular flowmeter for carbon dioxide, with a maximum flow rate of 2 l/min, includes a very small ball float made of stainless steel. The spring at the head of the tube is of exactly the same colour as the ball, and if the carbon dioxide control were inadvertently turned full on, the ball at the top of the tube could well escape notice, thereby perpetuating the danger mentioned on pp. 307–8. The use of a coloured ball would obviate this risk. Unfortunately the only coloured balls available are made of sapphire and are very expensive. One solution might be to redesign the head of the flowmeter tube with a nylon stop rather than a stainless steel one.

Flowmeters with ball floats rather than the rotating bobbin are not particularly more accurate, but ball floats are less likely to stick.

4

Piped Medical Gas and Vacuum Systems

The information given in this chapter refers mainly to the practice in Great Britain, though similar systems have been used for many years in other countries. In some of these other systems the nominal pressure is 45 lb/in^2 ($\sim$ 3 bar) rather than the British Standard of 60 lb/in^2 ($\sim$ 4 bar). In some systems a higher pressure is used for oxygen than for other services.

By virtue of the installation of a piped medical gas and vacuum (PMGV) system (Fig. 4.1) the need for provision of small 'duty' cylinders of oxygen and nitrous oxide on anaesthetic machines and similar items is obviated, and the number in 'reserve' may also be greatly diminished. The advantages of such a system are not only that there may be a reduction in the cost of the gases, but also that there is a saving of the cost of labour for transporting cylinders, a reduction in the introduction into the anaesthetic room and operating theatre of cylinders which may carry with them infection, and also a reduction of the incidence of accidents due to cylinders becoming exhausted. Much publicity has been given in recent years to the few accidents that have occurred in connection with piped medical gas supplies, but it is not easy to make a rational comparison between the incidence of accidents before and after the introduction of pipelines, owing to the great increase in the amount and complexity of work undertaken.

The PMGV services may be considered in five sections:

1. The bulk store or production plant.
2. The fixed distribution pipework.
3. The terminal outlets.
4. The flexible hoses, flowmeters and vacuum controllers which are detachable.
5. The connections between the flexible hoses and the anaesthetic machines.

Items 1 and 2 above may be considered as 'behind the wall' and it is usually felt that apart from broad strategy this is the province of the Engineering, Supplies and Pharmacy departments and the anaesthetist can take it on trust that the correct gases will be supplied. He cannot be held responsible for what goes on 'behind the wall'. In the case of items 4 and 5 above, the anaesthetist takes his share of responsibility to assure the maintenance of good standards, of checks and of tests and to prevent abuse. The terminal outlet is the interface between the two. The majority of the rare accidents that have occurred

have been between the wall and the patient, and possibly these could be deemed to be the most preventable — though several deaths have occurred in Great Britain and elsewhere due to cross connections (called 'confusion') which have led to gases, other than pure oxygen, being delivered from the oxygen outlet. It should be stressed that nearly all accidents have been caused by alterations or faulty repairs made by incompetent and sometimes unauthorized people rather than because the installation was that of one manufacturer or another or of a more modern or an older model, such as the BOC Mk 1 or Mk 4. Little benefit is to be gained by ripping out an older type of installation and replacing it with a more modern one just because new developments have been made. Indeed, the confusion that this could cause might add to, rather than diminish, the dangers. It has been suggested that if oxygen only were supplied by pipeline, there would be no possibility of confusion.

In most instances the cost of medical gases is reduced when they are delivered in large containers, and particularly in the case of oxygen when it is supplied in the liquid state. It should be noted, however, that the economy achieved in this manner is to some extent offset by the wastage that occurs during the use of a piped medical gas system. This wastage occurs at two points: mainly at the terminal outlet, which may be leaking or may be left running after the need for the supply has ceased, but also during the delivery of liquid oxygen, when a considerable volume is required to cool the delivery tube between the tanker and the vacuum insulated

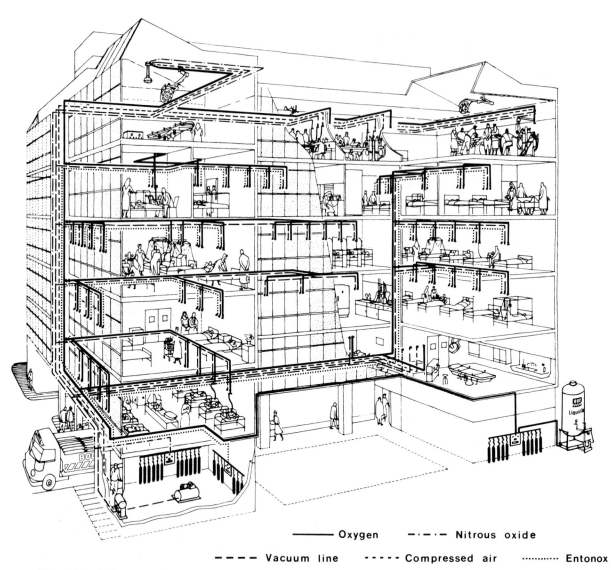

——— Oxygen   —·—·— Nitrous oxide

— — — Vacuum line   - - - - Compressed air   ·········· Entonox

Figure 4.1   A diagrammatical representation of a piped medical gas system.

evaporator (VIE) to below the critical temperature for oxygen (see pp. 1 and 33). Another small loss of oxygen from the liquid container occurs when there is little or no demand. In order to maintain a sufficiently low temperature, between 0.5 and 1.0% of the volume of liquid oxygen needs to evaporate daily so that the requirement of the latent heat of vaporization may offset the gain in heat owing to the inefficiencies in the insulation: if this vaporized oxygen is not drawn off into the pipeline it is voided to the atmosphere.

The 'gases' that are commonly supplied by pipeline are oxygen, nitrous oxide, Entonox (a nitrous oxide/oxygen mixture), compressed air and vacuum. Other gases such as helium and hydrogen are supplied in piped services to pathology laboratories and the like, but are not frequently used in direct connection with patients. They will not, therefore, be considered in this book.

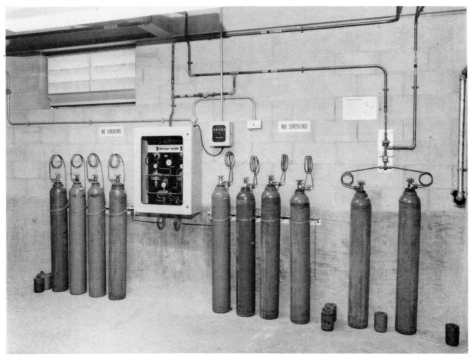

Figure 4.2   A major nitrous oxide manifold. Notice the coiled tail pipes, the indicator panel and the emergency supply cylinders on the right-hand side.

Bulk Store

Oxygen

In smaller installations oxygen is normally supplied and stored in cylinders as compressed gas. These are attached to *manifolds*, which consist of banks of several cylinders. There are usually two such banks, of which one is termed the 'duty' (or running) bank and the other the 'reserve' bank. The number of cylinders in each bank depends on the expected demand. The cylinders in each bank are all turned on and interconnected. However, the flow of oxygen from one cylinder to another is prevented by non-return valves. When the duty bank is almost exhausted the supply is automatically switched to the reserve bank. This now becomes the duty bank and an indication is given that this has occurred. The exhausted cylinders must now be replaced by full ones, and if this is not done before the second bank reaches a certain level of exhaustion, a compelling warning is given (see below). Figure 4.2 shows a

typical modern, automatic manifold for nitrous oxide, which operates in the same manner.

Figure 4.3 shows an emergency supply manifold, which may be used to continue the supply during periods of maintenance or repair, when the main manifold is out of action. Under these circumstances the pipeline is isolated from the main manifold by closing valve A and connected to the emergency manifold by opening valve B. Both of these latter operations are performed manually. Note that there is a pressure relief valve, which, like that on the main manifold, is vented to the outside rather than to an enclosed area where it might be dangerous. The valves on the cylinders of the emergency manifold may be kept open during periods of standby when valve B is closed, in order to show, by means of the contents gauge on the pressure regulator, that they are full, and by the regulated pressure gauge that the regulator is correctly set.

In many instances relatively small establishments such as dental clinics have piped gas installations with very few outlets. In Great Britain those employed by general dental practitioners are provided

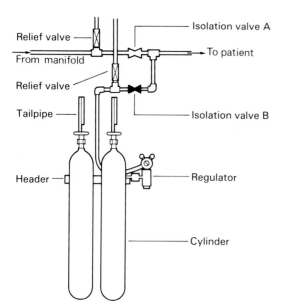

Figure 4.3   Emergency supply manifold. Note that valve A isolates the main manifold and valve B opens the emergency manifold.

and owned by individual practitioners and are not, therefore, subject to the regulations of the National Health Service or of Hospital Technical Memoranda. In the author's own town 'mini' pipelines such as that in Fig. 4.4 outnumber by at least 3 : 1 the larger and more sophisticated hospital installations. They include installations in which the pipework consists of ¼ inch (6 mm, ID) nylon tubing and there is a total absence of warning devices other than the pressure gauges on the regulators and the anaesthetic machines. Accidents associated with such systems are few and far between — possibly due to the ever reducing number of anaesthetics given in such clinics, due to the improvement in dental health! The visiting anaesthetist is well advised to inspect and test such installations before use. They are discussed further on p. 72–75.

LIQUID OXYGEN

In the case of larger consumers it may be found more economical to have deliveries of oxygen in the liquid form. Since the critical temperature of oxygen is about −119 °C if it is stored in liquid form, it must be kept at an even lower temperature. Liquid oxygen is transported in a specially insulated tanker and

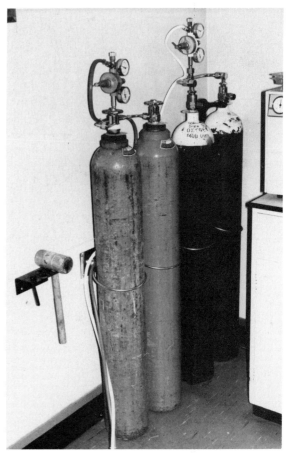

Figure 4.4   A small 'home-made' manifold, such as may be used in a dental operatory.

is delivered into a vacuum insulated evaporator (VIE) (Fig. 4.5). This consists of an inner shell of stainless steel, separated from an outer shell of carbon steel by a space which is kept at the greatest degree of vacuum possible and which also contains perlite powder. The temperature within the inner chamber is around −183 °C and, in that the container cannot be a perfect insulator, arrangements are made to maintain this very low temperature. There may be four connections to the inner cylinder. These are:

1. The filling port, through which fresh supplies of liquid oxygen are introduced.
2. A gaseous withdrawal line at the top of the cylinder, from which gaseous oxygen may pass via a restrictor plate and then a superheater

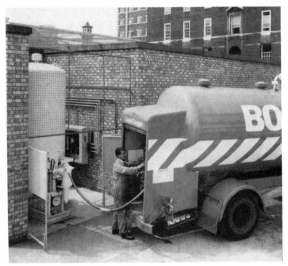

Figure 4.5 A vacuum insulated evaporator for storage of liquid oxygen.

(which consists of a length of copper tubing about 2.5 cm in diameter, on which are mounted metallic fins to conduct into it ambient heat), to the control system and distribution pipework. The purpose of the superheater is to raise the

temperature of the gaseous oxygen to that of the ambient air, for otherwise dangerously cold oxygen might be delivered to the terminal outlets in those parts of the hospital close to the VIE.

3. A liquid withdrawal line, which may withdraw liquid to enter the main flow downstream from the restrictor and upstream from the superheater, and,
4. A second liquid withdrawal line, which may pass through an evaporator and then either into the distribution network or back into the gaseous compartment of the container.

In older models there may be only two connections: one to the lower part, for the introduction and withdrawal of liquid, and the other at the top, for the withdrawal or reintroduction of gas.

Mode of operation of a liquid oxygen plant (Fig. 4.6) Since no insulation can be perfect, the inner container is continually receiving heat from the exterior, the effects of which are offset by the evaporation of liquid oxygen, thus helping to keep the latter at the appropriate temperature. If there is no demand for oxygen for a period of time, the pressure within the chamber may rise above normal (around 10.5 bar),

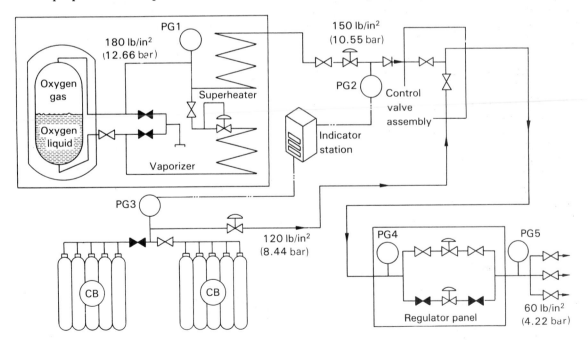

Figure 4.6 Schematic diagram of liquid oxygen plant. (See text for details.)

and at a predetermined, higher pressure a safety valve opens to allow the escape of some gas. The loss of oxygen owing to this venting is, as a rule, fairly small. Conversely, if the demand for oxygen is increased, there may be a fall of pressure within the vessel. In this case a control valve opens in the lower liquid withdrawal line and liquid passes through an evaporator and then either to the pipeline or to the gaseous compartment of the VIE until the pressure within it is restored to normal. In the event of an exceptionally high demand for oxygen, liquid may pass through the upper liquid withdrawal line directly to the superheater and via the control panel to the distribution system.

A cause of considerable waste is that during the delivery of fresh supplies of liquid, the hose between the tanker and the VIE needs to be cooled to below the critical temperature of oxygen before delivery can be effected. This is done by allowing liquid to escape from the tanker through it to the atmosphere. The oxygen delivered is metered at the tanker and on occasions it has been found that as much as one-quarter of the total delivery has been required for this pre-cooling.

The VIE rests on three legs, two of which are on hinged supports. The third rests on a simple steelyard weighing device with an appropriate counterweight. The contents of the VIE are expressed in weight and indicated on a dial.

The VIE is sited outside a building, within an enclosure which also houses two banks of reserve cylinders in a manifold similar to that described above (Fig. 4.7). The reserve cylinders automatically take over the load if the output from the VIE falls below a predetermined level. Being in the open, the VIE is subject to adverse weather conditions and it was once found that the weighing mechanism was immersed in water which had subsequently frozen into a solid block of ice. The estimation of the contents may well have been erroneous in this case.

Relative capacities of cylinders and the VIE
The pressure within a full cylinder of oxygen is 135 atm. Thus, when used on a pipeline, a cylinder can be expected to give approximately 130 times its capacity of oxygen at atmospheric pressure. Compared with this, one volume of liquid oxygen gives 842 times its volume of gas at 15 °C and normal atmospheric pressure. Since the VIE has a very much greater capacity than a cylinder, it will be obvious that it can deliver a far greater volume of oxygen than a whole manifold of cylinders.

Safety precautions
The manifolds for oxygen, nitrous oxide, Entonox and compressed air should be housed in a well-ventilated room constructed of a fire-proof material such as brick or concrete. The space within the room

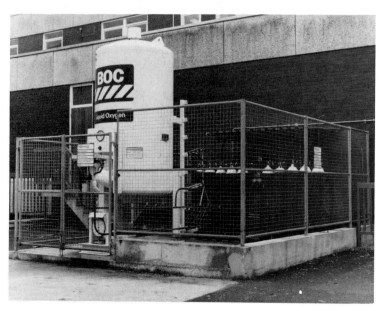

Figure 4.7   Banks of reserve cylinders for liquid oxygen plant.

should be adequate for handling trolleys carrying cylinders and for the unimpeded changing of cylinders on the manifold. All oils, greases and inflammable materials should be excluded from the room, as should pipes carrying town gas or oil. There should be no high-tension electric cables. The room should be well ventilated at high and low level and there should be no drains or gulleys in which gas could collect.

Cylinders of the gases used on the manifold may be stored in this room or in another location. They should preferably be sited where there is easy and close access from the delivery point by the supplier. The compressors and reservoir for the central vacuum plant and the plant for medical compressed air should not be housed in the manifold room. It should be impressed on all personnel that cylinders of compressed gas, particularly oxygen, can be dangerous, if mishandled. Provisions should be made for securing the cylinders to the wall.

Liquid oxygen plants should not be housed within a building. They should be sited in the open, a minimum distance of 6 m from any combustible material; no smoking should be permitted within this space. The ground surface should be of concrete or similar non-combustible material — and certainly not tar or asphalt, since they both form explosive mixtures when in contact with liquid oxygen. The plant should be surrounded by a fence of non-combustible material and there should be adequate access for the delivery tanker. There should be no overhead wires, nor drains or trenches within the prescribed area.

OXYGEN CONCENTRATORS

The desirability of the local manufacture of oxygen, obviating the need for the provision of cylinders or liquid oxygen, in the domiciliary and hospital scene, as well as in warplanes, has led to interesting new developments in the methods of separating oxygen from air. The principle of the oxygen concentrator (which is sometimes referred to as a molecular sieve) depends on the property of an artificial zeolite to entrap molecules of nitrogen. In Fig. 4.8 there are two steel chambers (A and B) containing the zeolite. To start with, A is charged with compressed air from the compressor, and while the nitrogen is retained in the zeolite, the remainder of the gases, of which over 90% is oxygen, passes on to a receiver and from there

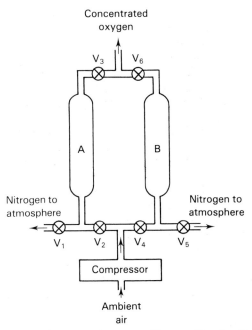

Figure 4.8   An oxygen concentrator. To start with, valves V_1, V_4 and V_6 are closed. Compressed air passes via V_2 into cylinder A, where the nitrogen is absorbed by the zeolite, and concentrated oxygen passes out via V_3. When the capacity of cylinder A is used up, valves V_1, V_4 and V_6 are opened and valves V_2, V_3 and V_5 are closed. Cylinder B then takes over the function, while nitrogen from cylinder A is discharged to the atmosphere.

to the patient. When the zeolite in A is calculated to have been fully charged with nitrogen there is an automatic change-over to B and a vacuum is applied to A to remove the nitrogen from it. The change-over is made on a time basis. The output provides at least 92% of oxygen, the other gases being nitrogen, argon and the other rare gases. Small oxygen concentrators are in regular use for the treatment, in their own homes, of patients with respiratory disease.

The whole of the equipment is encased in a small cabinet (Fig. 4.9), no larger than the average television set, and operates from the mains electric supply. Typically, the output might be 2–3 litres of oxygen per minute, which is the optimum for the patients for whom it is intended. Somewhat similar devices are used in military aircraft.

Very much larger oxygen concentrators may be used to supply a hospital. Of these there are currently two varieties: those with two large chambers, such as that shown in Fig. 4.10, and plants with multiple

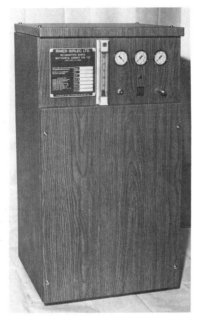

Figure 4.9   A small domiciliary oxygen concentrator.

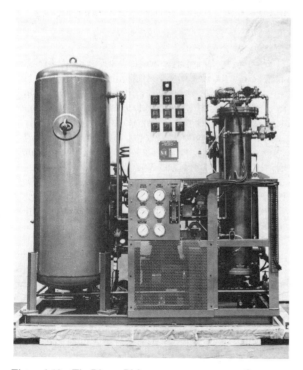

Figure 4.10   The Rimer–Birlec oxygen concentrator of sufficient capacity to supply a hospital.

air compressors and concentrators, such as that shown in Fig. 4.11. Not only is the latter system by MGI fully automated, but it is also capable of supplying medical compressed air.

The use of oxygen concentrators in hospitals is likely to increase, especially in those areas where reliable deliveries of oxygen in cylinders or liquid form may be impossible to guarantee. There may be prejudice by some physicians against the delivery of a gas which is not pure oxygen; however, the use of mixtures containing more than 90% oxygen is seldom vital.

The financial economy afforded by the use of oxygen concentrators greatly depends on the cost of oxygen supplied by other means. It should be pointed out, however, that there may be a considerable saving in labour in the delivery and handling of cylinders, a task which is sometimes beyond the capabilities of the domiciliary patient or his relatives. In domiciliary use the employment of an oxygen concentrator for a period of over one year has been shown to afford financial economy, but there is, as yet, insufficient experience to evaluate with certainty its use in hospitals.

Nitrous oxide

As stated on p. 32, nitrous oxide liquefies at room temperature when stored under pressure in a cylinder. It is therefore supplied to a piped medical gas system from a manifold of cylinders similar to those for oxygen, described above.

When considering the size and number of cylinders to be installed in each bank, thought must be given to the maximum demand that will be required. This is because nitrous oxide cools not only as it expands but also due to the latent heat required to vaporize the liquid. If a heavy demand is taken from a bank of small capacity, the gas may cool to such a low temperature that water vapour in the ambient atmosphere condenses, and may even freeze, on the surface of parts of the pipework and in particular the pressure regulators. In the days when nitrous oxide cylinders contained some water vapour, this used to freeze *within* the regulator, causing obstruction. For this reason a regulator heater, thermostatically controlled at 47 °C may be fitted to warm the gas and prevent condensation. Further details of cylinder manifolds are given in the caption of Fig. 4.2. There is not yet a practical method for the local manufacture of nitrous oxide, though progress in this field is being made.

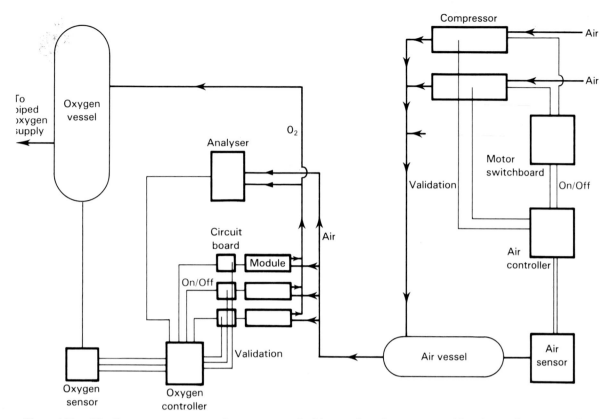

Figure 4.11 The Oxymaster oxygen cascade concentrator. In this a number of compressors, either alone or in company with others, take the load in turn. Similarly, there are multiple absorption vessels. One advantage of this system is that it may also supply medical compressed air as required.

Entonox (50% nitrous oxide + 50% oxygen)

This mixture is used for the administration of inhalational analgesia, principally in the obstetric department. The manifolds employed are essentially the same as those for nitrous oxide and oxygen, but additional safeguards are required in the handling of the cylinders. This is because the mixture has a pseudocritical temperature of approximately 6 °C and if the cylinder were allowed to cool below this point, the nitrous oxide and oxygen might separate out by a process known as lamination.

The large cylinders for Entonox manifolds have pin index outlets as shown in Fig. 3.3, and unlike smaller cylinders for this purpose, there is an internal tube from the valve block, leading down to within 10 cm of the bottom of the cylinder. The contents are supplied through this tube, the position of which would prevent the discharge of pure nitrous oxide if lamination had occurred. Excessive cooling of the cylinders is prevented by ensuring that there are a sufficient number of cylinders on the manifold and that all of them are turned on at the same time. No single cylinder should supply gas at a rate greater than 300 l/min.

Cylinders of Entonox should be stored for 24 hours after delivery before being connected to the manifold. There should be a special store for them and they should be kept in a horizontal position at a temperature between 10 and 38 °C.

There does not yet seem to have been much interest shown in the problems of atmospheric pollution arising from the use of Entonox analgesia. However, efficient scavenging would be difficult to achieve and this may, in the future, lead to a reduction in the popularity of a piped supply of this mixture.

Medical compressed air

Medical compressed air (CA) differs from industrial compressed air in that a greater degree of purity is required. Industrial CA may well contain not only water vapour but also an oil mist. Indeed, much industrial equipment operated by CA requires the addition of a lubricant. Medical CA may be administered to patients through both anaesthetic equipment and lung ventilators in the theatre and the

Intensive Therapy Unit and it is also employed to power some surgical instruments. Whereas a pressure of 4 bar ($\sim$ 60 lb/in^2) is sufficient for the former, many surgical instruments require a higher pressure of about 7 bar ($\sim$ 105 lb/in^2). Although the CA driving surgical instruments is not intentionally administered to the patient, it would, if not clean, contaminate the operating field. At first sight it might be thought that a 7 bar compressed air system would on its own be suitable to supply a hospital (this pressure being required for surgical instruments); however, it must be borne in mind that this might present difficulties in the Intensive Care Ward, where blenders are used for mixing oxygen with medical compressed air to achieve the appropriate mixtures for administration to patients. Where the use of surgical instruments is expected to be relatively infrequent, it might be considered better to install a piped medical CA system at 4 bar, and to use separate cylinders with the appropriate pressure regulators for a 7 bar supply. This would seem to be particularly appropriate since it is sometimes the practice of surgeons to vary the precise pressure of CA to suit the power tool in use and the speed at which it is required to run.

Piped medical CA may be supplied either from a manifold of cylinders, as described above for oxy-gen, nitrous oxide and Entonox, or by a compressor. A cylindered supply is relatively expensive, but the quality of the air can be assured. Since the cylinders of compressed air have the same right-hand thread on a bull-nosed outlet as oxygen, care must be taken in the storage of such cylinders to ensure that they are not accidentally interchanged. It is recommended that the storage bins be separated from each other, for example by a wall or partition, and that they be clearly marked.

In a larger hospital it may well be economical to install a compressor. In this case the air has to be both dried and filtered at the outlet of the compressor in order to achieve adequate quality. A scheme for such a compressed air plant is shown in Fig. 4.12.

Only too often in the past, it has happened that when a hospital was being built an industrial CA plant was installed and the air was found to be unsuitable for medical purposes. In one such instance the author found that the pipe run to an outlet in the basement was completely filled with condensed water which had gravitated there from the rest of the distribution pipework.

As was shown above, a single plant may be used both to provide medical CA and to run an oxygen concentrator.

In some instances it has been considered

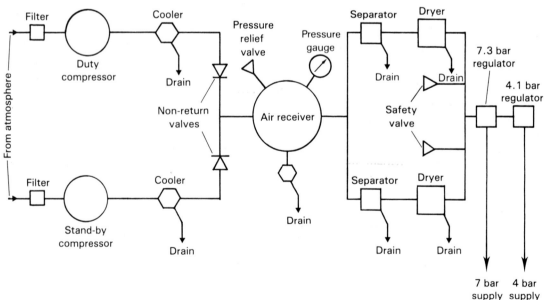

Figure 4.12   A simplified diagram of a medical compressed air plant.

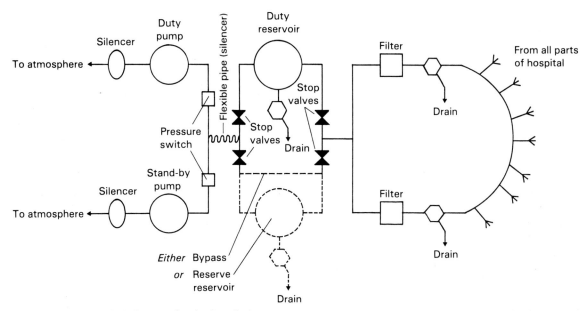

Figure 4.13 A simplified diagram of a piped medical vacuum plant.

appropriate to install a small local compressor for a particular department in order to save extensive pipework. If this is done, it is essential to ensure that there is adequate oil separation and filtration to suit the requirements of that department. This is often lacking in small compressors.

Piped medical vacuum

It is the author's view that this is the most advantageous of all the piped services. If the provision of vacuum is left to local suction machines throughout the hospital, there is only too often a disastrous delay, either because a particular machine is faulty or because the electric supply is not within reach. The most important limitation of the use of piped medical vacuum is the availability of an outlet point in close proximity to the patient for whom it is needed. The prompt use of suction, for example to clear the gastric contents from a patient's air passages, is of great importance, and in the author's experience the failure to provide this from small local suction machines is far more common than, for example, the exhaustion of an oxygen cylinder. More consideration of this will be found on p. 63, where the distribution of medical vacuum outlets is considered.

In Great Britain guidance on the design and in-

stallation of piped medical vacuum services is set out in British Standard 4957 of 1973 and Hospital Technical Memorandum (HTM) No. 22 as revised in 1977.

Fig. 4.13 shows the layout of a typical vacuum plant. The precise details of this may vary according to the type of pump in use.

The distribution pipework may take the form of a 'ring main', the two ends of which each pass towards the pump through a stop valve and then a drainage trap in which any aspirated liquid or condensed vapour, for example from body cavity drainage, may separate out and be removed. The pipes then pass through bacterial filters and from there to the vacuum reservoir. At the bottom of the reservoir is a drainage pipe, with a manual drain valve, to evacuate any liquid which may collect.

The connection between the reservoir and the vacuum pumps is made through flexible hoses in order to reduce vibration and the noise that this might transmit through the pipework. There are two pumps, each of which is adequate for the needs of the system. Thus one pump may be 'on duty', whilst the other is on standby or being serviced.

There are various types of vacuum pump, but particular mention should be made of those that are oil-lick lubricated. It has been suggested that if the vacuum system is employed for the purpose of

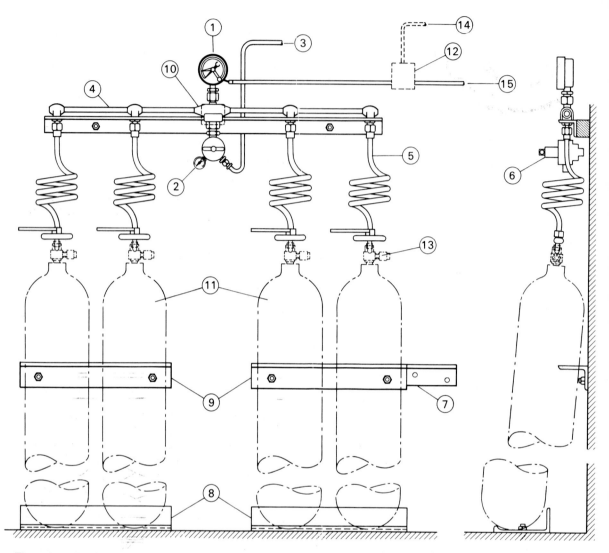

Figure 4.14   The BOC Minor manifold. Changeover from one bank of cylinders to the other is performed manually. The near exhaustion of one bank of cylinders is indicated by a warning signal which is ideally situated within view of the anaesthetist. 1, high-pressure gauge with contacts for the warning light; 2, regulated pressure gauge; 3, supply pipe; 4, header assembly; 5, tail pipe; 6, pressure regulator; 7, tool rack; 8 and 9, frames to secure cylinders; 10, header connection; 11, cylinder banks; 12, fused switch; 13, cylinder valves; 14, electric supply; 15, wiring to distant warning light.

scavenging waste anaesthetic gases, the vapour of halothane and other anaesthetic agents may be absorbed by the lubricating oil, and by reducing its efficiency may cause failure of the pump. However, this possibility is yet to be substantiated, and in the meantime frequent checks of the level and condition of the oil are called for.

The output of the pump passes through a silencer to be exhausted at a suitable point, such as above roof level, where the gases may be vented to atmosphere without risk of polluting the air breathed by staff or patients.

PERFORMANCE, LEVELS AND SPECIFICATIONS FOR A MEDICAL VACUUM

For Great Britain the specifications for a piped vacuum are laid down in BS 4957 of 1973. A few of these are quoted below, but for more complete information the full specifications should be consulted.

A vacuum of at least 400 mmHg (533 mbar) below standard atmospheric pressure (760 mmHg or 1013 mbar) should be maintained at the outlets, each of which should be able to take a flow of free air of at least 40 l/min; there should be at least two outlets per operating theatre, one per anaesthetic room and one per recovery bed.

The suction control units are described in Chapter 16 so that comparison may be made with other types of suction apparatus.

Indicators and alarms

The gauges and indicators that are an integral part of a major manifold are shown in Fig. 4.2. A typical arrangement has one green indicator marked 'running' or 'duty' and one red indicator marked 'empty' for each bank of cylinders. Thus when the first bank of cylinders becomes exhausted the green 'running' indicator on that side is extinguished and the red 'empty' indicator on that side is illuminated. At the same time the green indicator marked 'running' for the second bank will illuminate. The red indicator on the first bank stays lit until the cylinders have been replaced by full ones and have been turned on.

Since the manifolds are usually remote from the users and the members of staff responsible for changing the cylinders, repeater indicators may also be installed — for instance at the telephone switchboard or in the porters' lodge.

The above indicators may be expected to operate when the installation is running normally. Warning signals, which may consist of a red or orange flashing light, are given when there is some impending failure — for example if one bank is empty and the pressure in the cylinders in the other bank falls to a predetermined level, i.e. if there has been a failure to heed the indication that one bank of cylinders needs replenishing. Another warning may be given if the pressure in the output of the manifold falls below a predetermined level.

On smaller installations such as the 'Minor' mani-

fold (Fig. 4.14), on which the cylinder/s on one side are turned on manually, there are two indicator lamps per gas. A white one shows that the electric current is turned on and a red one that the cylinder pressure has fallen to a predetermined level.

The indicators for a liquid oxygen plant may show 'normal running', 'running from cylinders', 'first bank of cylinders empty' and 'low line pressure'.

Electric supply to PMGV systems

The pumps for compressed air and vacuum should be powered by the 'essential' supply, which is backed up by the emergency generator. If possible, the manifold controls and warning lights should also have their own emergency supply. Some manifolds are so constructed that if there is total power failure, the indicators and warning lights will fail, but all the cylinders, of both banks, are switched on so as to continue the supply. Other manifold controls have a manual override which may be used to switch from one bank to the other.

Distribution Pipework

For detailed information concerning the regulations and standards required for fixed distribution pipework, the regulations imposed by the appropriate Government or Health Ministries should be consulted. In Great Britain these are quoted in HTM 22 and its supplement, which refer to the 'permit to work' system, which lays down the procedures to be adopted when service maintenance, repair or alterations are to be effected.

In this chapter only a brief description can be given of the fixed pipework; since this part of the installation is 'behind the wall', it is more properly the concern of the hospital engineer rather than of the medical man. The anaesthetist should, however, be aware of the nature of the installation and should always be informed *and consulted* before any alterations to it are made.

The tubes used are copper, of a special degreased quality. Before they are delivered to the site, i.e. prior to installation, the ends are sealed so that there can be no ingress of dirt or other foreign material. The copper is also of a special alloy which prevents degradation of the gases. There is some relaxation of this in the case of the vacuum installation. The fittings are of degreased brass. Joints are made by brazing rather than with soft solder or compression fittings. Recently a system of brazing without the use of a flux has been developed and this results in a greatly reduced incidence of corrosion of both the surface and interior of the pipe and fittings. The diameter of pipe is determined by the demand that it will carry. Commonly it may start from the manifold with a diameter of 42 mm (1½ inch), but after branching to supply one or more areas pipes as narrow as 15 mm (½ inch) may be employed. 6 mm (¼ inch) pipework has been used for the final runs in many cases, but this is not now considered good practice for new work. In many instances a pipe of 6 mm diameter has been found to deliver gases at a perfectly satisfactory rate, and there is no valid reason for replacing it with pipes of a larger bore simply to comply with a new standard.

Large installations may be divided into sections, supplying various departments. Each of these sections may be isolated by valves. Each department or ward, or section thereof, may be further isolated by a valve that is readily accessible to the staff, which may be used to turn off the gas supply in case of fire, fracture or other catastrophe. In earlier installations the isolating valves were often placed in a position that was not readily accessible or known to the staff working in the department.

Area valve and service units (Fig. 4.15) may be installed in such positions as to protect a number of departments or wards. These consist of a locked box containing an isolating valve, upstream and downstream of which are branches with the appropriate NIST (non-interchangeable screw thread) unions. These latter are normally closed with a blanked off NIST union. When the blanking nut is removed a self-sealing valve within the union again closes it off. When the appropriate NIST connection is made, the self-sealing valve is reopened. These branches may be used to purge pipelines or to introduce a local supply during alterations or breakdowns. The box also contains a 'spade', which may be used to ensure absolute closure of the pipeline, irrespective of the action of the valve.

Regional flowmeters may be incorporated in piped medical gas systems to detect the section in which an excessive leak or wastage of gas is occurring. Moisture traps may also be installed.

The actual pipework should be identified by

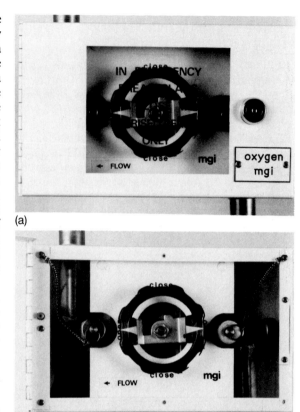

(a)

(b)

Figure 4.15   An area valve box: (a) with the door in the normal closed position; (b) with the door open, showing the NIST (non-interchangeable screw thread) connections.

labels placed upon it at regular intervals, in accordance with the identification code described in Fig. 4.16. Indeed, it is good practice for all pipework, whatever substances are carried, to be correctly labelled at regular intervals. The pipework may be hidden behind the wall or buried within the plaster on the one hand, or alternatively it may be mounted on the surface. The latter arrangement is not only aesthetically less attractive, but also less satisfactory from the standpoint of general hygiene and cleanliness.

There are two exceptions to the method of jointing: (i) isolating valves may be screw threaded in order to facilitate later replacement or alteration and to avoid damage during fitting; and (ii) a special type of compression joint, referred to as cold-jointing, may sometimes be used. A particular coupling

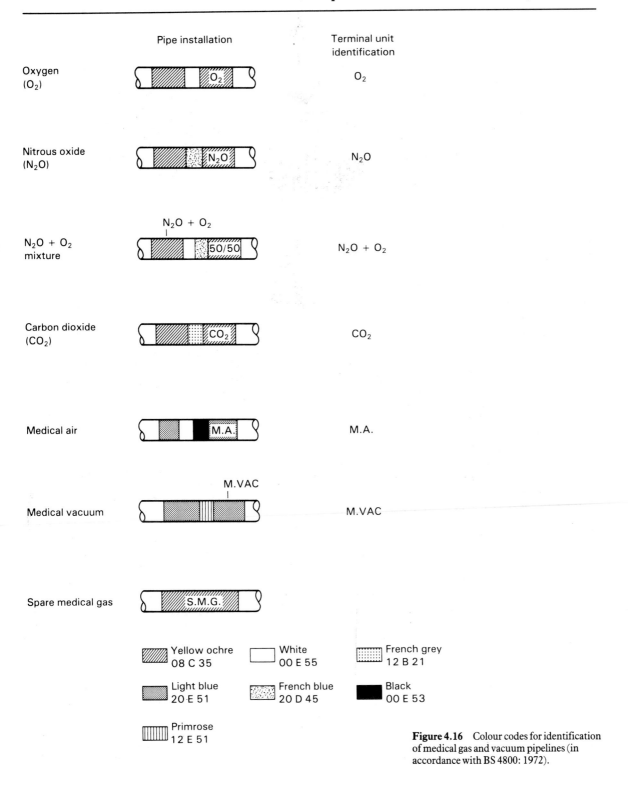

Figure 4.16 Colour codes for identification of medical gas and vacuum pipelines (in accordance with BS 4800: 1972).

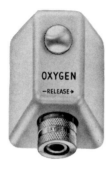
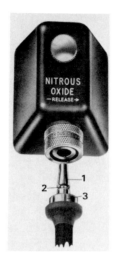
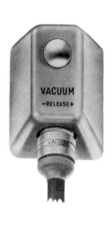

(a)

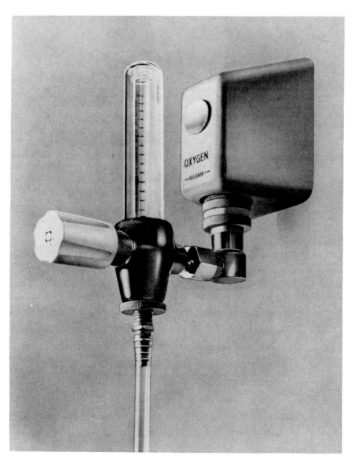

(b)

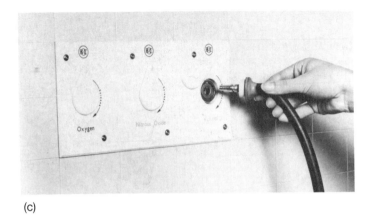

(c)

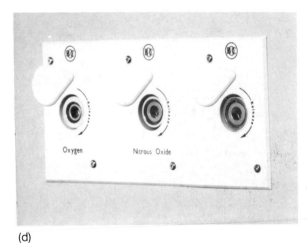

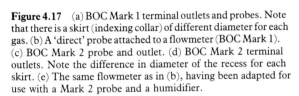

(d)

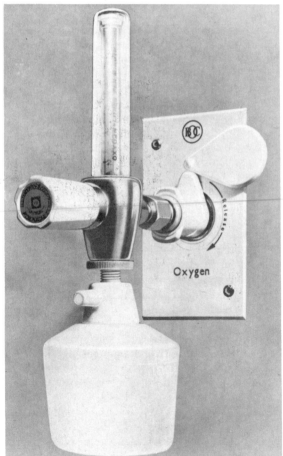

(e)

Figure 4.17   (a) BOC Mark 1 terminal outlets and probes. Note that there is a skirt (indexing collar) of different diameter for each gas. (b) A 'direct' probe attached to a flowmeter (BOC Mark 1). (c) BOC Mark 2 probe and outlet. (d) BOC Mark 2 terminal outlets. Note the difference in diameter of the recess for each skirt. (e) The same flowmeter as in (b), having been adapted for use with a Mark 2 probe and a humidifier.

manufactured by Hydroculpin is specified in HTM 22.

The pipework for medical gases and a vacuum, and their fittings, should be separated from other pipework so as to avoid confusion. The isolating valves should be clearly labelled and situated in such a location that they may be closed by the retreating staff in the event of a fire.

Terminal Outlets

The distribution pipework terminates in outlets that are in the form of self-closing sockets. Into each of these sockets one may introduce a probe attached either to a terminal unit such as a flowmeter or to a hose that is, in turn, connected to an anaesthetic machine. By virtue of their design, each terminal outlet will accept only the probe appropriate to the gas for which it is intended, as can be seen in Figs. 4.17 to 4.21. This is therefore a non-interchangeable system. In the ideal situation, non-interchangeability would be continued right back to the bulk supply of the gas concerned. Tubes and fittings of diameters unique to each gas might be used, as is the case in the pipeline kit offered to dentists by Nesor (see Fig. 4.29). Unfortunately this ideal is not yet universally achieved, but in more recent practice steps are being taken to prevent a terminal outlet for one gas being attached to the base fittings for another. For example, in the BOC Mark 4 conversion kit, a locating pin in a position specific to each gas, prevents the assembly of inappropriate parts (Fig. 4.22) The author found that, unfortunately, this locating pin may be displaced easily and this defeats the object of the exercise.

Although several systems have been used in Great Britain, there is now a British Standard, No. 5682 of 1978, for outlets and probes, which is very similar to BOC Mark 4.

It is quite obvious that in all new installations the best and most up-to-date equipment should be installed. However, the policy of some hospital authorities to replace all previous types by the latest, simply because the Standard has been more recently published, should be viewed with caution. For example, it is the author's belief that although BOC Mark 1 outlets have some disadvantages and potential dangers, before these are all removed and re-

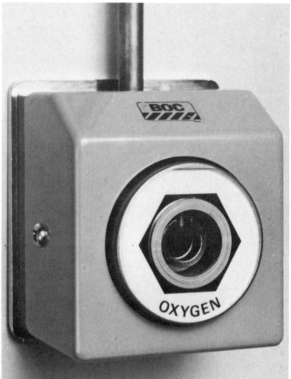

Figure 4.18   BOC Mark 3 terminal outlet. (The probe used is similar to that for the Mark 4 terminal outlet, shown in Fig. 4.18.)

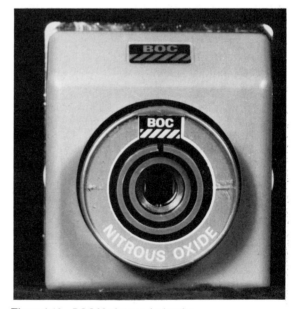

Figure 4.19   BOC Mark 4 terminal outlet.

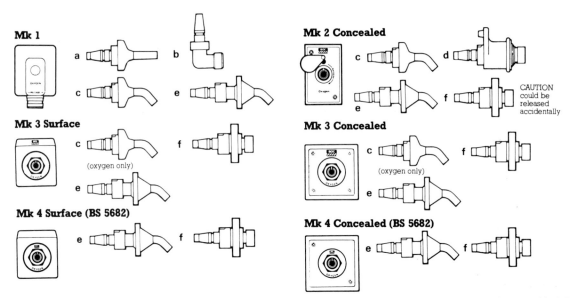

Figure 4.20 Profiles of BOC Mark 1, 2, 3 and 4 terminal units and probes. Probes: (a) Mark 1 remote; (b) Mark 1 direct; (c) Mark 2 remote; (d) Mark 2 direct; (e) Mark 3 and 4 remote (BS 5682); (f) Mark 3 and 4 direct (BS 5682).

placed with the latest model, one should consider carefully whether:

1. The financial outlay is justified; and
2. All the disturbance caused by the building work involved is justified. The very fact that changes are being made could lead to accidents.

It is considered that a much more realistic attitude should be taken with regard to the implications of the publication of a new Standard or Code or Practice than has been the case with some hospital authorities.

In the ideal situation there would be only one pattern of probe throughout the world, with absolute non-interchangeability of all components of the system, including those 'behind the wall'. In the meanwhile a single standard should be sought for each hospital or hospital group: alterations being made only after considerable deliberation and consultation, and all engineering work and maintenance being carried out by staff who are properly trained for the purpose.

Flexible Hoses

The hosepipe connecting the terminal outlet of the fixed pipeline installation to the anaesthetic machine is the section of the system in which damage and wear are most likely to occur, and which is most accessible to well-meaning but ignorant members of staff who may attempt to make repairs or alterations. Originally the hosepipe for each gas was constructed of the same black, reinforced rubber or neoprene tubing, identified only by a short length of coloured sheath at each end. This predisposed to accidents when, during repairs, cross-connections were made. More recently characteristically coloured tubing has been used for each gas. The development of such self-identifying tubing was unfortunately delayed by the difficulties involved in manufacturing it with the necessary antistatic (electrically conductive) properties.

Several accidents have been caused by the connection, or reconnection, of the probe for one gas at the upstream end of such a hose, but the socket or union for another at the downstream end. On the commissioning of one hospital, the author found that a pair of hoses intended for the supply to an anaesthetic

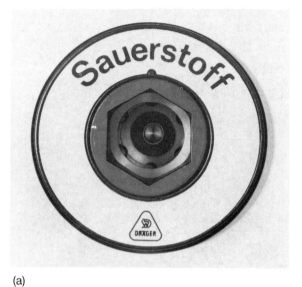

(a)

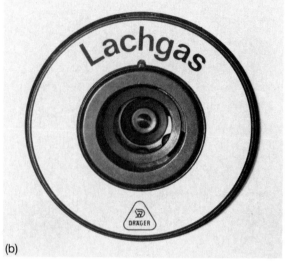

(b)

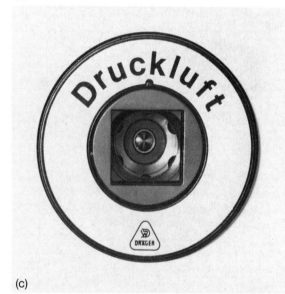

(c)

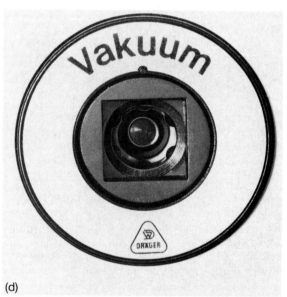

(d)

machine had been supplied, as new, by the manufacturer with the oxygen and nitrous oxide probes and sockets reversed.

The incidence of such accidents should be reduced by the current practice of most manufacturers to produce hoses, complete with the appropriate connections, in different factories or different areas of one factory. Furthermore, it is now a recommended practice that a damaged hose should not be repaired on site, but should be returned in its entire-

ty to the manufacturer in exchange for a factory-made service replacement.

The connections between the hose and fittings must be secure. Originally a fairly thin ferrule was used. This could be crimped on by a special pair of pliers or a purpose-made crimping clamp (Fig. 4.23). These ferrules could be removed without difficulty by using a pair of wire cutters. 'O' clips (see Fig. 2.12) have also been used, but these are equally vulnerable to tampering. An improved fer-

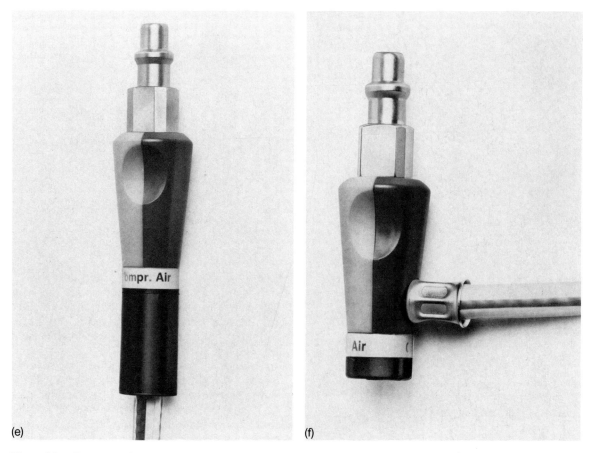

(e)   (f)

Figure 4.21   Dräger terminal units. Note that the sockets have a profile specific to each service. (a) Sauerstoff = oxygen. (b) Lachgas = nitrous oxide. (c) Druckluft = compressed air. (d) Vakuum = vacuum. There are (e) direct and (f) right-angled probes.

rule (Fig. 4.24), manufactured by MIE, is made of stainless steel and is of much greater thickness; it is applied by a 30 ton press and is sufficiently robust to defy all but the most determined attempts at removal.

Under no circumstances should one use devices such as the deservedly popular Jubilee clip (see Fig. 2.11), which can be released and retightened easily and repeatedly.

The development of the attachment of the hose to the anaesthetic machine requires some consideration. When PMGV systems were originally installed they were commonly connected to anaesthetic machines designed to be supplied by cylinders. It was often required to retain the facility to return to a cylindered supply without difficulty. The hoses,

therefore, terminated in a pin index block which resembled the valve block of a pin indexed cylinder. The block had either a tail (Fig. 4.25a) onto which the hose could be directly attached (and secured by a ferrule), or a probe which fitted an appropriate terminal outlet, which is in turn was attached to the end of the hose (Fig. 4.25b).

This system was safe so long as no one tampered with it. If it became damaged, it could be safely replaced by an entire assembly — provided that such an assembly was available. Lack of spare parts often led to 'on the spot' repairs, some of which turned out to be disastrous.

In 1973 the DHSS drew attention to the dangers, and among other recommendations advised that the connection of the hose to the anaesthetic machine be

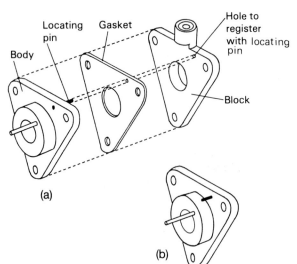

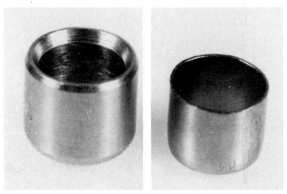

Figure 4.24 An improved ferrule manufactured by MIE, with an old-type ferrule for comparison.

Figure 4.22 (a) Locating pin in BOC Mark 4 conversion kit. (b) The pin displaced.

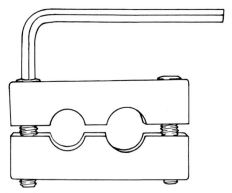

Figure 4.23 A purpose-made crimping clamp.

'made permanent'. However, the varying interpretations of this gave rise to problems. If the hose were ferruled onto a spigot on the machine, this would encourage the very type of repair that it sought to prevent. A more satisfactory solution was the employment of a nut and liner (Fig. 4.26) for a gas-specific non-interchangeable connection to a branch of the regulated pressure pipework of the machine extra to the usual complement of cylinder yokes. Provided that an appropriate spanner and an adequate stock of spare hose assemblies are to hand, such a system should be safe. To this end anaesthetic machines are now manufactured with the appropriate fittings (Fig. 4.27). In the case of other models

where a cylinder yoke is to be used, it is recommended that the pin index block with the hose ferruled directly to a tail be used and that the tommy bar of the yoke be replaced by an Allen screw (Fig. 4.28), the appropriate wrench for which is available with the spare hose assemblies.

In addition to the above, and probably even more important, proper arrangements should be made for planned preventive maintenance by suitably qualified engineers, and one named member of the medical staff should be appointed to act in a supervisory and advisory capacity.

Pipeline Kits for Installation by the Owner

Nesor offers three kits (Fig. 4.29). Kit A consists of the cylinder mountings, coupling assemblies, regulators and so forth, and enough tubing and fittings to provide one operatory with a pair of nitrous oxide and oxygen outlets. It also includes the hoses from the wall outlet to the anaesthetic machine. Kit B is an extension for another operatory, and up to three extra operatories can be done with one Kit B for each. Kit C, as an alternative, consists of regulators and flexible hoses for attaching the anaesthetic machine to cylinders on the wall of the operatory itself. The copper tubing and fittings for nitrous oxide and oxygen are of different diameters throughout, to prevent the possibility of confusion.

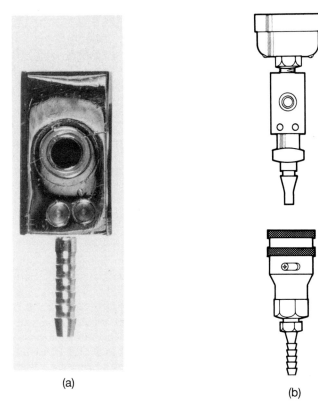

(a)

(b)

Figure 4.25   (a) A pin index block with a tail for a flexible hose. (b) A pin index block fitted with a BOC Mark 1 spigot; a Mark 1 terminal fitted to the end of a flexible hose. Such systems are now discouraged owing to the increased risk of mistakes being made during repairs which could lead to the confusion of gases.

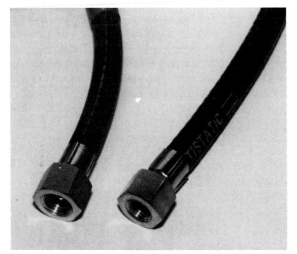

Figure 4.26   Nut and liner union to an anaesthetic machine. The threads are non-interchangeable and gas-specific.

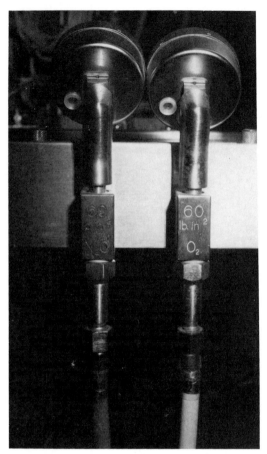

Figure 4.27   Hosepipe union block.

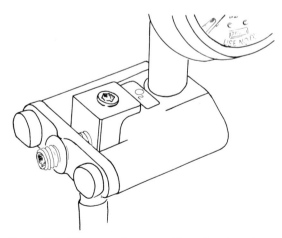

Figure 4.28   The tommy-bar removed from the yoke and replaced by an Allen screw.

McKesson supply a similar kit but with nylon tubing. That for oxygen is white and of 10 mm outside diameter, while that for nitrous oxide is self-coloured blue and 8 mm outside diameter. An offer is made to test an installation that has been assembled by the owner himself. Although nylon tubing is less robust and fireproof than copper tubing, it has the advantages that it may be threaded through narrow spaces and that there are far fewer joints.

Before a decision is made to install a piped system using nylon rather than copper tubing, it should be confirmed that this would not invalidate the owner's fire insurance policy.

Tests and Checks for PMGV Systems

The anaesthetist should be held responsible for checking only that part of the PMGV system between the terminal outlet and the patient. He should be able to take for granted the quality and unfailing supply of gases.

Quality control is usually considered to be the province of the hospital pharmacist, who should make or have made tests to confirm the identity of the gas, its purity and composition, and freedom from contaminants, including solid particulate matter. Compressed air should be examined for water vapour and oil mist. The pharmacist is usually responsible for maintaining adequate supplies of cylinders.

The engineering department is responsible for organizing both planned preventive maintenance and emergency repairs.

The portering staff are usually responsible for changing cylinders and holding a store of portable oxygen cylinders with flowmeters and suction equipment for use in emergencies or during shutdown for maintenance and alterations.

The anaesthetist is responsible for the correct insertion of his pipeline probes and any necessary adjustments. A fuller description of 'cockpit drill' is given on pp. 117–120, but at this point two simple tests may be recommended:

1. Plug in the oxygen probe *only* and check that on opening the oxygen flow control valve oxygen flows — and that no gas flows through the nitrous

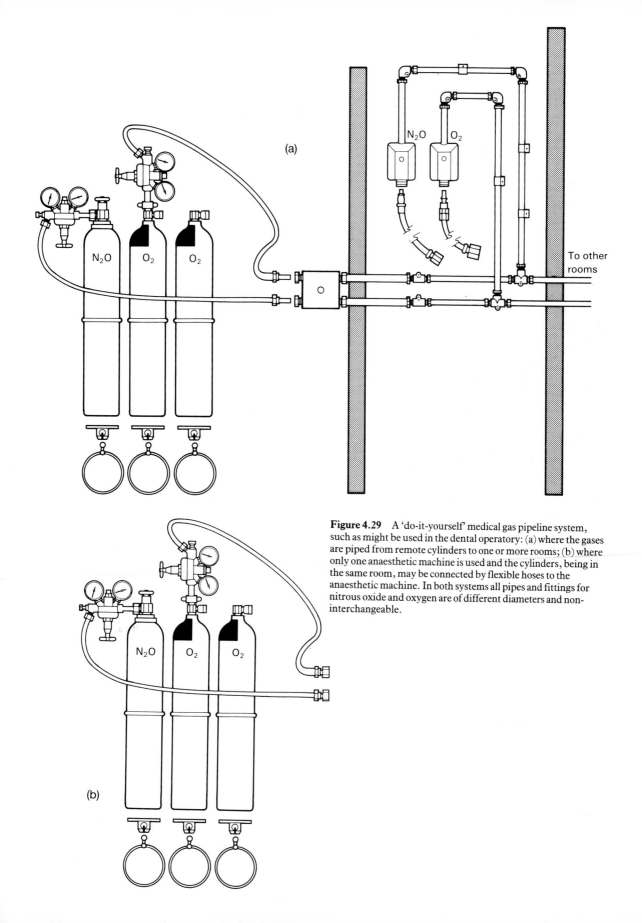

(a)

N₂O O₂

To other rooms

N₂O O₂ O₂

Figure 4.29 A 'do-it-yourself' medical gas pipeline system, such as might be used in the dental operatory: (a) where the gases are piped from remote cylinders to one or more rooms; (b) where only one anaesthetic machine is used and the cylinders, being in the same room, may be connected by flexible hoses to the anaesthetic machine. In both systems all pipes and fittings for nitrous oxide and oxygen are of different diameters and non-interchangeable.

N₂O O₂ O₂

(b)

PERMIT TO WORK ON PIPED MEDICAL GASES

AHA...   SERIAL   N⁰   79025

PART 1   LEVEL OF HAZARD – HIGH/MEDIUM/LOW   ....

Authorised Person

The Piped Medical Gas System supplying (state gases)..

....to...

may be taken out of service for a period of approximately........................ days / hours at.......................(time) on................(date).
without hazard to patients.

Medical Officer or
....Authorised Nurse   ....date ....time

---

PART 2   SPECIFICATION No........................ DRAWINGS No........................   DATED...............

The system(s) is/are isolated as follows at..

....

....

....

The following work shall be carried out..

....

....

....

....

Other associated Permits to Work in use are...issued to......................date...............

....issued to......................date...............

.........................Authorised Person.............................date.........................time.

.........................Authorised Person.............................date.........................time.
(taking over)
NO OTHER WORK SHALL BE CARRIED OUT

PART 3

I accept responsibility for carrying out the work as indicated above. No attempt will be made by me nor by any person under my control to work on any other part of the installation. I am fully conversant with the relevant fire and safety precautions required.

....Competent Person...date.........................time

....Competent Person...date.........................time
(taking over)

PART 4 (*Initial in spaces to indicate actual tests completed)

I declare that the work described in Part 2 is now complete. Valve tightness/   */pressure/   */anti-confusion/   */ flow rate and delivery pressure/   */alarm/   */tests have been successfully carried out. The system(s) is/are internally clean/   */purged/   */and ready for identity and purity tests. No additional fire hazards exist due to this work. All modifications have been recorded in ink on the pipework, valve, and alarm system "As Fitted" drawings.

.... Authorised Person...date.........................time

FOR COMPLETION AFTER HIGH HAZARD WORKS ONLY

PART 5 (*Initial in spaces to indicate actual tests completed)

Identification tests have been undertaken for O_2...........*N_2O...........*N_2O/O_2...........* Air...........*Vacuum...........*

Purity tests have been undertaken for O_2...........*N_2O...........*N_2O/O_2...........*Air...........*

The installation may be taken into use.

....Authorised Person   ....Suitably Qualified Person

....date   .... date

PART 6   FOR COMPLETION AFTER MEDIUM OR LOW HAZARD WORKS ONLY

The installation may be taken into use...Authorised Person   .... Date

---

Original – to Competent Person. Duplicate – to Suitably Qualified Person. Triplicate retained in Book for permanent record and retained for at least two years.
On completion the original should be filed by the Hospital Engineer for a period of at least six months.

(Right-hand margin labels:)
Level of hazard
Approval of doctor or nurse
Description of work
Acceptance of responsibility by competent person
Declaration of completion and testing of work
Purity and confusion tests (high-hazard work only)
Completion of medium- and low-hazard work

Figure 4.30   A 'permit to work' form.

oxide flowmeter when its flow control valve is opened.

2. When all probes are plugged in, give each a short, sharp tug to make sure that they are correctly engaged. It is possible for a probe to be retained in a socket, even vertically, without proper connection having been made: no gas will flow.

The supplement to HTM 22, which should be consulted for further details, describes a 'permit to work' system. Essentially this is a code of practice in which the engineer discusses with the appropriate people the nature of the work to be done so that services such as oxygen and vacuum independent of the PMGV system may be made available as required. Only too often there has been a lack of communication between the medical, nursing and engineering staff, invariably because no one named person has been specified for responsibility in each discipline. The 'permit to work' document (Fig. 4.30) with no less than six parts to be completed (depending on the degree of hazard), may at first seem to be yet another proliferation of the already burdensome paperwork in hospitals. It does, however, increase safety and improve the relationships between departments.

5

Vaporizers

Many inhalational anaesthetic agents are liquids under normal conditions and require to be vaporized before they can be administered to the patient. They are not used as pure vapours, but are diluted by a vehicle such as nitrous oxide and oxygen mixtures, pure oxygen or air.

For some agents such as halothane, where too high a vapour concentration would be dangerous, one needs a vaporizer in which the concentration of vapour can be controlled and in which the calibration takes account of changes of temperature and the level of the liquid agent within the vaporizer. However, agents such as diethyl ether may be used safely with more simple apparatus, in which the vapour concentration is not known, since there is less risk arising from overdose.

Not only are some agents more volatile than others, but there is also a considerable variation in the concentration of each that is required to produce safe and efficient anaesthesia. For instance, halothane is seldom used above 4%, whereas diethyl either may be needed in as high a concentration as 20%.

This chapter describes the general principles of the construction of vaporizers, though obviously not all types can be discussed in detail. The maintenance required for a particular vaporizer is stated by the manufacturer, and it should be remembered that when an anaesthetic machine as a whole is routinely serviced by the maintenance engineer of one company, he may not necessarily check a vaporizer made by another, and separate arrangements should be made for this. Most manufacturers recommend that temperature-compensated vaporizers be returned to them each year for cleaning and recalibration, and they provide a service exchange system.

Vaporization in Air

Open-drop method

The earliest method of vaporizing anaesthetic agents such as ether and chloroform was to pour the liquid drop by drop into a napkin which was placed close to the patient's mouth and nose. The vapour concentration was gradually raised by increasing the number of drops per minute. The napkin was later replaced by devices such as the Schimmelbusch mask (Fig. 5.1). There are several varieties of the mask, but in essence it consists of a metal frame over which gauze or lint is spread. In the case of ether the liquid is dropped evenly over the whole area of the gauze, whereas with chloroform it is restricted to one-half of it in order to ensure that air may be freely drawn without too high a concentration of the vapour. For ether, sixteen layers of gauze are put on the mask, whereas for ethyl chloride or chloroform twelve layers of gauze or one of lint are used. When ether is being used its high rate of vaporization requires so much latent heat that the mask becomes cool and water vapour from the exhaled air may condense on it and eventually freeze. This not only causes resistance to air passing through the gauze,

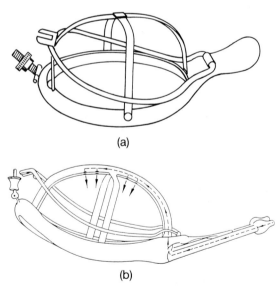

(a)

(b)

Figure 5.1 (a) The Chadbourne modification of the Schimmelbusch mask. (b) Another modification, in which oxygen or anaesthetic gases may be delivered via the two perforated tubes.

but also reduces the rate of vaporization. For this reason a second mask or a fresh supply of gauze is required during a long administration.

When using the Schimmelbusch mask it is customary to cover the patient's face with a piece of gamgee about 25 × 20 cm and to cut (or tear) in this a central hole to expose the patient's nose and mouth (Fig. 5.2). The gamgee is utilized primarily in order to prevent vapour or liquid from entering the patient's eyes, but it also reduces the amount of air drawn in by the patient between the mask and his face. Sometimes a similar piece of gamgee is used to cover the mask.

'Open-drop' administration has little place in modern anaesthesia, and anaesthetic vapours are usually supplied by vaporizers operated by gases under pressure.

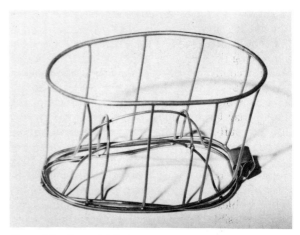

Figure 5.3 Ogston's inhaler.

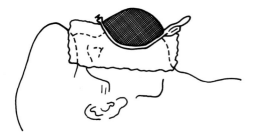

Figure 5.2 A layer of gamgee over the patient's face protects his eyes during open-drop administration.

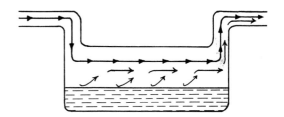

Figure 5.4 The principle of the plenum vaporizer.

Semi-open-drop method

In this technique a mask somewhat similar to the Schimmelbusch was used, but this mask, the Ogston's inhaler, was surmounted by a wire frame round which a napkin or some gauze could be erected in order to 'keep the ether in' (see Fig. 5.3). Note that the use of the term 'semi-open' to describe the method used in breathing systems such as the Mapleson A is incorrect, though only too often used.

Vaporizers Intended to be Used in Conjunction with Gases Under Pressure

Figure 5.4 shows a metal box with an inlet port at one end and an outlet port at the other. As the gases pass through it a certain amount of anaesthetic vapour is carried with them. The concentration of this vapour varies with the temperature (which drops as vaporization proceeds), the level of the liquid, and the rate of gas flow. This is known as a Plenum vaporizer.

In practice the vaporizer is controlled by providing two channels, one of which passes through a vaporization chamber, while the other is a bypass through which the gases flow without coming into contact with the liquid anaesthetic agent. In the 'off' position all the gases pass through the bypass: in the 'on' position some or all flow through the vaporization chamber (Fig. 5.5).

Figure 5.6 shows various methods of increasing the rate of vaporization. In (a) a wick is immersed in the liquid and draws it up, thereby considerably increasing the area over which vaporization occurs and also compensating for a fall in the liquid level. In (b) the Boyle's bottle (see also Fig. 5.8), the degree to which the gases impinge on the surface of the liquid may be controlled by a cowl. If the cowl is lowered sufficiently, the gases are made to bubble through the liquid, causing the maximum degree of vaporization. In (c), the 'copper kettle' and Halox vaporizers, the gases are broken up into small bubbles by being passed through a sintered diffuser. The bubbles, being very small, present the maximum possible area of contact between the gas and the liquid. In (d) the type of low-resistance ether vaporizer used on a circle absorber, baffles ensure that the gases repeatedly impinge on the surface of the liquid.

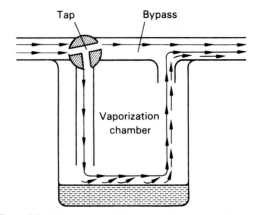

Figure 5.5   The tap controls the proportion of the mixed gas flow that passes through the vaporization chamber, as compared with that which passes through the bypass and does not come into contact with the liquid anaesthetic agent. In the 'off' position the whole of the fresh gas flow passes through the bypass.

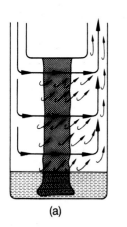
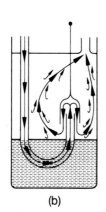

(a)   (b)

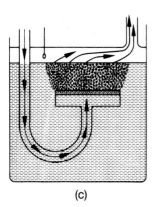
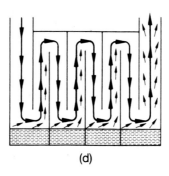

(c)   (d)

Figure 5.6   Methods of increasing the vaporization rate in a vaporizer. (a) The liquid anaesthetic agent is drawn up a wick, thus presenting a greater surface area for vaporization. (b) The mixed gas flow is directed onto the surface of the liquid anaesthetic agent by a cowl. (c) The mixed gases are broken up into a large number of small bubbles which pass through the liquid anaesthetic agent, thus presenting the maximum possible surface area to the liquid. (d) A series of baffles repeatedly redirect the mixed gas flow onto the surface of the liquid anaesthetic agent.

Factors Influencing the Vaporization Rate of Volatile Anaesthetic Agents

The rate of vaporization depends on:

1. The volatility of the liquid.
2. The temperature of the liquid.
3. The temperature of the gases flowing over the liquid.
4. The flow rate of the gases.
5. The area of contact between the gas and the liquid.
6. The shape and volume of the space above the liquid.

Methods of Minimizing Changes of Vapour Concentration Due to Changes in Temperature

1. By attaching a large mass of metal or liquid such as water, a considerable reservoir of heat can be provided and the temperature drop in the anaesthetic liquid can be reduced to a minimum. This method is used in the 'copper kettle' vaporizer (see Fig. 5.20).

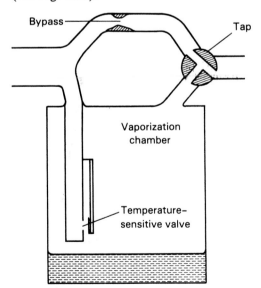

Figure 5.7   A temperature-sensitive valve further controls the proportions of gas passing through the bypass and the vaporization chamber.

2. Variable bypass (Fig. 5.7). The proportion of gases passing through the vaporization chamber is varied not only by the control knob selecting the appropriate vapour concentration but also by a second, automatic, thermostatic valve.

Examples of Vaporizers

The Boyle's vaporizer

The Boyle's vaporizer (Fig. 5.8) and similar types of 'bottle' are commonly used to vaporize ether, methoxyflurane (Penthrane) and trichloroethylene (Trilene). It is neither calibrated nor temperature or level compensated.

When the control lever is in the 'off' position, the mixed gas flow passes entirely through the bypass, as shown in Fig. 5.9a. As the lever is turned progressively towards the 'on' position, a steadily increasing proportion of gases is passed through the bottle. In the fully 'on' position all the gases pass through the bottle. The 'natural' path the gases would take is straight from the end of the U-tube to the outlet O. They may be diverted, however, by lowering the cowl C over the end of the U-tube, so that they impinge on the surface of the ether, as shown in Fig. 5.9b. With the cowl fully down, Fig. 5.9c, they are forced to bubble through the liquid itself, thus producing the maximum rate of vaporization. The position of the cowl is adjusted by the plunger P, which passes through a gland to maintain a gas-tight seal. The working parts of this vaporizer are best seen in an exploded diagram (Fig. 5.10). The control drum rotates inside the body of the vaporizer, and is positioned laterally by the adjusting and locking rings at each end. Special grease is used to maintain a seal and yet allow free rotation; there is spare grease in the grease injector cap and by turning this it can be fed into the seating of the drum. As gases and vapours pass through the vaporizer, even when it is turned off, the grease tends to be slowly washed away and this results in stiffness if extra grease is not added. In order to remove the drum for cleaning, the actuating lever is first unscrewed and then the locking and adjusting rings are removed from the inlet end. If the drum is so tight that it cannot be easily withdrawn, it can be pushed through by screwing inwards the adjusting ring at the other end.

Bypass — Tap — Vaporization chamber — Temperature-sensitive valve

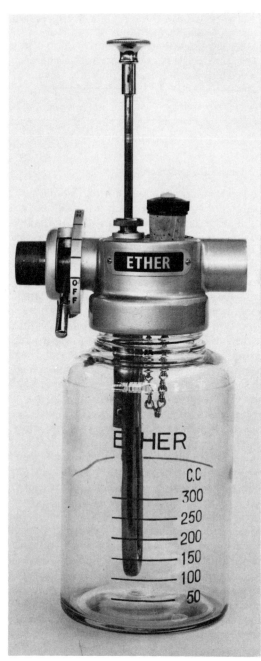

Figure 5.8   The Boyle's vaporizer

Note that in some instances the drum is conical and can be withdrawn only from one end. This operation is usually carried out by a service engineer.

After long service the plunger may become loose and tend to fall down on its own. This can be corrected by tightening the gland nut. Eventually the packing in the gland will need to be replaced. This usually consists of cotton, but in some of the more modern vaporizers the cotton is replaced by neoprene or nylon, which should not wear out. The cork stopper in the filling orifice should be a good fit, and is normally retained by a small chain. In some vaporizers the metal anchor for this chain passes through the cork. Should the chain be broken, this metal core to the cork could act as a sparking-plug if somebody who was charged with static electricity were to touch the metal cap (see Fig. 5.11a). For this reason it is important that the chain is intact. Sometimes the top of the cork is insulated so as to prevent this hazard.

The bottle sealing washer is usually made of cork, sometimes with a canvas or metal insert. It often becomes brittle and damaged and may fall out. This allows a leak of anaesthetic gases and vapour. There may also be a leak if the top of the bottle is chipped. This leak can assume considerable proportions and may lead to a situation where the gas flow reaching the reservoir bag is very much less than that indicated by the flowmeters and much of the volatile agent escapes (Fig. 5.11b). Rebreathing by the patient ensues, and this leads to difficulties during the induction and maintenance of inhalation anaesthesia.

It will be noticed that in some vaporizers the metal parts within the bottle are not plated but are left as bare copper. The reason for this is that copper is an anticatalyst that prevents the decomposition of ether. Some bottles are made of dark glass, either brown or green, to prevent the decomposition of anaesthetic agents by light. Two sizes of bottle are commonly used, a broad one for ether and a narrow one for other volatile agents. In the case of chloroform and trichloroethylene a sufficient concentration is produced by turning the control knob fully on without depressing the plunger at all. Indeed, by doing so a dangerously high concentration would be produced. The concentration of vapour depends on the temperature (which drops as vaporization proceeds), the level of the liquid anaesthetic agent in the bottle and the rate of gas flow.

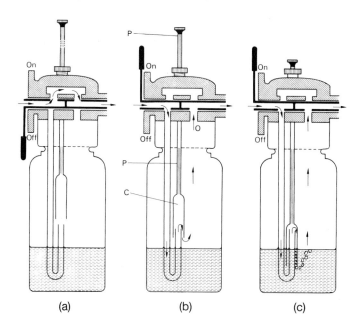

Figure 5.9 Three diagrams of the Boyle's vaporizer showing (a) the control lever in the 'off' position, (b) the control lever fully 'on' and the cowl C lowered so as to cause the gases to impinge on the surface of the liquid, and (c) the cowl C further lowered so as to cause the gas to bubble through the liquid.

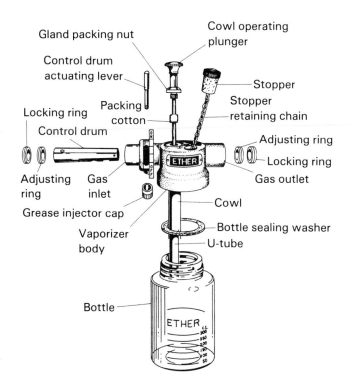

Figure 5.10 Exploded diagram of the Boyle's vaporizer.

PRACTICAL USE OF THE BOYLE'S VAPORIZER

The graduations for the control lever are entirely arbitrary and as a rule the vaporizer begins to operate when the lever is at about the second mark. When using ether the lever should be turned on very slowly. A common practice is to advance it one-quarter of a division after each four consecutive regular breaths.

The bottle may be charged with as much as 10 oz (~ 270 ml) of ether, which fills the bottle to nearly half full. In the case of trichloroethylene and chloroform only about 1 cm depth of the anaesthetic agent is used. Note that the Boyle's vaporizer is not particularly suitable for methoxyflurane because of the difficulty of producing a sufficiently high concentration of this agent for the induction of anaesthesia.

Because ether is so volatile, a vapour pressure tends to build up in the bottle when it is turned off, especially if the anaesthetic machine is kept in a warm environment. If this has happened, there is a surge of high-concentration ether vapour when the vaporizer is turned on. This undesirable effect can be prevented by turning the vaporizer on and running a small quantity of mixed gases through it immediately prior to the anaesthetic being commenced, or simply by removing the cork from the filler orifice for an instant.

Volatile anaesthetic agents used in the Boyle's vaporizer should be removed from the bottle after use, and preferably be discarded in order to prevent a risk of their being poured back into the wrong bottle. It is desirable that all agents should be characteristically coloured, but such an ideal has yet to be realized.

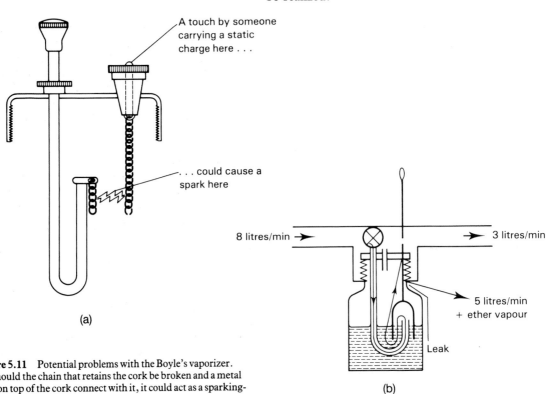

Figure 5.11   Potential problems with the Boyle's vaporizer. (a) Should the chain that retains the cork be broken and a metal stud on top of the cork connect with it, it could act as a sparking-plug if touched by someone charged with static electricity. (b) A leak from the jar could result in the loss of much of the carrier gas and all the ether vapour.

Temperature-compensated vaporizers

From the foregoing it will be appreciated that the output concentration of a simple vaporizer may alter considerably from time to time, depending on flow rates, the length of time the vaporizer has been in use and the type of anaesthetic agent used. With some agents it is important that the vapour concentration be kept constant. Examples of how this may be achieved are shown in Figs 5.12 to 5.16.

The *Fluotec Mark 2* vaporizer is shown in Fig. 5.12. In this vaporizer the gases pass through the vaporizer by two channels, one leading through a bypass and the other through the vaporization chamber. The proportion of gases passing through the bypass is determined by the calibrated control knob M, which operates the portions F and G of the valve, which are individually adjusted both by the manufacturer and during servicing. The fraction of gas passing through the vaporization chamber is varied not only by the position of this valve but also by a bimetallic thermostatic valve H, inside the vaporization chamber, where a series of wicks, saturated with halothane, present a very large area from which it evaporates. This ensures that the gases passing through the vaporization chamber are saturated with vapour. The percentage of halothane vapour at the outlet depends on the amount of vapour-laden gases that are mixed with the fresh gases passing through the bypass. As the temperature within the vaporization chamber falls (and therefore the vapour concentration in the gases passing through it also falls), the thermostatically operated valve opens wider and a greater proportion of the total gas flow passes through the chamber; by this means the vapour concentration in the output of the 'Fluotec' is kept constant.

FACTORS INFLUENCING THE ACCURACY OF
TEMPERATURE-COMPENSATED VAPORIZERS

Flow rate

The graphs of the performance characteristics (Figs 5.12 to 5.16, all of which are published by the manufacturers) show that by no means all vaporizers give an accurate vapour concentration under all conditions. The most significant factor is the flow rate of the carrier gases. For example, the *Halothane 4* vaporizer (Fig 5.15) gives lower concentrations at flow rates below about 3 *l*/min, while the Fluotec Mark 2 may give higher concentrations at the same flow rates (Fig. 5.12).

Liquid level

Although the wicks in vaporizers such as the *Abingdon* (Fig. 5.16) and *Vapor* (Figs. 5.17 and 5.18) can compensate for the level of the liquid, they can only do so within limits. Some vaporizers have 'high' and 'low' marks on the level sight window. In fact, when a survey of vaporizers was made, it was discovered that with Fluotec Mark 2 vaporizers there was a slightly higher concentration of vapour when they were a quarter or half full than after they had been filled to the 'full' mark with halothane at the same temperature. This was probably due to the larger area of wick presented to the gas when the level of liquid in the vaporizer was low.

Extremes of temperature

It is obvious that temperature-compensating mechanisms can operate only within a reasonable temperature range. At too low a temperature, vaporization will be low, and it may be uncontrollably high when it is too hot. In the case of the Emotril obstetric analgesia apparatus the temperature is indicated on a dial which shows whether the ambient temperature is within 'safe' limits.

Pumping effect

When gas-driven ventilators of the 'minute volume divider' type, such as the Manley or Howells' are employed, or even when manually assisted or controlled ventilation is used, there is a 'back pressure' exerted on the vaporizer. This back pressure is intermittent or variable, and causes an alternating pressure in the vaporization chamber, increasing the vapour concentration. This effect is particularly important with low fresh gas flow rates. Edmonson has shown how this effect can be prevented by installing a pressurizing valve (Fig 5.19) downstream from the vaporizer and so preventing the transmission of back pressure. (In theory at least, the flowmeters should be recalibrated at this pressure.)

Gas direction

With some vaporizers a higher concentration of vapour is given if, by misconnection, the gas is made to pass through in the reverse direction.

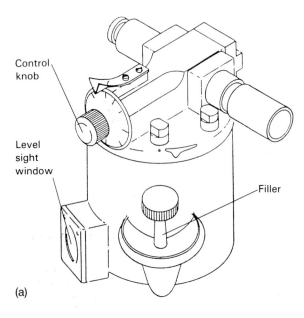

Control knob

Level sight window

Filler

(a)

Figure 5.12   (a) The Fluotec Mark 2 vaporizer. (b) Cutaway diagram showing how in the 'off' position all the gases are channelled through the bypass. (c) Cutaway diagram showing how in the 'on' position a carefully metered proportion of the gases pass through the vaporization chamber. (d) Performance characteristics. N.B. This vaporizer is now obsolete, but so many are still in use that it is included here.

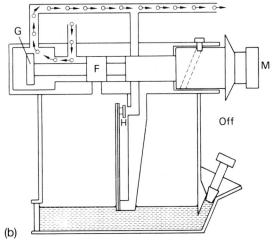

(b)

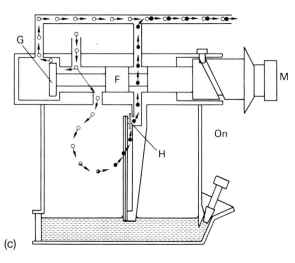

(c)

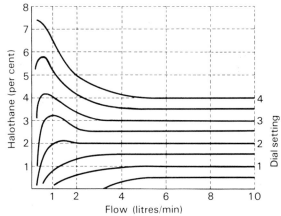

(d)

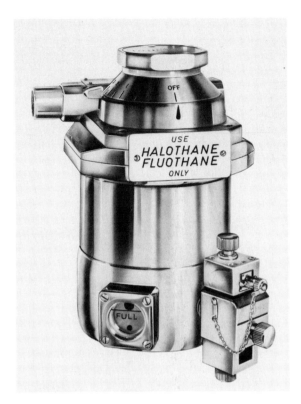

Figure 5.13   (a) The Fluotec Mark 3 vaporizer, which operates in much the same way as the Mark 2 but incorporates several refinements. (b) Working principles. For simplicity, the control valve has been omitted. In the 'off' position, the carrier gas passes through two passages, a simple bypass and a second bypass in which the flow is regulated by a temperature-sensitive valve. In the 'on' position, the first bypass is closed but the second remains open, and the gas also passes through a passage leading to the vaporization chamber, the valve for which is opened to a degree according to the vapour concentration required. Note that in this vaporizer the carrier gas passing through the vaporization chamber is fully saturated owing to the large area of wicks from which the liquid evaporates. The pathway by which the vapour-laden gas leaves the vaporization chamber may be in the form of a relatively long tube to help overcome the 'pumping effect' (see p. 85. (c) Performance characteristics.

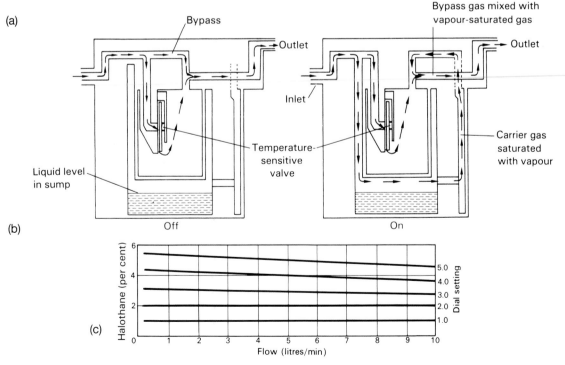

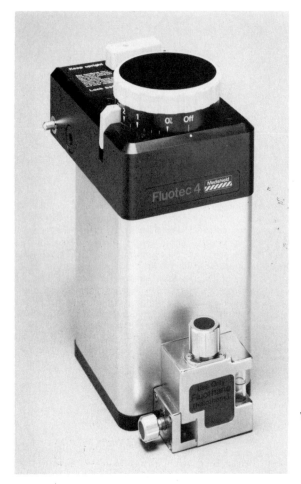

(a)

Figure 5.14 (a) The Fluotec Mark 4 vaporizer. (b) Working principles. Although this vaporizer is in a different housing from the Mark 3, it contains many of the features of the latter and functions in much the same way. Added features are that if it is accidentally inverted, the liquid agent will not spill into the bypass, and that in one model, if two vaporizers are mounted side by side on the appropriate back bar, a push-rod mechanism prevents their both being turned on at the same time. The author prefers a single hook-on mounting, being the simplest and least expensive. (c) Performance characteristics.

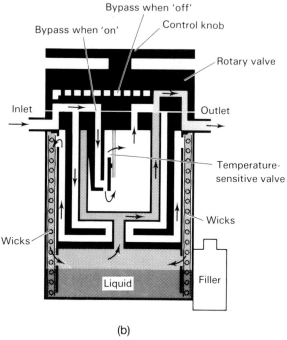

(b)

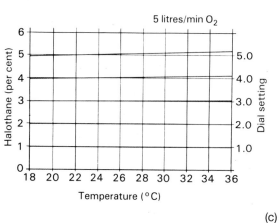

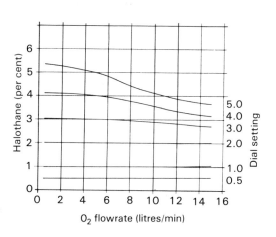

(c)

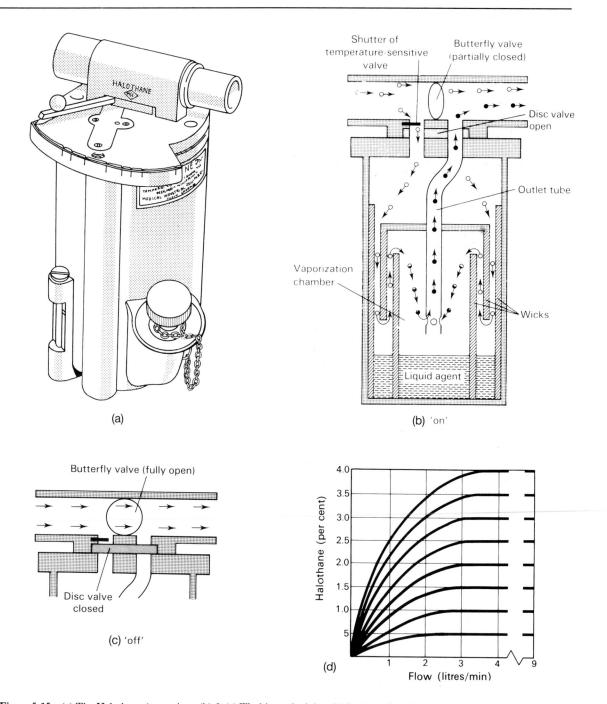

(a)

(b) 'on'

(c) 'off'

(d)

Figure 5.15 (a) The Halothane 4 vaporizer. (b) & (c) Working principles. (b) In the 'on' position a proportion of the carrier gases passes via the partially closed butterfly valve to the outlet. The remainder passes through the disc valve, the aperture of which is partially closed by the shutter of a temperature-sensitive valve, past several wicks to the vaporization chamber, from where it enters the outlet tube to rejoin the rest of the carrier gas. (c) In the 'off' position the inlet and outlet to the vaporization chamber are both closed and the carrier gases pass from the inlet to the outlet via the fully open butterfly valve. (d) Performance characteristics.

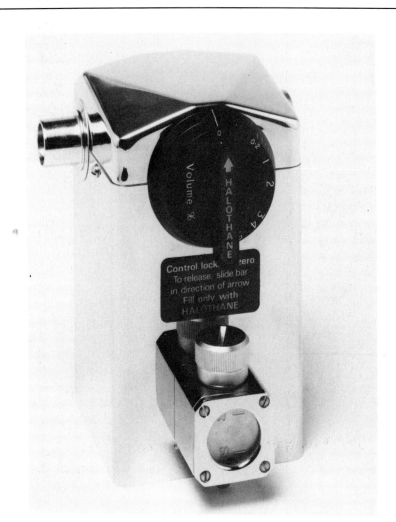

(a)

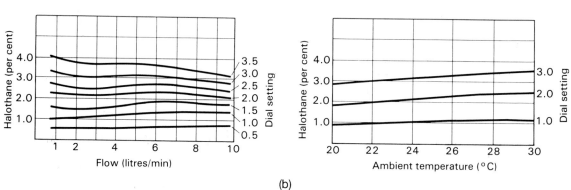

(b)

Figure 5.16 (a) The Abingdon vaporizer. (b) Performance characteristics. The wicks and vaporization chamber of this vaporizer may be cleaned by the owner. Space does not permit full details here, but well-illustrated instructions may be obtained from Penlon (see Appendix 2 for address).

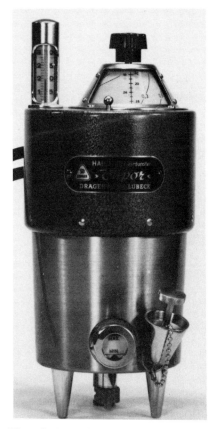 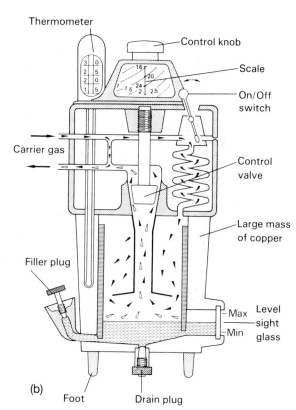

(a) (b)

Figure 5.17 (a) An early model of the Dräger Vapor temperature-indicated, level compensated vaporizer. (b) Working principles. Note the large mass of copper, which acts as a heat sink.

Stability
A fatal outcome occurred when a vaporizer was accidentally overturned. Liquid halothane ran into the bypass, and from there into the patient's respiratory tract. Even if the agent spilt in the breathing attachment did not reach the patient as liquid, the vapour concentration could be so high as to have fatal results.

The 'copper kettle' vaporizer

This type of vaporizer (Fig. 5.20) depends on maximum vaporization of the anaesthetic agent in a small volume of the carrier gas. A separate supply of oxygen from an extra rotameter passes through the vaporizer. The oxygen is broken up into a large number of very small bubbles by a diffuser made of 'Porex' or sintered bronze. These bubbles are so

small that they present an enormous surface area as they pass through the liquid anaesthetic agent and are totally saturated with its vapour. For halothane at 20 °C, this saturation is about 33%. As its name implies, the vaporizer contains a large mass of copper which, in conjunction with its attachment to the anaesthetic machine as a whole, provides a sufficient reservoir of heat to prevent a great fall in temperature as the halothane is vaporized.

The oxygen, now saturated with the anaesthetic agent, is added to the fresh gas flow via a mixing chamber. A calculation is necessary to determine the required flow rate of oxygen through the vaporizer, as compared with that of the main mixed gas flow, to achieve the desired concentration of anaesthetic agent in the final mixture.

The *Halox* vaporizer as shown in Fig. 5.21 has been developed from the 'copper kettle'. In this the

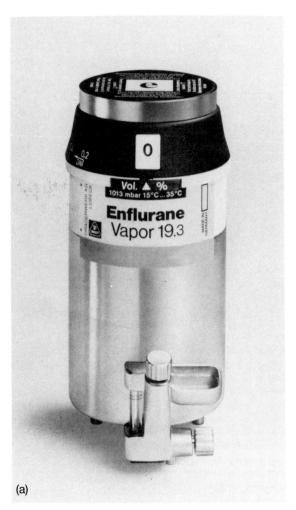

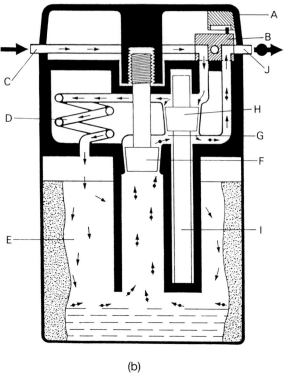

(b)

Figure 5.18 (a) A recent model of the Dräger Vapor vaporizer, which is now both temperature and level compensated. (b) Working principles. A, vapour concentration control; B, on/off switch (actuated by A); C, inlet; D, pressure compensator; E, vaporization chamber; F, control valve; G, mixing chamber; H, vaporization chamber bypass valve; I, expansion element of temperature-compensation sensor; J, outlet. (c) Performance characteristics.

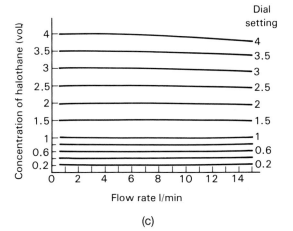

(c)

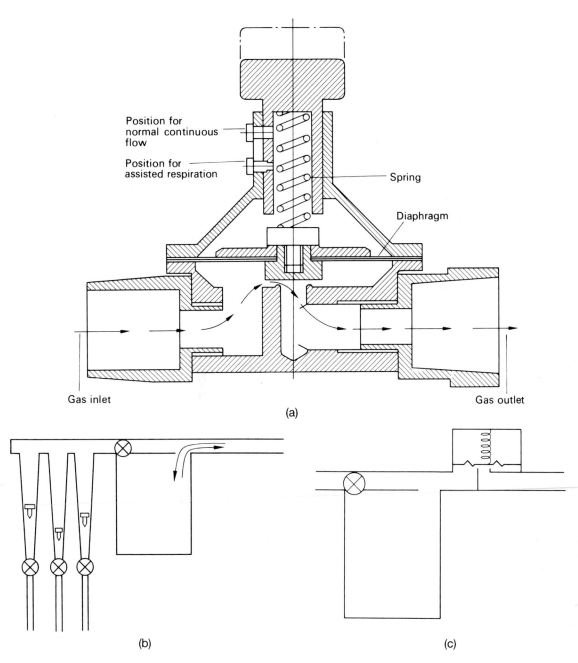

Figure 5.19 A pressurizing valve for the back bar. This is fitted downstream from a temperature-compensated vaporizer in order to protect it from the effects of fluctuations in back pressure when controlled ventilation by hand or automatic ventilator is used. The valve operates when the knob is depressed, as shown in (a), but presents no resistance when the knob is free. (b) The 'pumping' effect that may occur if there is no pressurizing valve. Variations in pressure in the breathing system may cause fluctuations in pressure in the back bar, and even reciprocal gas flow, and excessively high concentrations of the anaesthetic vapour may be generated due to gases re-entering the vaporization chamber. (c) The spring maintains the valve closed in the absence of a higher pressure upstream.

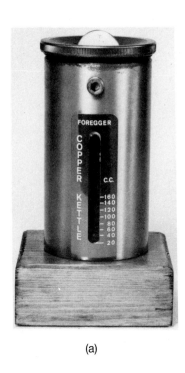

(a)

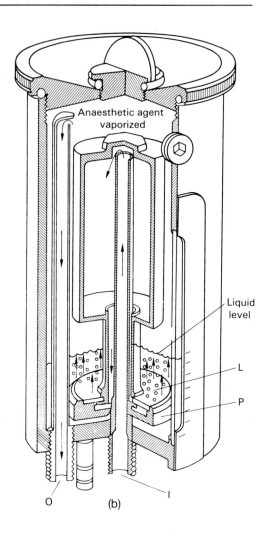

Anaesthetic agent vaporized

Liquid level

L

P

O   (b)   I

Figure 5.20   (a) The 'copper kettle' vaporizer. (b) The carrier gas (oxygen) enters via the inlet I, is broken up into very small bubbles by the Porex diffuser P, and passes through the liquid agent L, becoming saturated with the vapour. It then passes out via the outlet O, to join the main fresh gas flow. (c) The position of a 'copper kettle' vaporizer in the back bar. Note the extra oxygen flowmeter, the gas from which is saturated with the anaesthetic agent before being added to the mixed gas flow.

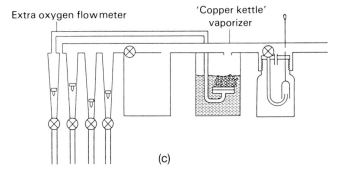

Extra oxygen flow meter   'Copper kettle' vaporizer

(c)

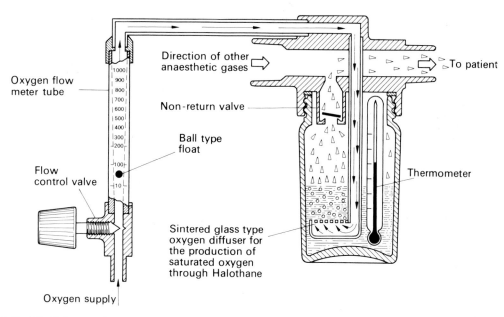

Figure 5.21   The Halox vaporizer.

diffuser is made of sintered glass, and the large mass of copper is replaced by a glass container (for simplicity and to enable the level of halothane liquid to be observed). Since the vapour concentration of halothane required for anaesthesia is low, and therefore only a relatively small amount of liquid halothane needs to be vaporized, the fall in temperature is much less than is the case when ether is vaporized in the original 'copper kettle'.

At the outlet of the vaporizer there is a non-return gravity disc valve, which prevents halothane vapour entering the gaseous pathway of the back bar when the Halox is turned off, and also prevents the pumping action due to back pressure when positive-pressure ventilation is employed. There is a thermometer in the vaporizer, and a slide-rule is provided for the necessary calculations.

A danger of both the 'copper kettle' and Halox vaporizers is that, should the total gas flow be diminished (for example if the nitrous oxide cylinder runs out), a high and possibly dangerous concentration of halothane vapour will be delivered to the patient in a situation where, owing to a reduced fresh gas flow rate, rebreathing, hypoxia and hypercarbia may occur. To new users of the 'copper kettle' or Halox, the necessary calculations must seem to be a disadvantage. However, those anaes-

thetists who have used it routinely do not find them an undue burden.

The *Heidbrink Kinet-O-meter* unit contains a number of flowmeters of the rotameter type, and a separate 'copper kettle' type of vaporizer for each volatile agent. The vaporizers are fitted with electric heating coils and thermostats, and their temperature is maintained at about 24 °C. The maintenance of a constant temperature has the advantage of eliminating the need for calculations of temperature drop, and also gives an adequate vapour concentration of methoxyflurane (Penthrane), which cannot easily be achieved at lower temperatures. There are two oxygen flowmeters (one for low and the other for high flow rates), and from these the oxygen passes to a special 'bypass' valve, which diverts part of the flow to the vaporizer. The amount of oxygen diverted to each vaporizer is controlled by a fine adjustment valve and is indicated on a flowmeter labelled for the particular volatile agent in question. The flowmeter is calibrated in actual flow rate of *vapour* per minute, and does not include the oxygen passing through the vaporizer. The accuracy of this calibration depends on the vaporizer being at the correct operating temperature, which is indicated by a thermometer and also by the illumination of only one of two pilot lights in the heating circuit for the vaporizer. The vapour-laden oxygen and the main oxygen stream from the bypass valve both join the mixed gas flow.

The concentration of the anaesthetic vapour may be determined by the following formula:

$$\frac{\text{Vapour}}{\text{concentration}} = \frac{\text{ml vapour/min} \times 100}{\text{total gas and vapour flow/min}}\%$$

For example, with the following flow rates:

Oxygen	= 1880 ml/min
Nitrous oxide	= 2000 ml/min
Oxygen to halothane vaporizer	= 120 ml/min

The vapour concentration would be:

$$\frac{120 \times 100}{1880 + 2000 + 120} = \frac{12000}{4000} = 3 \text{ per cent}$$

The original 'copper kettle' vaporizer included two important features:

1. A small, carefully measured fraction of the oxygen flow is saturated with anaesthetic vapour, so that a predetermined *amount* of the latter is added to the system per minute — a different concept from a mixed gas flow containing a specific *percentage* of vapour regardless of absolute quantity. The 'copper kettle' is therefore rather more applicable to closed circuits with low fresh gas flow and where reduction of pollution and economy are important.
2. The provision of a large 'heat sink', by virtue of the great mass of copper, minimizes the fall in temperature by supplying sufficient heat to replenish that lost by the latent heat of vaporization. This is of particular importance when ether is being used.

It is regrettable that the term 'copper kettle' is associated with both these otherwise unrelated principles.

Level-compensated vaporizers

In the Boyle's vaporizer, even if the flow rate of gases through the bottle and the temperature are kept constant, there is a fall in the concentration of anaesthetic vapour as the level of liquid in the bottle drops. If a wick, part of which is immersed in the liquid, is used in a vaporizer somewhat similar to the Boyle's but without the plunger, it is possible to obtain a more constant vapour concentration for any given temperature, provided that the level of anaesthetic liquid in the vaporizer is within reasonable limits. An example of this is the *Loosco* TILC (temperature-indicated, level-compensated) vaporizer (Fig. 5.22a and b). Provided that the level of halothane is between the 15 and 75 ml mark, there is compensation for the level. A built-in thermometer is incorporated and by reference to the graph supplied (Fig. 5.22c) the halothane concentration can be adjusted to that required.

TILC vaporizers may be rather more difficult to use than temperature compensated ones, but their results can be very accurate. In the case of the *Dräger Vapor* a very large mass of copper is included to prevent rapid temperature changes (Fig. 5.17).

The Boyle's 'Fluothane' vaporizer

This adaptation of the original Boyle's vaporizer was devised when halothane was first introduced and there was a great shortage of vaporizers for this agent. The characteristics of the drum are changed, the cowl is removed and a single tube with a side port is substituted for the U-tube (Fig. 5.23a). The calibration of the larger scale which replaces the usual graduation does not represent a precise percentage of halothane, and, in fact, this vaporizer is neither temperature nor level compensated. There are several variants of the Boyle's vaporizer, each with its own characteristics. For a typical Boyle's Fluothane vaporizer the graph in Fig. 5.23b shows the percentage output of halothane (Fluothane) by volume with the vaporizer filled with 50 ml of halothane at 20 °C and a flow rate of 4 to 8 *l*/min. In practice there are several variables, in particular the level of liquid and the temperature. The 'calibrations' given on this vaporizer are of use simply to prevent an overdose.

Low-resistance vaporizers

All the vaporizers described in the foregoing pages offer resistance to the gas flow. For this reason the gases have to be driven through them and it is not, therefore, possible to install them in the actual breathing system. As will be seen in Fig. 5.24 there are various positions in which the vaporizer may be installed. If it is situated within the breathing system, it should have a negligible resistance. A vaporizer

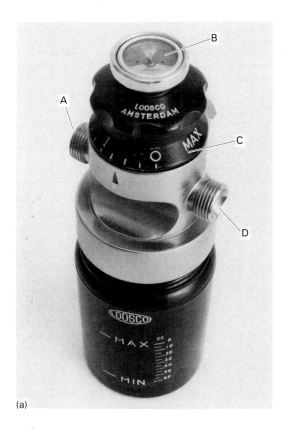

(a)

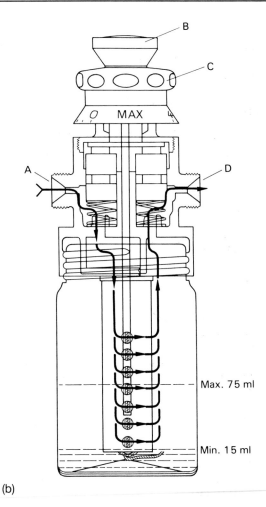

Max. 75 ml

Min. 15 ml

(b)

Figure 5.22   (a) The Loosco TILC vaporizer. (b) Working principles. Note that the pathways for the carrier gas are arranged so as to present the greatest possible area for vaporization to the gas. A, inlet; B, thermometer; C, control knob; D, outlet. (c) Performance characteristics at 20°C. (Conversion factors for 15 °C and 25 °C are 0.8 and 1.23 respectively.)

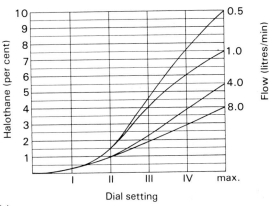

(c)

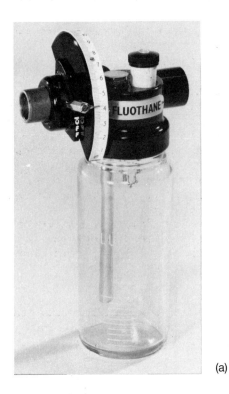

(a)

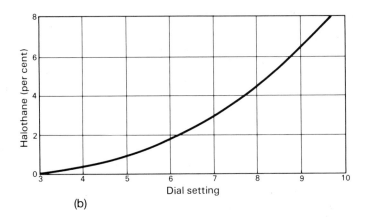

(b)

Figure 5.23   (a) The Boyle's Fluothane vaporizer.
(b) Performance characteristics. Note that these are approximate
only, since there is no temperature or level compensation.

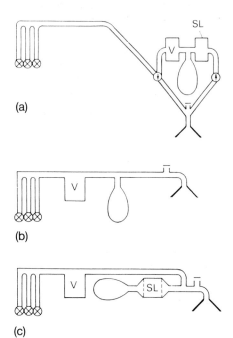

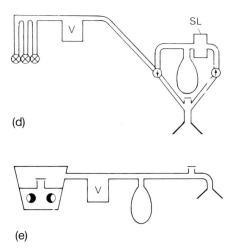

Figure 5.24   (a) VIC ('vaporizer in circle'). (b), (c) and (d) VOC
('vaporizer out of circle'). V, vaporizer; SL, soda lime.
(e) Vaporizer in breathing system (as used in intermittent flow
and draw-over anaesthetic equipment).

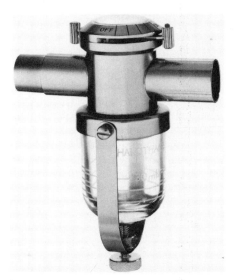

Figure 5.25   The Goldman halothane vaporizer.

in the position shown in Fig 5.24a is referred to as 'VIC' ('vaporizer in circle'); vaporizers used in the positions shown in Fig 5.24b, c and d are referred to as 'VOC' ('vaporizer out of circle').

In the case of a VIC (Fig. 5.24a) the patient's expired air passes through the vaporizer. This is of importance since not only will the concentration of volatile agents be increased by the repeated passage of the gases through the vaporizer, but also the vaporizer must be of a type that does not have any cloth wicks, since these could become sodden with water condensed from the expired air.

Table 5.1   The Goldman vaporizers

Drum position	Gas flow rate		
	2 *l*/min	8 *l*/min	30 *l*/min
Halothane			
1	0.03	0.03	0.03
2	0.41	0.74	0.92
3	0.73	2.21	1.31
On	0.74	2.08	1.21
Trichloroethylene			
1	0.01	nil	0.01
2	0.16	0.44	0.35
3	0.47	0.68	0.52
On	0.45	0.70	0.45

Halothane and trichloroethylene percentages by volume, liquid levels 20 ml at 21°C after 1 minute.

Typical examples of low-resistance vaporizers are mentioned below.

The Goldman halothane vaporizer (Fig. 5.25) is a small, simple and inexpensive vaporizer which is used for halothane in relatively low concentrations, when it is introduced as an adjuvant to nitrous oxide and oxygen anaesthesia; it is commonly used in dental anaesthesia. It is neither temperature nor level compensated and its output is somewhat influenced by the gas flow rate. Typical performance figures are shown in Table 5.1. Since the resistance to gas flow is small, this vaporizer may be used within the breathing system.

The McKesson and Rowbotham vaporizers are somewhat similar, the latter having a wire-gauze wick (see Figs. 5.26 and 5.27 and Tables 5.2 and 5.3).

Table 5.2   The McKesson vaporizer

Dial reading	Halothane (per cent)
1	0.05
2	1.05
3	1.84
On	2.80

These are performances on a particular occasion with the halothane at 20°C, gas flow at 8 l/min and a pressure of 5 mmHg.

Table 5.3   The Rowbotham vaporizer

Setting	Gas flow rate	
	4 *l*/min	8 *l*/min
Top mark		
Full on	3.10	2.50
¾	2.10	1.95
½	1.40	1.55
¼	0.60	0.65
Blue mark		
Full on	1.10	1.40
¾	0.65	1.00
½	0.40	0.65
¼	0.30	0.25

Halothane percentages by volume at 20°C.

Draw-over vaporizers

In the case of these, air or anaesthetic gases are drawn over or through the vaporizer by the effort of

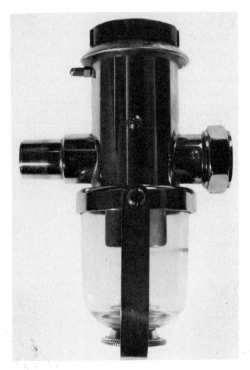

Figure 5.26   The McKesson vaporizer.

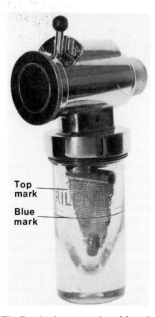

Top
mark

Blue
mark

Figure 5.27   The Rowbotham vaporizer. Note that there is a wick made of wire gauze.

such as the AE Fluothane vaporizer, which is designed for use with intermittent-flow dental anaesthetic equpment and also emergency field equipment, have wicks within them and for the reasons stated above are not suitable for use VIC.

The Blease Universal vaporizer (Fig. 5.28) can be used in any system. It has interchangeable control knobs calibrated for a number of different agents. It is for the individual anaesthetist to weigh the advantages of having a single calibrated vaporizer capable of being used for a variety of agents, with the dangers that might accrue from the possibility of using one agent with the control knob intended for another. Although this is a temperature and level compensated vaporizer, the accuracy of the calibration under certain circumstances has been questioned.

The Oxford Miniature vaporizer (Fig. 5.29) is primarily used with portable anaesthetic equipment and has the advantage that it may be drained of one anaesthetic agent and charged with another. Detachable scales are available for several agents. It is very simple to use and needs little in the way of servicing.

It is not temperature compensated, but there is a sealed compartment, filled with water plus antifreeze, which acts as a heat sink to minimize changes of temperature. The triservice version is described on pp. 350–351.

Vaporizers for the administration of vinesthene (divinyl ether)

Vinesthene is seldom, if ever, used now but was very popular at one time. The difficulties in its use arise from its very high volatility and are of sufficient interest to include in this chapter. Attempts to use it by the open-drop method failed, but it could be thus employed as a mixture with diethyl ether; in proportions of 25% divinyl ether, 75% diethyl ether the agent is known as 'VAM' (vinesthene aether mixture). On its own it was used either in a drip-feed device as shown in Fig 5.30 or, for short procedures, in a closed system with a rebreathing bag and a vaporizing chamber in which there was a sponge onto which a few ml of vinesthene were poured shortly before the induction of anaesthesia. This type of inhaler was also used with ethyl chloride, sometimes with dramatic and frightening results!

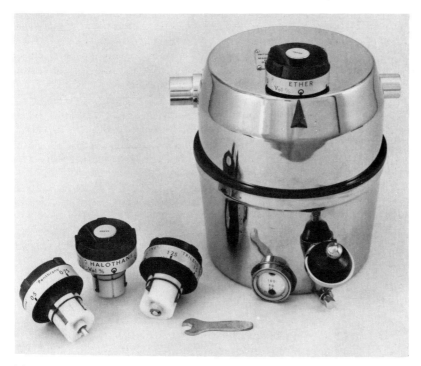

(a)

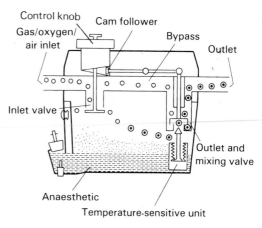

Figure 5.28 (a) The Blease Universal vaporizer. (b) Working principles. Whether it is used as a draw-over or as a plenum vaporizer, carrier gases enter via the inlet and leave via the bypass to the outlet. The proportion of gases that pass through the vaporization chamber depends on the degree of opening of the inlet valve and of the 'outlet and mixing' valve. These two valves are linked mechanically and their action is determined by a cam which is part of the control knob. For each agent there is a control knob with a cam of suitable gradient. There is also a temperature-sensitive valve. This vaporizer may be emptied of liquid and, after 'blowing through' to remove all vapour, charged with another agent.

(b)

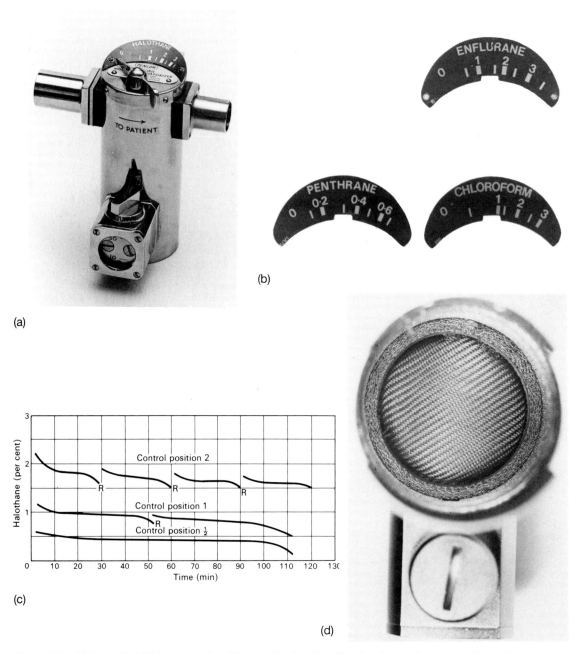

Figure 5.29 (a) The Oxford Miniature vaporizer. Note that the direction of flow is indicated. On some models the flow to the patient is from right to left. Note also that the scale is fixed by two screws and is detachable. It may be replaced by scales for other anaesthetic agents, shown in (b). (c) Performance characteristics. Note that there is no temperature compensation, but a mass of water in the base of the vaporizer acts as a heat sink and reduces temperature changes during use. The letter R indicates refilling of the vaporizer. (d) The wick within the vaporizer is constructed of wire gauze and may therefore be cleaned by rinsing the vaporizer with ether, draining it, and then blowing air or other gases through it, until all the ether has been eluted.

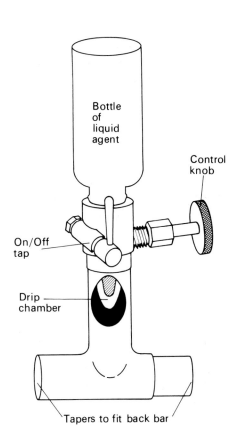

Improvised vaporizers

Under primitive conditions improvisation is sometimes necessary. Flagg described a metal can with holes pierced in the top, through which the patient inhaled, through an endotracheal tube, air enriched with ether vapour. More recently a somewhat more sophisticated version, using an instant coffee jar, was described by Boulton (see Fig. 5.31).

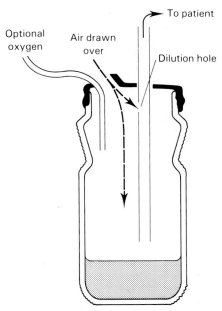

Figure 5.30   This device (now obsolete) was used for vaporizing vinesthene, which is highly volatile. The rate of administration could be observed by counting the drops as they passed through the observation chamber.

Figure 5.31   Improvised vaporizer made from a 4 oz (125 g) coffee jar. For further details refer to Boulton, T. B. (1966) Anaesthesia under difficult conditions. (3) General anaesthesia — technique. *Anaesthesia* Vol. 21, No. 4. pp. 529–34.

6

The Continuous-Flow Anaesthetic Machine

Figure 6.1 shows a typical anaesthetic machine. There are two cylinders of oxygen and two of nitrous oxide (one of each 'running' and the others 'in reserve'), and there may be one each of carbon dioxide and cyclopropane. Each cylinder (except the one for cyclopropane) is connected via its yoke to a regulator. Each oxygen cylinder is also connected to a pressure (contents) gauge which indicates the contents of the cylinder. Often there is also a pressure gauge for each nitrous oxide cylinder, but as explained in Chapter 1 the reading on it does not necessarily give a true indication of the contents of the cylinder. There is rarely a gauge fitted for carbon dioxide, but when there is the same reservations are required in reading it as for nitrous oxide. Connections between the cylinder yoke, the inlet of the pressure regulator and the contents gauge are made of high-pressure metal tubing. The outputs of the two oxygen regulators are connected together, and to the flow-control (fine-adjustment) valves on the oxygen flowmeter, with either metal or rubber tubing. Rubber tubing is now rarely used, but where it is, special non-interchangeable connections (described later in this chapter) are required. A similar low-pressure tube connects the outputs of the two nitrous oxide regulators with their flow-control valve and flowmeter.

The gases pass through their individual flowmeters, the flow rate being adjusted by the flow-control valves. They are mixed in the top of the flowmeter block and from there pass via the vaporizers to the outlet.

The components of the machine are usually mounted on a table with wheels, but sometimes they are mounted on a portable stand instead. (Some small portable machines have only one cylinder each of nitrous oxide and oxygen.) Carbon dioxide and cyclopropane are not always fitted.

This type of machine is commonly called a 'Boyle's' machine, named after the anaesthetist who originated it. However, the term 'Boyle's' is actually a trade mark of the British Oxygen Company, and, strictly speaking, should be used only in connection with their apparatus.

Components of Anaesthetic Machines

Cylinder yokes

On modern machines the cylinder yokes are bolted on to the side of the frame, but there still remain a number of older machines with a low (regulated) pressure of 5 to 11 lb/in^2, the cylinders being supported in 'baskets', the yokes of which are attached to the regulators, and clamped on to the valve blocks of the cylinders, and rubber low pressure tubing is used. The pressure gauge is also connected directly to the cylinder yoke (Fig. 6.2).

Pressure (contents) gauges

Pressure gauges are described elsewhere in this book (pp. 8–10). They are usually either fitted with a $1/8$ in. BSP parallel thread and sealed with a non-inflammable washer or PTFE tape, or are fitted with a conical union with no washer. The entry to the pressure gauge contains a constriction to prevent sudden surges of pressure from damaging the mechanism. Each pressure gauge is marked for the gas for which it is intended and may be colour coded.

One manufacturer calibrates the contents gauge simply at 'full', 'half', 'quarter', etc., and has a segment coloured red and marked 'change' at the lower end of the scale. At present there is a great variation in the units in which gauges are calibrated, but most older units are calibrated in bar or lb/in^2. Recently the adoption of kPa has been accepted.

One satisfactory arrangement is to have nitrous oxide gauges calibrated at one point, 54 kPa × 100, and carbon dioxide gauges similarly at 57 kPa ×

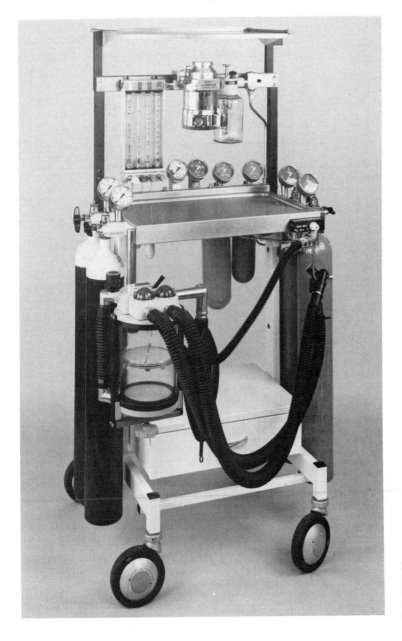

Figure 6.1 A typical modern anaesthetic machine, complete with circle absorber. Soda lime has been omitted so that the division between the two ends of the canister can be seen.

100. In each case this is the pressure in a full cylinder at average operating-room temperature.

On machines used from the pipeline, a pressure gauge may be mounted on the pipeline inlet to the machine. In this respect it is important to understand that in one version of the 'Boyle's International' machine (BOC) there are a pair of gauges mounted close to the pipeline hose connections, labelled 'Circuit'. This does not refer either to the pipeline pressure or to the pressure in the breathing attachment, but to regulated pressure, whether the machine is operating on pipeline or cylinders.

On a similar machine, for cylinders only, there are two nitrous oxide yokes, with a single contents

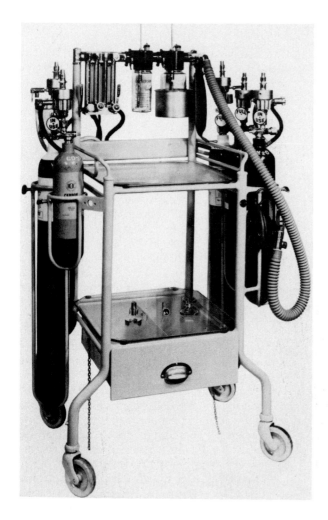

Figure 6.2 An old fashioned 'basket' Boyle's machine. Notice the water jacket on the ether vaporizer. Although now obsolete in the United Kingdom, many of these are still giving useful service around the world.

gauge mounted on one of them. This gauge is connected to both yokes, and could therefore give a false impression that the cylinder mounted on the same yoke is full when it is, in fact, empty.

High-pressure tubing

High-pressure tubing is invariably of metal, and the joints are either cap and liner unions, or brazed rather than soft-soldered. They are constructed of heavy-duty materials, since they have to withstand not only a pressure of up to 120 atm, but also sudden surges of pressure when a cylinder is turned on.

Low-pressure tubing

In modern anaesthetic machines low-pressure tubing is usually constructed of metal. Connections are made by means of compression couplings such as the 'Simplifix' (see p. 15), or may be soft-soldered. The low-pressure oxygen line frequently has branches to power items such as an injector suction unit, a sphygmomanometer, or a ventilator.

Where the low-pressure tubing is made of rubber or plastic, and is detachable, all connections are made with non-interchangeable connections (Fig. 6.3). The rubber is of the antistatic variety and each

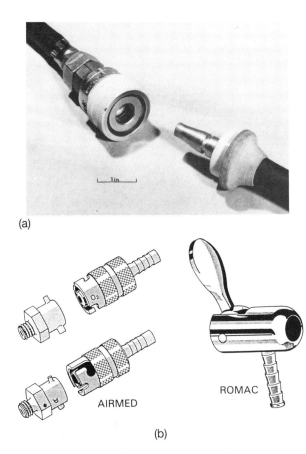

(a)

(b)

AIRMED

ROMAC

Figure 6.3   (a), (b) Various non-interchangeable connections.

Pipeline connections

The method of attaching pipeline hoses to the anaesthetic machine is important. There have been accidents, some fatal and others resulting in brain damage, due to the crossing over of hoses, so that nitrous oxide has been delivered via the oxygen flowmeter and vice versa. These are considered on p. 69 et seq.

Pressure regulators

Pressure regulators have been described in Chapter 3. In many anaesthetic machines, especially older ones, they are set to give an output of approximately 5 lb/in² (~ 34 kPa). In later machines a pressure of around 12 lb/in² (~ 80 kPa) is employed, while on most modern British machines pressure regulators are set at 60 lb/in² (~ 400 kPa). The latter coincides with the pressure of the piped supply, so that when piped gases are used, regulators may be replaced by flow restrictors. (This refers to Great Britain: in many other countries the regulated and pipeline pressure is 45 lb/in².) It is common practice to set the regulators for oxygen at a slightly higher pressure than those for nitrous oxide to assure the supply of the former. Except in special circumstances, however, both regulators for each gas should be set at the same pressure so that when a change is made from one cylinder to another the flow rate is not altered. The Adams regulator is attached either directly to the cylinder yoke, or to a block by which it is secured to the frame of the anaesthetic machine. It has a nut-and-liner union with a Bodok or other non-inflammable sealing washer. The fittings and the new BOC regulators are shown in Fig. 6.4. Regulators are labelled with the gas for which they are intended to be used. This is because a special alloy is required for the seating for each gas in order to prevent corrosion.

end is colour-coded for the gas it carries. (Recently some countries have considered relaxing the regulations regarding the use of antistatic materials, but this has not as yet been universally accepted.) The connection at each end is secured by a ferrule applied using a special crimping tool (Fig. 4.23, p. 72).

Supply of cyclopropane

Because of its relatively low pressure in the cylinder, and the small flow rate used, no regulator is fitted for cyclopropane. If metal tubing is used, a flow-control valve may be fitted to the flowmeter block, but where the tubing is of rubber there is none, and the flow rate is controlled by the cylinder valve. This is because not only is there a danger of rupture, but also cyclopropane under pressure tends to cause rubber to perish or may even diffuse through it.

Non-return valves

Sometimes a single regulator and contents gauge are used for both the running and reserve cylinders. When one cylinder runs out, its valve should be closed before the other is turned on, since gas could flow from one cylinder to the other, resulting in the two being partially filled. This can be prevented by fitting non-return valves, as shown in Fig. 6.5. Not only will this prevent the empty cylinder being

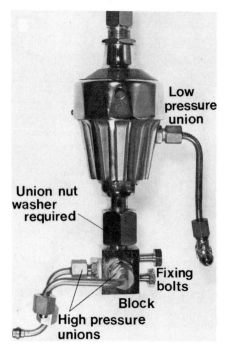

(a)

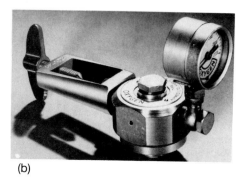

(b)

Figure 6.4   Different methods of mounting pressure regulators. (a) A special block is fitted to the frame of the anaesthetic machine by one or two bolts. The block contains unions for connections to the cylinder yoke, the pressure (contents) gauge and the pressure regulator. Such blocks are usually used for mounting the regulators underneath or behind the working surface of the anaesthetic machine. (b) Alternatively, a regulator may be mounted directly on a pin-index cylinder yoke. (c) If unions of a sufficiently robust nature are used, regulators may be mounted underneath the worktop of an anaesthetic machine.

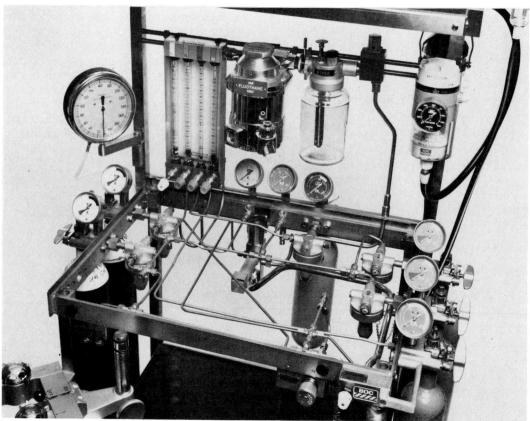

(c)

refilled from the full one, but it will also enable its removal and replacement when the reserve has been turned on, without interrupting the supply of gas. Unfortunately these valves tend to leak, so when an empty cylinder is removed it should be replaced promptly, in order to prevent the loss, via the empty yoke, of gas from the second cylinder.

Flow-control (fine-adjustment) valves

Flow-control (fine-adjustment) valves are needle valves, and in some modern anaesthetic machines they may be removed completely from the flowmeter block by detaching the 'cartridge' (Fig. 6.6). The gland of the flow-control valve on older machines is filled with a packing material such as cotton and may need occasional tightening, but on modern machines nylon or neoprene stuffing is used. Occasionally it is found that it is impossible to completely close a flow-control valve and the gas flow cannot be completely stopped. This may be because the gland nut has become loose and has

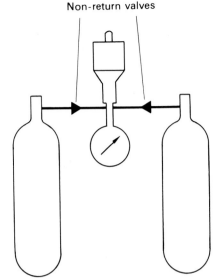

Figure 6.5 Non-return valves fitted to cylinder yokes, where two cylinders share one regulator.

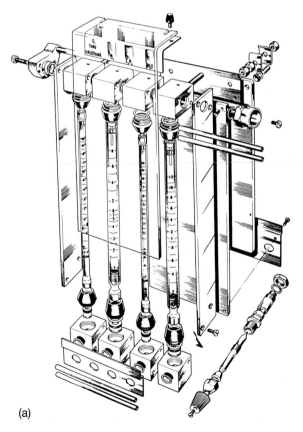

(a)

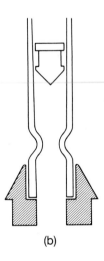

(b)

Figure 6.6 (a) An exploded diagram of a modern flowmeter block. Note that the needle valve is in the form of a cartridge which may be removed from the block. Note also the manner in which the flowmeter tubes fit into rubber, nylon or neoprene sockets, as shown in (b).

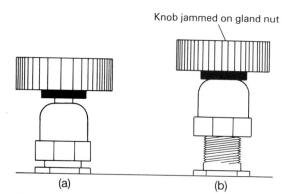

Knob jammed on gland nut

(a)   (b)

Figure 6.7   Failure of a flow-control valve to close. In (a) the gland nut is correctly tightened, while in (b) it has worked loose and has unscrewed so much that the control knob impinges upon it before the needle valve is closed.

unscrewed so much that it has jammed against the control knob (Fig. 6.7). Gentle retightening of the gland nut will cure this fault. The valve may also fail to close completely because the seating has been damaged by rough usage or by grit.

ROUTINE MAINTENANCE OF FLOW-CONTROL VALVES

If the flow-control valve becomes too free-running or loose, because the gland nut is not sufficiently tightened, the gas may escape past the spindle. Provided that the valve is fitted upstream of the flowmeter, this will not lead to inaccuracy, but the knob may accidentally be turned by the slightest touch, causing an unintentional change in flow rate. Indeed, at least one fatal incident has occurred where the oxygen supply was accidentally interrupted: an investigator found that the valve was so loose that it could be turned 'at the touch of a feather'. In order to prevent such accidents, the tightness of the gland nut should be regularly checked. If it does need retightening, this should be done gently, and it should be ascertained whether the stuffing needs renewing.

Flowmeters ('Rotameters'*)

The flowmeters for the various gases are usually joined together in a block. It has been customary to

* As already mentioned, 'Rotameter' is strictly speaking the trade name used by one particular manufacturer, but in practice it has become synonymous with flowmeter.

mount them always in the same sequence in order to prevent confusion, the order being (from left to right): oxygen, carbon dioxide, cyclopropane and nitrous oxide. However, as mentioned in Chapter 18, there is no international standard, and, indeed, in a single hospital one may find anaesthetic machines with the flowmeters set in different order. This is most regrettable, and has already been the cause of at least one death. In the past one single flowmeter was sometimes used for both cyclopropane and carbon dioxide. (In this case two sets of calibration had to be shown — an obviously undesirable arrangement!)

The flowmeter block is secured to the back bar of the anaesthetic machine by one or more bolts. It is constructed in such a way as to minimize the risk of damage to the flowmeter tubes. In older models the flowmeter tube is secured and made airtight by means of a screw in the top of the block which compresses two sealing washers (Fig. 6.8). In mod-

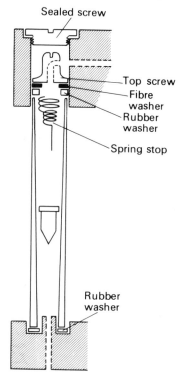

Sealed screw

Top screw

Fibre washer

Rubber washer

Spring stop

Rubber washer

Figure 6.8   Part of an older type of flowmeter block, in which the tubes are secured by means of screw in the top of the block which compresses two sealing washers. Caution should be exercised when tightening the top screw, so as to prevent a fracture of the tube.

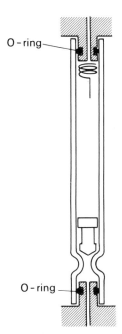

Figure 6.9 Part of a modern flowmeter block, in which the tubes are secured by means of O-rings.

ern machines this is replaced by neoprene sockets or by O-ring fittings (Fig. 6.9). These modern innovations make dismantling the tubes for cleaning and replacement much easier, and also tend to prevent damage when the block is reassembled. Figure 3.24a (p. 47) shows what might happen if the carbon dioxide or cyclopropane tubes were fractured. Some manufacturers now mount their flowmeter blocks on the right-hand side of the anaesthetic machine so that the gases may be led off from the 'oxygen end' of the block. An alternative method to prevent this accident has been suggested (Fig. 3.24b). As stated above, the reversal of the order of the flowmeters is undesirable.

It was a common practice to fit an oxygen bypass valve adjacent to the oxygen fine-adjustment valve, but it is now more usual to mount it at the downstream end of the back bar. Oxygen passing through a bypass in the former position may enter the rotameter itself, in which case the bypass flow is indicated, or it may enter the top of the rotameter block and not be indicated. Bypass levers tend to work loose and therefore care must be taken to see that they do not fall into the 'on' position unnoticed. The oxygen bypass should give a flow of at least 35 l/min.

A second oxygen rotameter may be fitted, for example where a Halox or 'copper kettle' vaporizer is fitted.

Back bar

That part of the frame of an anaesthetic machine that supports the flowmeters, vaporizers and various other components is known as the back bar. (In some contexts the term 'back bar' includes the flowmeters and vaporizers also.) It may consist of a pair of metal rods or bars and Fig. 6.10 shows its typical dimensions. Flowmeter blocks and vaporizers are connected to each other by tapered fittings and are bolted onto the back bar. There are two common positions in which they may be mounted, referred to as BOC and MIE mountings. In many cases it is possible to fit a flowmeter block or vaporizer with an adaptor to enable it to be used for the alternative mounting. The diameters of the tapers for the inlets and outlets of vaporizers and other units differ. BOC use a taper that is larger than that on MIE components. The British Standard 22 mm taper was introduced to replace both of these, but more recently the 23 mm 'Cagemount' standard has been reintroduced. There remains, therefore, a lack of standardization. Adaptors can usually be obtained to interconnect components of different manufacture. On British anaesthetic apparatus it is customary, but not universal, for the flowmeter block to be mounted on the left-hand side of the back bar.

There are three factors to consider when deciding the order in which to mount the vaporizers. First, and most importantly, temperature compensated vaporizers should be mounted upstream. This is because they contain wicks which absorb a considerable amount of anaesthetic agent. They cannot,

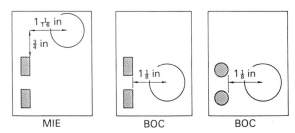

Figure 6.10 Dimensions of the back bar. Notice that in the case of MIE fittings the gas passages of the components are higher than the back bar, while in BOC fittings they are at the same level.

therefore, be emptied completely and cleaned after each time they are used. Consequently, if there were two such vaporizers mounted in series, the one downstream could become contaminated to a dangerous degree with the agent for the one upstream.

Undoubtedly the safest arrangement is to have only one temperature-compensated, calibrated vaporizer on the back bar. This has been facilitated by the development of the 'Selectatec' range of vaporizers, which can be individually hooked onto or removed from the back bar at the touch of a catch. Their use may lead not only to economy in capital outlay, but also to considerable versatility of the anaesthetic machine. For agents that are seldom used there is no need to buy a specific vaporizer for each machine. Older anaesthetic machines may be converted for the use of these vaporizers by installing a 'compatibility kit' (Fig. 6.11a) on the back bar. These kits are available for both BOC and MIE mountings and various tapers. Figure 6.11b shows a similar 'off-line' hook-on system by Penlon.

A development which seems less conducive to safety is a back bar that can carry two Selectatec vaporizers together, but with a tap between them so that only one may be used at a time. Although the pollution of one vaporizer by the other is avoided, the addition of an extra control, which could be overlooked, could lead to a misadventure.

If a vaporizer containing wicks does become contaminated with an agent for which it is not intended, it should be washed out several times with the agent for which it is to be used, drained, and then blown through with oxygen or air until all smell has been eliminated. In the case of the Boyle's vaporizer the jar can easily be removed, emptied and cleaned, and contamination is not a serious problem.

The second consideration is the order in which temperature-compensated, calibrated vaporizers should be mounted if there is to be more than one in series. At one time it was recommended that the one for the more volatile agent should be mounted upstream. Later, when the danger of a vaporizer for methoxyflurane (Penthrane) being contaminated with halothane was pointed out, it was considered prudent to mount that for the most volatile agent

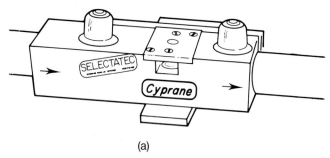

(a)

Figure 6.11   (a) The Selectatec compatibility block, and (b) the Penlon 'off-line' block.

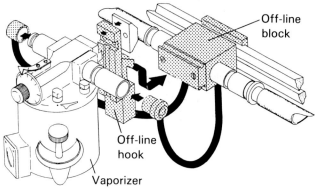

(b)

downstream. The rationale for this is as follows. If an upstream vaporizer for halothane were turned 'on' at the same time as a downstream one for methoxyflurane, halothane could be dissolved in (or absorbed by) the liquid methoxyflurane. (The vaporizer for the latter is constructed so that when fully 'on' the bypass is closed and all the carrier gas passes through the vaporizing chamber.) When the methoxyflurane vaporizer was next used a high concentration of halothane could be given off, the saturated vapour concentration of halothane at room temperature being of the order of 30%. Bearing in mind the advent of other volatile agents, perhaps one should consider the ratio between the saturated and highest clinically safe vapour concentrations and mount the vaporizer for the agent with the lowest ratio upstream and the highest, downstream.

The third consideration is that the trichloroethylene (Trilene) vaporizer is normally mounted next to the outlet so that one or another of the various devices to prevent its vapour from entering the circle absorber may be used (Fig. 6.12). (It will

be remembered that if trichloroethylene vapour comes into contact with warm soda lime, it may be decomposed, forming toxic substances.)

At the end of the back bar there may be one or more of the following:

1. An angled outlet.
2. A non-return valve (Fig. 6.13). This is considered to be important when using ventilators such as the Howells' or Manley, which produce 'back pressure' (see note below). A non-return valve prevents any possibility of back pressure on the vaporizer causing a high vapour concentration.
3. An oxygen flush (bypass) (Fig. 6.14). Mounting the oxygen flush in this position has an advantage over fitting it on the flowmeter block in that

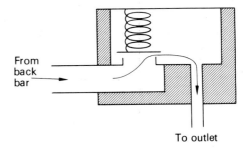

Figure 6.13 Non-return valve in the back bar.

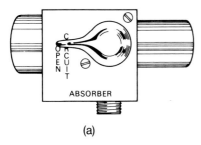

(a)

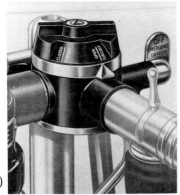

(b)

Figure 6.12 (a) The trichloroethylene (Trilene) safety bypass control MIE. (b) The Trilene safety interlock combined with a tap to direct the fresh gas flow to either the Magill attachment or the absorber. There is also an oxygen emergency flush control.

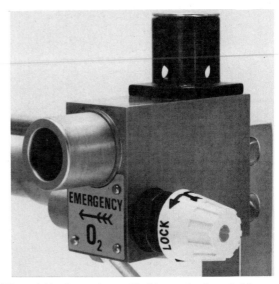

Figure 6.14 Oxygen bypass (flush) control at the end of the back bar.

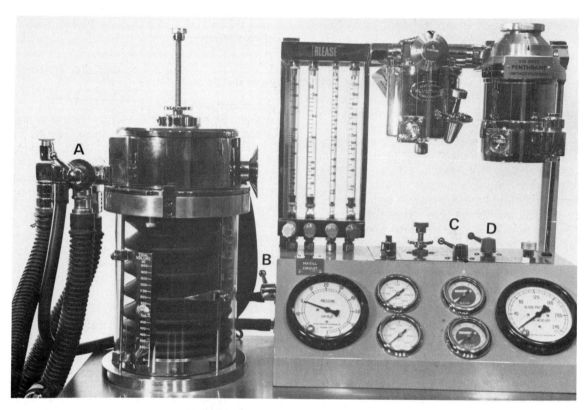

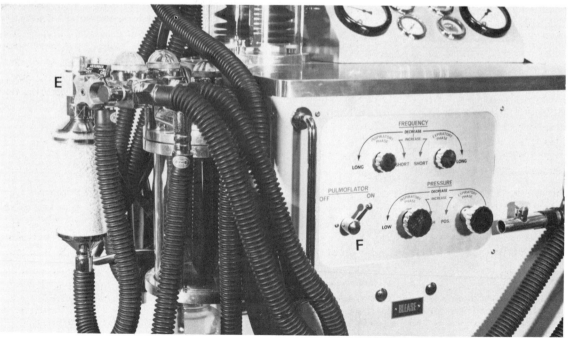

when it is operated, even if the vaporizers are turned on, the patient will receive pure oxygen, uncontaminated with nitrous oxide, carbon dioxide or volatile agents. It has the disadvantage that if it is accidentally turned on unobserved, this will not be indicated by the flowmeters, and the patient may not be adequately anaesthetized. The oxygen flush should give at least 35 l/min, and this usually makes sufficient noise to prevent its being overlooked.

4. The back bar may terminate in a valve which, turned in one direction permits the use of a semiclosed breathing attachment, and in the other passes the gases to a circle absorber (Fig. 6.13). This unit is sometimes combined with a 'Trilene safety interlock', which prevents the trichloroethylene vaporizer being turned on when the closed circuit is in use. A similar valve on an anaesthetic ventilator may direct the fresh gas flow either to the ventilator or to an attachment for spontaneous breathing. The danger of its misuse is shown in Fig. 6.15.

5. There may be a tube taking the gases to a 'Cardiff' swivel outlet (Fig. 6.16) on the front of the anaesthetic table.

6. On anaesthetic machines with a regulated pressure of 45 or 60 lb/in^2 ($\sim$ 300 or 400 kPa) there may be a relief valve which opens at 5 lb/in^2 ($\sim$ 34 kPa) to prevent the risk of damage to the vaporizers and flowmeters by their being subjected to a higher pressure if the outlet is obstructed (Fig. 6.17).

7. A blow off valve set at 40 mmHg ($\sim$ 5 kPa) may be fitted to protect the patient from pressure surges, particularly in paediatric use. With a valve opening at such a low pressure it is not possible to operate minute volume divider ventilators such as the Manley or East–Freeman Automatic Vent.

Note that the term 'back pressure' is sometimes thought to mean that gases pass back from the ventilator and through the vaporizer again. This is not the case. What happens is simply that because the ventilator requires power from the gas flow to

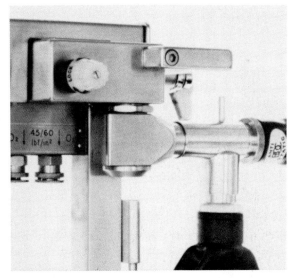

Figure 6.16 The Cardiff swivel.

operate it, there is a resistance to the flow. This acts in exactly the same way as if the outlet of the anaesthetic machine were partly obstructed, and pressure builds up in the back bar. Back pressure in the back bar is not prevented by a simple non-return valve, but its effects can be prevented by installing a pressurizing valve to maintain a higher pressure. It not only may affect vaporizers, but will introduce an inaccuracy in the calibration of flowmeters by increasing the density of gas flowing through the annulus. This could be prevented by installing the flow-control valve downstream from the flowmeter (see p. 47), but this is not usual in anaesthetic machines.

Portable Anaesthetic Machines

Whereas most anaesthetic machines can be described as transportable, in that they can be moved by suitable conveyance, and with some difficulty, from one place to another, there are also portable machines which can easily be carried by the itinerant

Figure 6.15 The multiplicity of controls on an anaesthetic ventilator may lead to accidents when a control such as B is turned to the wrong direction, resulting in a patient being ventilated with expired air rather than fresh gases. A, manual/automatic selector; B, tap diverting fresh gas to either the ventilator or the Magill attachment; C, patient triggering on/off switch; D, oxygen flush. E, absorber; F, on/off control. Controls such as A and E may inadvertently be altered by accidentally draping across them objects such as rubber tubing, etc.

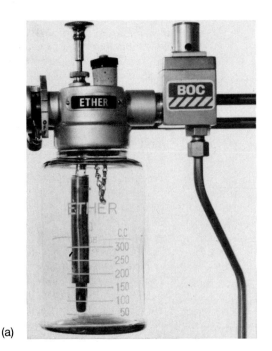

(a)

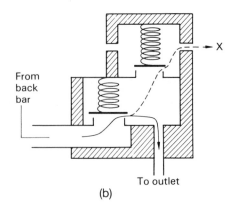

(b)

Figure 6.17   (a) Combined non-return and pressure relief valve at the end of the back bar. (b) If the outlet is obstructed, the gases escape at X, so protecting the back bar from overpressure. A low-pressure relief valve is also available to protect the patient.

anaesthetist in his own car. These work in precisely the same way as the continuous flow machine mentioned above. An example is the *Enderby* portable anaesthetic machine (Fig. 6.18).

'Quantiflex' Machines

There is a range of continuous-flow machines for different purposes, all of which embody safety devices to prevent the administration of mixtures of gases containing less than a predetermined amount of oxygen. The Quantiflex MDM is described below, and the Quantiflex RA in Chapter 9. Note that the oxygen flowmeter is usually on the right and nitrous oxide flowmeter is on the left.

The Quantiflex 'Monitored Dial Mixer' (MDM) surgical anaesthetic machine (Fig. 6.19)

The flow rates of nitrous oxide and oxygen are indicated by the two flowmeters, but the combined flow rate is controlled by a single knob. The relative percentages of nitrous oxide and oxygen are determined by the mixture control wheel, which is calibrated in steps of 10% from 30% to 100% oxygen.

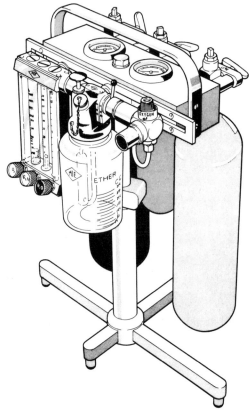

Figure 6.18   The Enderby portable anaesthetic machine. Note that with modern anaesthesia one would require a halothane vaporizer in the breathing system.

Thus never more than 70% nitrous oxide can be given. A carbon dioxide flowmeter and fine adjustment valve may be provided as an 'add-on' unit, but works independently of the flow rate and mixture controls.

Maintenance of Anaesthetic Machines

In the United Kingdom, it is recommended that all anaesthetic machines are serviced by competent engineers every three months, and that ventilators are serviced every six months. This service consists of cleaning all parts of the machine, including the flowmeter tubes, checking flowmeters, regulators and all other parts such as corrugated tubing and breathing bags, and the cleaning and regreasing of the drums of vaporizers, circle absorbers, etc. It does not, however, usually include attention to the temperature-compensated vaporizers, which are serviced by the appropriate manufacturer. Thymol, a normal constituent of Fluothane, tends to collect in vaporizers, and most manufacturers advise that temperature-compensated vaporizers be returned to their factory once a year for an overhaul. It is usually possible to obtain a service exchange or other vaporizer on temporary loan while the original is away at the factory.

Besides maintenance by service engineers it is wise for the anaesthetist to carry out his own checks in a manner such as the following 'cockpit drill' (the details of which will obviously vary depending on the type of machine).

'Cockpit drill'

1. *Supply of gases*

Check that the cylinders are in position.

Turn on the 'reserve' oxygen cylinder and see that it registers full on the gauge.

Close the reserve cylinder, open the oxygen bypass or flow-control valve to empty the system and then close it. Open the 'running' oxygen cylinder and check that its contents are sufficient. If they are not, replace the cylinder; leave it turned on.

In the case of pipeline machines, check the flow as with the 'running' cylinder, unplug the hose at the pipeline terminal and note that the flow through the appropriate flowmeter ceases; recon-

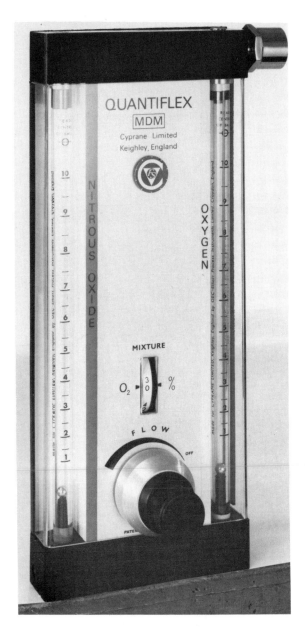

Figure 6.19   The Quantiflex MDM anaesthetic machine. The lower knob controls the flow rate and the wheel above it adjusts the percentage of oxygen. Notice that 30% is the minimum amount of oxygen in the mixed gas flow. Note also that the nitrous oxide and oxygen flowmeters are in the reverse sequence to that which is customary in Great Britain.

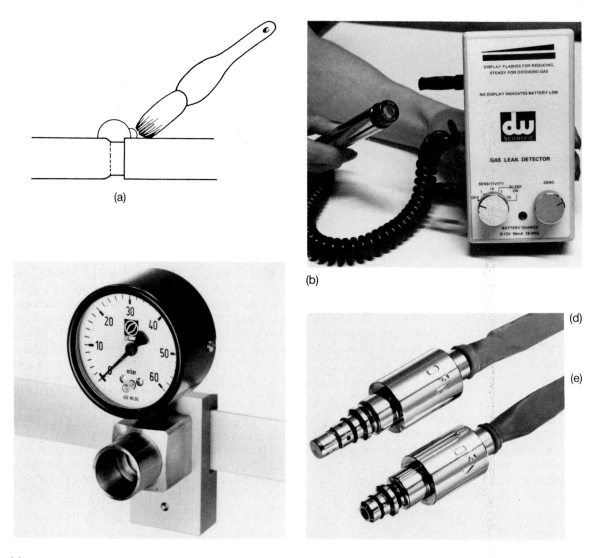

(a)

(b)

(c)

(d)

(e)

Figure 6.20   Testing for leaks. (a) A crude method. A very weak solution of soap or detergent, such as Hibitane, is applied liberally with a pastry brush. Bubbles indicate a leak. The remaining solution should be cleaned off after testing. A proprietary brand of bubbling leak detector, Snoop, is supplied in a squeezable bottle with an applicator. The manufacturers claim that no traces remain, and cleaning is not required. (b) The DW Scientific gas leak detector. Its principle of operation relies on the differing thermal conductivity of various gases (as is the case with the Bedfont gas discriminator, which is described on p. 261). A flashing display indicates the presence of reducing gases and a steady display of oxidizing gases (though these terms should not be taken as literal descriptions of their chemical properties). The machine will readily detect small leaks of oxygen, nitrous oxide or other gases or vapours from an anaesthetic machine. It is battery operated and requires 10–20 min to warm up and stabilize after it has been turned on. (c) The Dameca gauge for 'tightness control'. This may be mounted on a rail or onto the back bar of an anaesthetic machine and is connected to a 22 mm ISO female taper. A breathing system may be connected directly to it and then pressurized. The rate of fall of pressure, as shown by the gauge, will indicate the amount of leakage from the breathing system. (d)–(g) The Dameca 'balloon method' for detecting leaks at pipeline terminal outlets, in this case those manufactured by AGA. Special probes, referred to as A and B (shown in (d) and (e)) test the end and side seals respectively. If, 1 min after engagement the balloon is still only partially inflated (f), there is no significant leak, but if it inflates fully (g), the outlet requires servicing.

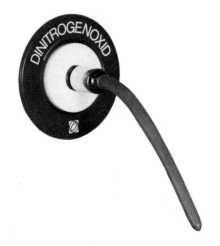

(f)

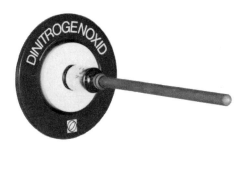

(g)

nect the hose, give it a short sharp pull to establish that it is fully engaged and check the flowmeter again. (The tug test).

Repeat this procedure with the nitrous oxide cylinders or pipeline.

Check that the cylinders are correctly labelled 'full', 'in use', etc.

Open the carbon dioxide cylinder and check that it is not empty; leave it turned on.

Open the cyclopropane cylinder (if fitted) and having checked that it is not empty close it.

Open the oxygen bypass to check it and to expel the carbon dioxide and cyclopropane from the machine.

Close the bypass.

Finally leave the cylinder key on the top of the anaesthetic machine. It is a good idea to attach it by a chain in order to prevent unauthorized 'borrowing'. You are lost without it!

2. *Vaporizers*

Check all temperature-compensated, calibrated vaporizers such as those for halothane and refill them as required. It has been recommended that halothane and other volatile agents be emptied out and discarded once a fortnight, and this may be conveniently done when the vaporizer is not too full, so as to reduce wastage. This may prove rather too expensive where vaporizers are used infrequently.

The Boyle's vaporizer. If any agent remains from the previous day discard it and wash out the jar. Refill as required, but do not overfill. If a colourless anaesthetic agent is used, the jar should be labelled appropriately. Make sure that the cork sealing washer is intact. Leave the vaporizer with the plunger up and the lever turned off.

3. *Check for leaks*

Machines with low regulated pressure. With the vaporizers turned off, turn on the oxygen to 5 *l*/min. Obstruct the outlet of the machine with the palm of the hand and observe the oxygen rotameter which should fall to below 200 cm³/min (a small leak of below 200 cm³ is permissible). *Note* that this test cannot be done on machines that have pressure relief valves on the back bar.

Machines with high regulated pressure and those with pressure relief valves set at 5 lb/in² (~ 34 kPa) should be tested as follows. Remove the reservoir bag and reconnect the hose to the outlet of the machine. Remove or close the expiratory valve. Turn on oxygen to 5 *l*/min. Allowing the corrugated hose to hang in a loop, occlude the open end. The hose should be seen to increase in length by a centimetre or so before the relief valve is heard to open.

If a leak is suspected in either the anaesthetic machine itself or the ventilator, or in one of the breathing attachments or piped medical gas hoses connected to them, it may be located by listening carefully for a hissing sound. Leaks of small magnitude, however, are sometimes difficult to hear. They may be located using one of the methods shown in Fig. 6.20.

The possibility of there being a leak is often not considered at first when a problem arises during anaesthesia and therefore the leak is not detected as quickly as it might have been.

4. *Breathing attachments*
Semi-closed systems. Check the reservoir bag, hose and expiratory valve. Make sure that there is an elbow and an endotracheal adaptor (catheter mount). Check for leaks by occluding the open end, closing the expiratory valve and squeezing the bag while fresh gases are flowing.

Closed circuits. Check the rebreathing bag and expiratory valve. Remove the corrugated hoses and hang them vertically to make sure that there is no condensed water in them. Replace them. Check for leaks and that the soda lime is fresh. When the system is in use check that both unidirectional valves are operating correctly.

5. *Check for leaks*
With all the flow-control valves and the oxygen bypass turned off, listen carefully for leaks, especially from cylinder yokes.

6. *Earthing*
Check the earthing of the machine. The wheels will have a yellow mark on them if the castors are antistatic, or, in some very old machines, will be fitted with earthing chains, at least three links of each of which should be in contact with the floor. (Whereas ordinary trolleys require only one earthing chain, it is standard practice to fit two to anaesthetic machines.) An earthing chain must be electrically connected to the frame of the machine.

7. *Accessories*
Check that the following either are on the anaesthetic machine or are immediately available nearby:
Cylinder key
Facepieces
Airways
Elbow
Harness and ring
Catheter mounts
Endotracheal tubes and connectors
Laryngoscopes
Syringe and forceps or Mitchell's inflator
Adhesive tape
Bandage
Mouth gag
Tongue forceps
Swabs
Laryngeal spray (filled and tested)
Lubricant
Scissors

The Anaesthetic Machines of the Future

The anaesthetic machine has developed in a haphazard manner, and is not a good example of ergonomic design. At the same time, various safety devices have been added to prevent the recurrence of accidents which had previously happened. By the very proliferation of these devices, the machine has become more complicated — both for the anaesthetist and the maintenance man.

In some centres new machines are in the process of development which show a completely new approach. On the one hand there is the relocation of components with which we are familiar, on the other the machine has a microprocessor at its centre, with what to some anaesthetists will be a bewildering number of options for the selection of vapours and breathing systems.

If such machines are to be employed in areas where more complicated techniques are used, there is still a need for more and more simple machines for the situations where short, uncomplicated anaesthetics are administered — in fact for the gross numerical majority of cases.

The need is therefore for two continuous-flow machines: the *major* of which will replace the present anaesthetic ventilator, such as the Blease Deansway and Cape Waine, and the *minor* of which will retain the features of the present minor machine, with few frills, but possibly its components arranged in a more logical manner, perhaps on a rack system.

The function of the major machine and the selection of all its modes may well be supervised by a microprocessor — the programming of which will prohibit selection of a mode or vapour or gas concentration that could harm a patient.

The needs of developing countries and of establishments where few and simple techniques are used will dictate that the trainee must become conversant with the use of the minor machine before going on to use the more complex equipment.

7

Breathing Attachments and their Components

The breathing attachment is defined as that part of the anaesthetic apparatus downstream from the back bar, in which the gases are at or close to atmospheric pressure and from which the patient inhales and into which he may exhale. It includes reservoir or rebreathing bags, or the bellows of a ventilator.

Breathing attachments may be classified into three groups: those in which the rebreathing of gases is prevented, those in which it does not occur during correct use, and those in which partial or total rebreathing is intended.

There has been considerable misuse of the terms 'breathing circuit', 'breathing system' and 'breathing attachment'. The term *breathing system* should be used in the abstract, and describes the method by which the gases are delivered to the patient. A *breathing attachment* refers to the actual group of interconnected components used to achieve this. The term *circuit* should refer only to a system in which gases pass through various channels and some or all of them return to the point from which they came. This is analogous to an electric circuit or to a motor-racing circuit where the cars go round and round the same track. The term *circle* also refers to such a circuit.

There is also much variation in the interpretation by anaesthetists of the classification of breathing systems according to their mode of operation. Confusion could be avoided if the following classification were used:

Mapleson A, B, C, D or E (where there is no provision for carbon dioxide absorption).

Non-rebreathing (as with the Ambu-E or Ruben valve).

Closed (circle or 'to-and-fro'), with or without a leak (where there is provision for carbon dioxide absorption and rebreathing of alveolar gas is intended).

Draw over (usually with air).

Open drop.

The following terms are commonly used and should be employed (if they must!) as follows:

Open: an 'open-drop' mask which does not fit the face. There is free access of air (see Fig. 5.2).

Semi-open: 'open drop', but with a mask which fits the face or is made to do so with gamgee, etc. and has an enclosure above it to promote partial rebreathing (see Fig. 5.3). This seldom, if ever, is used today.

Semi-closed: systems such as the Mapleson A, the Magill attachment, where rebreathing at least of alveolar gases is not intended. Nevertheless, it could occur as a result of misuse.

Closed: where total or partial rebreathing is intended. There is provision for carbon dioxide absorption. Some fresh gas flow is necessary to allow for oxygen utilization and unavoidable losses. Usually a considerable degree of 'spill' or leak is intended, the fresh gas flow rate being correspondingly higher, though recently there has been more interest in totally closed systems.

Assisted: in which some device such as a venturi or circulating fan is used to promote the flow of gases along the pathways of the system.

Note that in ventilators the term 'open' is used when all the expired gases are voided and 100% fresh gases are delivered at each stroke, and 'closed' when part or all of the exhaled gases are returned to the inspiratory side of the ventilator. As in the closed system above, provision is made for carbon dioxide absorption.

Dead space: This is discussed on pp. 136–138.

Scavenging: the removal of used or waste gases.

This, and the components required to achieve it, are discussed in Chapter 15.

Non-rebreathing Systems with Valves

The Magill attachment (Mapleson A) (Fig. 7.1a)

This is the most commonly used of all breathing

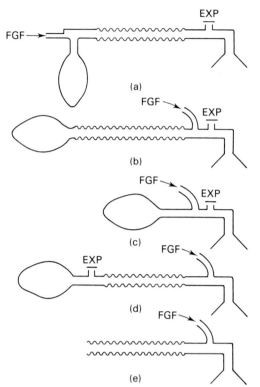

Figure 7.1 Mapleson's classification of semi-closed breathing systems. (a) This is the Magill attachment. The fresh gas flow (FGF) rate can be slightly less than the patient's minute volume without functional rebreathing occurring. In (b), (c) and (d) rebreathing will occur even if the fresh gas flow rate exceeds the patient's minute volume. (e) is the T-piece system, which is described elsewhere (p. 130). Note that (d) is, in fact, also a T-piece system. EXP = expiratory valve.

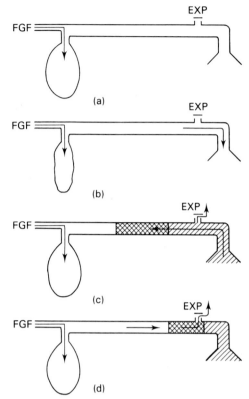

Figure 7.2 The Mapleson-A system used with spontaneous breathing (see text). FGF = fresh gas flow. EXP = expiratory valve.

systems. It consists of a reservoir bag (*not* rebreathing bag, since the patient's exhaled gases should never get back to it), a corrugated hose (of adequate length, usually 42 in., ∼ 110 cm) an expiratory valve (EXP)* and a connection to either a facepiece or an endotracheal tube. It is an extremely efficient system for spontaneous ventilation and a fresh gas flow (FGF) of rather less than the patient's minute volume is sufficient to prevent rebreathing of alveolar gases. This is explained by the fact that during spontaneous ventilation there are three phases in the

cycle: inspiratory, expiratory, and expiratory pause.

If in Fig. 7.2a the reservoir bag has been filled by the FGF and the patient is about to take a breath, the whole system is full of fresh gas. As the patient inhales, he draws the gases at a rate greater than that of the FGF, so the reservoir bag partially empties, as shown in Fig. 7.2b. In Fig. 7.2c the patient has begun to exhale and because the reservoir bag is not full the exhaled gases are breathed back up the corrugated hose, pushing the fresh gases in the hose back into the reservoir bag. However, before the exhaled gases can pass as far as the reservoir bag, the latter has been refilled by the fresh gases from the corrugated hose plus the continuing FGF from the anaesthetic machine. The point is reached when the reservoir bag is again full and as the patient is still exhaling the remaining exhaled gases have to pass out through the expiratory valve, which now opens.

The next stage is the expiratory pause. The fresh gas flow now drives the exhaled gases, or some of

---

* According to British Standard no. BS 6015 this should now be termed an 'adjustable pressure limiting valve' (or APL valve), but the author feels that the term expiratory valve is more suitable when it is intended that all the expired gases pass through it.

them, out of the expiratory valve. It will be seen, therefore, that the expiratory pause is important to prevent the patient's rebreathing of exhaled alveolar gases that occupy part of the hose at the end of expiration (Fig. 7.2d).

The first portion of exhaled gases to pass up the corrugated hose from the patient during expiration was that occupying dead space, and therefore, apart from being warmed and slightly humidified (a satisfactory state of affairs), they are unaltered. They have not taken part in respiratory exchange. During the expiratory pause all the alveolar gases and some of the dead space gases are expelled from the corrugated hose through the expiratory valve by the continuing FGF. Thus during the next inspiratory phase the gases inhaled will be fresh gases plus some of the dead space gases from the previous breath. As explained above, these dead space gases may be reinhaled without detriment to the patient. The FGF rate may, therefore, be rather less than the patient's minute volume. Functional rebreathing is still prevented.

Various modifications of the Magill attachment have been described and evaluated by Mapleson (Fig. 7.1b–e). In all of these there is a tendency towards rebreathing of alveolar gases unless the FGF rate is greater than the patient's minute volume.

A disadvantage of systems in which an expiratory valve is required is that it invariably causes a slight resistance to expiration. Manufacturers have attempted to design expiratory valves with the lowest possible resistance, and methods by which it can be further diminished are shown on pp. 140 and 246. This problem has also been tackled by Samson in his 'valveless' breathing system (Fig. 7.3).

THE MAGILL ATTACHMENT AND CONTROLLED VENTILATION

The mechanical aspects of the Magill attachment (Mapleson A) as described above refer to its use during spontaneous breathing. However, if controlled or assisted ventilation is used, i.e. if the patient is inflated by means of squeezing the reservoir bag, a different state of affairs occurs. The expiratory valve has to be kept almost closed, and at the end of the inspiratory phase, with the anaesthetist still squeezing the bag, the excess of fresh gases are blown out of the valve. At the end of inspiration the reservoir bag may be completely empty and as soon as the anaesthetist relaxes his pressure on it the patient exhales into the corrugated hose. On this occasion both dead space and alveolar gases may pass right back to the reservoir bag. (The capacity of the standard 42 in. corrugated hose is about 550 ml.) There is a natural tendency to allow no expiratory pause, so that when the anaesthetist squeezes the bag again the first gases

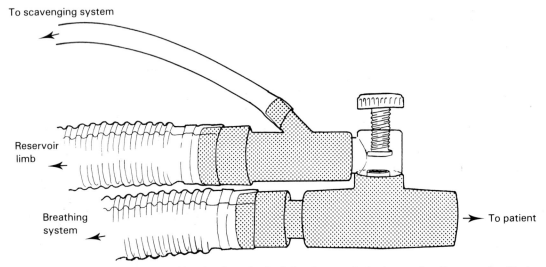

Figure 7.3 The Samson breathing system. Note that the spring-loaded expiratory valve has been replaced by a port, the effective orifice of which may be varied.

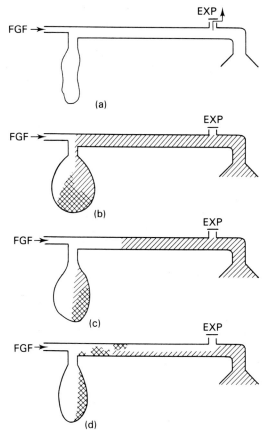

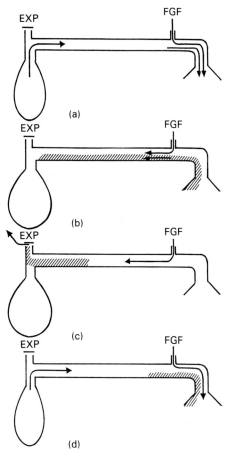

Figure 7.4   A Mapleson-A system with assisted or controlled ventilation (a) at the end of inspiration; (b) at the end of expiration; (c) during subsequent inspiration; (d) at the end of the subsequent inspiration. Note that much rebreathing takes place (see text). FGF = fresh gas flow. EXP = expiratory valve.

Figure 7.5   The Mapleson-D system with spontaneous ventilation (see text.) FGF = fresh gas flow. EXP = expiratory valve.

to enter the patient's lungs will be the exhaled alveolar gases. When the expiratory valve eventually opens it is fresh gases that escape. Under these circumstances there is considerable rebreathing (Fig. 7.4). An attempt to use the Magill attachment for controlled or assisted ventilation in order to initiate an anaesthetic technique, would therefore seem to be rather unsatisfactory, and its prolonged use dangerous.

The Mapleson-D system

THE MAPLESON-D SYSTEM WITH SPONTANEOUS VENTILATION

During the first inspiration the patient breathes fresh gases (Fig. 7.5a). During expiration the ex-

haled gases, mixed with the FGF, pass down the tube to the reservoir bag (Fig. 7.5b), and when this has been refilled a mixture of FGF and exhaled gases are voided via the expiratory valve. Of the expired gases, it is those from the dead space that are voided first, followed by alveolar gases.

During the expiratory pause, the FGF passes down the tube, displacing some of the mixture of FGF and exhaled gases, which are voided through the expiratory valve (Fig. 7.5c). At the next inspiration the inhaled gases consist of the FGF plus the mixture of any FGF and exhaled alveolar gases that remain in the tube (Fig. 7.5d). Functional rebreathing occurs unless (i) the FGF is at least twice the patient's minute volume and (ii) the expiratory pause is sufficiently long for all the expired gases in the tube to be voided. The tube must be of such a length that the volume of gas in it, when augmented by the volume of the fresh gas flow being delivered *during inspiration*, is no less than that of the patient's tidal volume.

It is worthy of note that the Mapleson-D system is, in fact, a T-piece.

THE MAPLESON-D SYSTEM WITH CONTROLLED OR ASSISTED VENTILATION

During the first inspiration the FGF and fresh gases in the tube pass to the patient and at the same time some gases from the reservoir bag are lost through the partially open expiratory valve (Fig. 7.6a). At the end of the first inspiration a mixture of FGF and exhaled gases pass down the tube and eventually enter the reservoir bag, the latter having been deflated during inspiration by the amount of both the patient's tidal volume and the volume of gases lost through the expiratory valve (Fig. 7.6b). Provided that there is an expiratory pause, the FGF passes

down the tube and drives the mixture of fresh and exhaled gases out via the expiratory valve. Again it is the dead space portion of expired gas that is voided first. At the next squeeze of the reservoir bag, (Fig. 7.6c) the FGF plus the fresh gas from the tube, plus any expired (alveolar) gases that remain in the tube, pass to the patient, while some of the mixed gases within the bag escape via the expiratory valve. The cycle then repeats itself. Thus to prevent rebreathing in the Mapleson-D system, both during spontaneous and controlled ventilation, the FGF must be greater than the patient's minute volume, and there must be a sufficient expiratory pause.

Figure 7.6d shows how the Mapleson-D system may be employed with an automatic ventilator. The reservoir bag is removed and replaced by a standard length of corrugated hose of sufficient capacity to accommodate the air that is delivered by the ventilator and prevent its reaching the patient in place of the intended anaesthetic gases.

In Chapter 15 the equipment for scavenging waste anaesthetic gases is described. Its use requires pro-

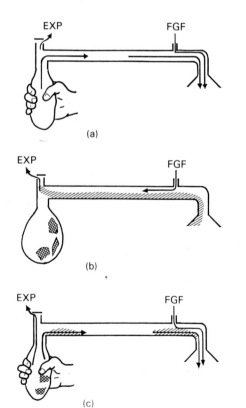

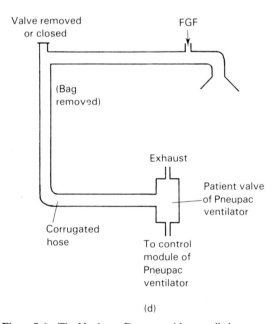

Figure 7.6   The Mapleson-D system with controlled ventilation. (a) to (c) With manual ventilation (see text). (d) With the employment of a ventilator such as the Pneupac. Note that in this case a standard length of corrugated hose (capacity approximately 500 ml) is required to prevent mixing the driving gas from the ventilator with the anaesthetic gases in the breathing attachment. FGF = fresh gas flow. EXP = expiratory valve.

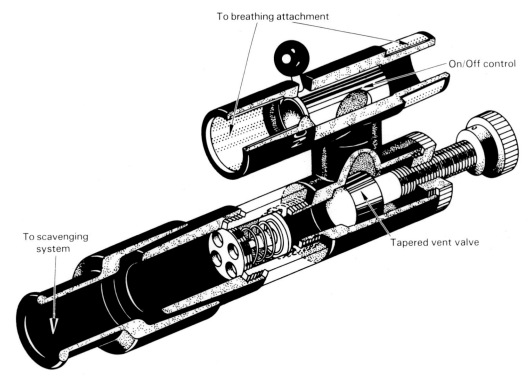

Figure 7.7   The Enderby scavenging valve.

vision for collecting, in some way, the gases emerging from the expiratory valve. This is usually done by a form of shroud which surrounds it. Earlier types, such as that of Enderby (Fig. 7.7), were installed at the patient end of the corrugated hose and their weight, plus that of the extra hose for scavenging, proved a nuisance. Modifications were therefore made to the Mapleson-A and -D systems, two of which are described below:

The Bain attachment (Fig. 7.8)

The Bain attachment is no different from the Mapleson-D system, except that the FGF is carried by a tube within the corrugated hose. In the earlier models in particular, there was a risk that the inner tube could become disconnected at the machine end, and if this happened there was a very big dead space! It could also become kinked — so cutting off the supply of fresh gases. The tubing is intended to be 'disposable'.

The Lack attachment (Fig. 7.9)

The Lack attachment is a coaxial version of the Mapleson A. The inner tube, which carries the expired gases, is of larger bore than that of the Bain attachment, and less likely to kink. It is constructed of more robust materials and is intended for repeated use.

Both the Bain and the Lack attachments are particularly convenient to use in cases where the patient's head and neck are covered by drapes and not accessible to the anaesthetist. The Bain, in particular, is lightweight and longer than the standard Mapleson A. This is an additional advantage when the anaesthetist is remote from his patient. The expiratory valve, being at the machine end, renders this arrangement far more convenient for scavenging than systems in which it is at the patient end.

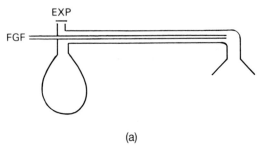

(a)

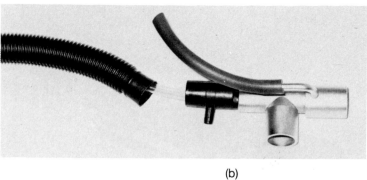

(b)

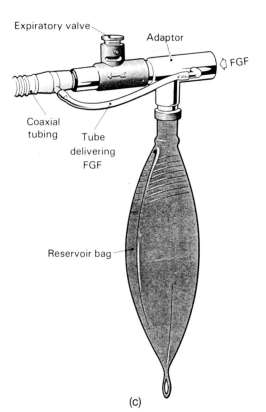

Expiratory valve

Adaptor

◊ FGF

Coaxial
tubing

Tube
delivering
FGF

Reservoir bag

(c)

Figure 7.8   The Bain attachment. (a) Working principles. (b) A Bain attachment in which the corrugated tube has been pulled away from its correct position of attachment to its adaptor in order to show the internal tube. This is the point at which accidental detachment may occur if tension is put upon the outer tubing. (c) An adaptor which may be used to mount the Bain attachment onto a 22 mm male outlet. FGF = fresh gas flow. EXP = expiratory valve.

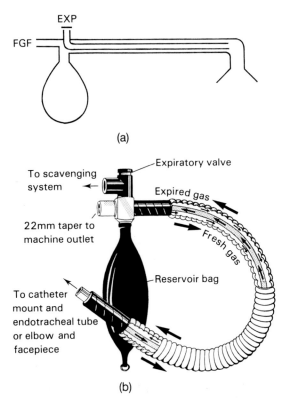

(a)

(b)

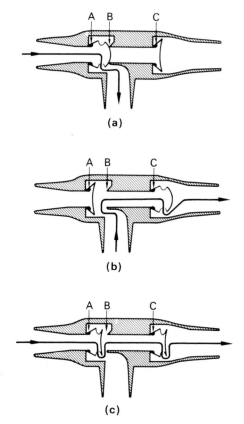

(a)

(b)

(c)

Figure 7.9   The Lack attachment. (a) Working principles. (b) The actual assembly. Note that the outer corrugated hose is partly transparent so that the inner tube may be seen to be intact. The expiratory valve EXP is fitted with a shroud having a 30 mm outlet so that it may be attached to a scavenging system. No adaptor is required as is the case with the Bain attachment (Fig. 7.8). FGF = fresh gas flow.

Figure 7.10   The Ambu-E valve. (a) During assisted inspiration. Note that the port B is closed by the pressure of the head of the 'mushroom' valve A. (b) During expiration. (c) During the expiratory pause excess gases may pass straight through the valve so preventing excessive build up of pressure.

The Ambu-E and Ruben valves

These expiratory valves, which are made of plastic, may be used in place of the Heidbrink valve in the standard Magill attachment. They are designed to positively prevent rebreathing, even with controlled ventilation.

In the Ambu-E valve (Fig. 7.10) the fresh gases from the reservoir bag flow to the patient via the corrugated hose, through the first elastic non-return valve A. During inspiration, which may be either spontaneous or passive as in controlled ventilation, valve A is open. This valve is so constructed that when it opens to admit inspiratory gases to the patient it also presses against port B, thus closing the expiratory limb. During the expiratory phase valve A closes and a second valve, C, opens to allow the expired gases to pass to the atmosphere. It will be

noted that during inspiration valve C remains closed, preventing any air being drawn in. The two valves, A and C, are identical and easily replaced. If the reservoir bag becomes overfilled, both valves open partially, allowing excess gases to escape into the atmosphere.

The Ambu-E valve can be dismantled for cleaning and the makers point out that it cannot be reassembled incorrectly. There is a low resistance to both inspiration and expiration. It is quiet in operation, but some anaesthetists find that they miss the reassuring 'hiss' of the Heidbrink expiratory valve. In the author's experience rebreathing is not altogether eliminated by the Ambu-E valve during quiet respiration.

The Ruben valve, which is shown in Fig. 7.11, is somewhat similar to the Ambu-E valve. It depends

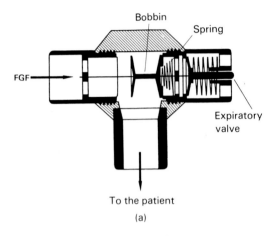

To the patient

(a)

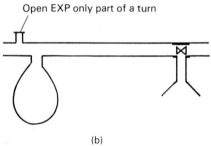

Open EXP only part of a turn

(b)

Figure 7.11   (a) The Ruben valve. (b) An arrangement used by some anaesthetists to prevent excessive overpressure if the bobbin sticks due to excess moisture from condensation of the expired gases. The expiratory valve EXP fitted adjacent to the reservoir bag should be opened only part of a turn. FGF = fresh gas flow.

for its operation, however, on a bobbin which moves against the tension of a light spring. It is not un-known for the bobbin to stay in the inspiratory position, resulting in overpressure being applied to the patient. Some practitioners incorporate a Heid-brink valve, partially screwed down adjacent to the reservoir bag, as a protection. However, this will only ameliorate the danger and will not prevent it altogether.

Non-rebreathing valves in a bag mount

In varying (intermittent) flow machines such as the McKesson, Walton Five and AE, there is no indica-tion of flow rate. The latter could therefore be too low to prevent rebreathing unless special arrange-ments were made. One way to overcome this is to include a non-return valve immediately downstream from the reservoir bag. Further discussion of this

will be found in Chapter 8. Such a valve completely prevents rebreathing and is very satisfactory when the patient is breathing spontaneously. Unfortu-nately it makes controlled or assisted ventilation difficult, since the expiratory valve has to be con-tinually readjusted.

Non-rebreathing Systems without Valves

The T-piece system

However efficient an expiratory valve may be, it is bound to offer some resistance to exhalation, which

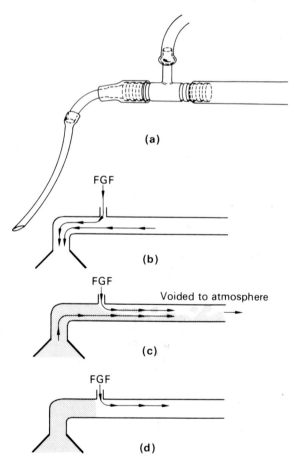

(a)

FGF

(b)

FGF   Voided to atmosphere

(c)

FGF

(d)

Figure 7.12   (a) The Ayre's T-piece connected to an endotracheal tube. (b) During spontaneous inspiration. (c) During expiration. (d) During the expiratory pause.

may not be acceptable in certain anaesthetic techniques. To avoid this resistance the T-piece system may be used. In Fig. 7.12 the fresh gases are supplied via a small-bore tube to the side arm of an Ayre's T-piece. The main body of the T-piece is within the breathing system and must, therefore, be of adequate diameter. One end of the body is connected by the shortest possible means to the patient. (This limb represents apparatus dead space.) The other end is connected to a length of tubing, which acts as a reservoir.

The fresh gas flow (FGF) rate must be high in the case of spontaneous ventilation. During inspiration the peak inspiratory flow rate is higher than the FGF, so some gases are drawn from the reservoir limb. During expiration both the expired air and the fresh gases, which continue to flow, pass into the reservoir limb and are expelled to the atmosphere. During the expiratory pause it flushes out and refills the reservoir limb. The dimensions of the reservoir limb and the FGF rate are governed by the following considerations:

1. The diameter of the reservoir limb must be sufficient to present the lowest possible resistance. For example, not less than $0.75 \, cmH_2O$ for a neonate and not less than $2 \, cmH_2O$ for an adult.
2. The volume of the expiratory limb should be approximately the same as the patient's tidal volume — too great a volume would matter only in that the greater length would lead to increased resistance. Too great a diameter would lead to mixing of the fresh gases with alveolar gas and to inefficiency of the system. For an adult an ordinary 42 in. length of corrugated hose is satisfactory.
3. The optimum FGF rate depends not only on the patient's minute volume but also on the capacity of the reservoir limb. If the latter is at least that of the patient's tidal volume, then a rate of two-and-a-half times the patient's minute volume is sufficient. This is the most satisfactory arrangement. However, if the capacity of the reservoir is reduced, the flow rate must be increased. If the capacity of the reservoir is reduced to zero, the flow rate must be in excess of the peak inspiratory flow rate.

The shape of the T-piece is also important. Normally the side arm is at right angles to the body. If it is at an angle pointing towards the patient, there is continuous positive pressure applied which would act as a resistance during expiration; similarly, if the gases were directed towards the reservoir, a subatmospheric pressure would be caused by a venturi effect.

CONTROLLED VENTILATION WITH THE T-PIECE

Unlike the Magill attachment, the T-piece is equally efficient during spontaneous and controlled ventilation, which may be effected by intermittently occluding the end of the reservoir limb with the thumb. This should be done with care, since when the outlet is occluded the full pressure supplied by the anaesthetic machine is applied to the patient. It would seem prudent to include, in infant systems at least, a blow-off valve set to about $40 \, cmH_2O$ pressure; but this is seldom done. A limitation in its use arises from the fact that the peak inspiratory flow rate is limited to that of the FGF. This is overcome in the Rees T-piece, described below.

The T-piece system is particularly suited to neonates and infants, where an expiratory valve presents a significant resistance. The scaling down of a system suitable for adults does not lend itself to paediatric anaesthesia.

A disadvantage of the T-piece system is that it is not easy to observe the patient's respiration without the reassuring whistle of the expiratory valve. This can be overcome by attaching to the open end of the reservoir limb a small wisp of cotton wool, which can be seen to wave in the breeze, or by the use of an indicator devised by Marshall (Fig. 7.13).

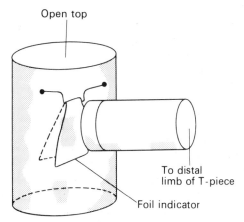

Figure 7.13 Marshall's indicator.

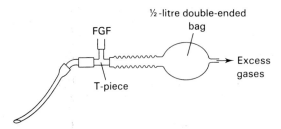

Figure 7.14   The Rees T-piece. FGF = fresh gas flow.

THE REES T-PIECE

A great improvement to the T-piece was made by Rees, who added a small double-ended bag to the end of the reservoir limb (Fig. 7.14). Note that the tubular portion of the limb should still approximate to the patient's tidal volume or rebreathing could occur as a result of the mixing of expired and fresh gases. During spontaneous ventilation small movements of the semi-collapsed bag demonstrate the patient's breathing. During controlled ventilation the open end of the bag is partially or totally occluded by the anaesthetist's little finger during the inspiratory phase, while the bag is squeezed between his other fingers and thumb. The little finger is relaxed during expiration. This simple system is extremely efficient for infants and small children.

Other paediatric breathing systems are described in Chapter 12.

T-PIECE FOR ADULTS

This is not employed as often as it was in the past, but it is still favoured by some anaesthetists for operations such as thyroidectomy where expiratory resistance, and therefore venous pressure, is to be kept as low as possible. It may be arranged simply as follows. Take a 'double tube and T-piece' from a circle absorber. Connect one of the tubes to the outlet of the anaesthetic machine, and the T-piece to the patient as usual, closing the expiratory valve if there is one. Place the open end of the other tube in a convenient position for observation, and attach a small wisp of cotton wool or other indicator as mentioned above. The indicator will be seen to move during changes in the phase of breathing.

Systems in which Rebreathing is Intended

Systems in which the patient continually rebreathes the same gases were devised in order to effect economy in anaesthetic agents, in particular cyclopropane which was, and remains, expensive. Other advantages include the reduction of pollution of the atmosphere of the operating theatre, the reduction of the risk of explosion when employing inflammable agents, the maintenance within the system of moisture and heat, and the ease with which the ventilation may be assisted or controlled.

'Closed' systems may be kept completely closed, merely the patient's basal oxygen requirement being added, with perhaps an increment of anaesthetic vapour, or be 'closed-with-spill', in which an excess of fresh gas flow is added and there is a continuous loss via the expiratory valve. The latter, although lacking in economy, is the more efficient, since in the former the concentration of oxygen and anaesthetic vapour is difficult to assess, and the mixture of gases contains nitrogen which is voided from the patient's plasma during the early stages of anaesthesia. Also, complete elimination of carbon dioxide is difficult to ensure. Completely closed systems with air, oxygen and halothane or totally intravenous anaesthesia are now being advocated by some anaesthetists in order to avoid the problems of atmosphere pollution. It is advisable to include monitors for halothane and oxygen with such a system, but this entails extra complication and expense.

Carbon dioxide absorption

In any system where there is functional rebreathing, whether total or partial, provision must be made for the removal of the carbon dioxide that would otherwise accumulate. The usual absorbent used is soda lime. This consists of calcium hydroxide with 5% sodium hydroxide and sometimes a small percentage of potassium hydroxide. Silicates are usually included to make granules which are less likely to disintegrate into powder. The size of granule is important: if it is too big, there are large voids between the granules, leading to poor contact with the gases, and therefore poor absorption; and if too small, the soda lime canister becomes clogged with dust and there is resistance to gas flow. Some moisture is also required for efficient absorption.

However, even if the soda lime is dry to begin with, moisture is obtained not only from the patient's expired gases but also from the reaction between the soda lime and carbon dioxide, viz:

$$2NaOH + CO_2 \rightarrow Na_2CO_3 + H_2O$$

Various brands of soda lime contain indicators which change colour when it is 'exhausted'. If exhausted soda lime is allowed to stand for some hours there may be some degree of 'regeneration', as the carbonate on the surface moves to the interior of the granule and the hydroxide from within migrates to the surface.

Soda lime should be stored in sealed containers and handled with care to avoid the granules being reduced to dust. The last remains in the container usually have to be thrown away because of dust. Baryta lime, another absorbent, based on barium hydroxide, is not so commonly used, but acts in the same way as soda lime.

The lifespan of soda lime depends on the amount of rebreathing permitted, the fresh gas flow rate and whether all the expired gases pass through it. In a completely closed system, 1 lb (0.45 kg) of soda lime, which is the capacity of the standard canister, cannot be expected to last for more than four hours, and, in fact, becomes inefficient after two hours. Larger canisters are described below.

Closed systems

'TO-AND-FRO' ABSORBERS: THE WATERS' CANISTER (Fig. 7.15)

Here the patient breathes in and out of a closed bag, which is connected to the face-piece or endotracheal tube via a canister containing soda lime. The part of the system between the patient and the soda lime is dead space and therefore its volume must be kept to a minimum. This means that the soda lime canister must be close to the patient's head, and this leads to mechanical difficulties. A length of wide-bore tubing may, however, be interposed between the canister and rebreathing bag without detriment. The fresh gases are introduced at the patient end of the system, and the expiratory valve is usually mounted close by, though it may equally well be put at the bag end. The canister is usually placed in the horizontal position for convenience, and it is most important that it is well packed, since if there were a void above the soda lime, 'channelling' would occur and absorption would be incomplete (Fig. 7.16). The soda lime may conveniently be compressed to prevent gaps by the insertion of a nylon pot scourer at one end. When the canister is closed the sealing washer should be checked to ensure that it is in the correct position. Any soda lime on the threads of the canister or the sealing washer should be carefully removed. The whole system should be tested for leaks before use.

Apart from being cumbersome, the 'to-and-fro' system has the disadvantage that the patient could inhale soda lime dust. The anaesthetist may prove this by taking a few breaths through a canister himself. Cotton wool filters may be inserted in the patient end of the canister to prevent this.

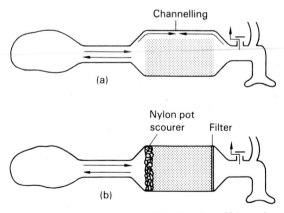

Figure 7.16 (a) Channelling in a Waters' canister. If the canister is not completely filled with soda lime and is placed in a horizontal position, the gases can pass through the void at the top and therefore fail to come into adequate contact with the soda lime. (b) The prevention of channelling by the insertion of a nylon pot scourer to compress the soda lime. Note also the filter at the patient end which prevents particles of soda lime reaching the patient.

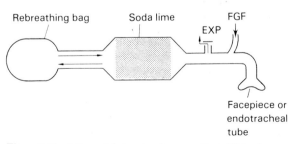

Figure 7.15 A 'to-and-fro' system incorporating a Waters' canister. FGF = fresh gas flow.

One of the advantages of the 'to-and-fro' system is that it is easy to sterilize after an infected case. If the canister is made of metal it may be autoclaved; if it is made of Perspex it may be disinfected by chemical means. Boiling is not advisable for Perspex, since it may become distorted.

CIRCLE ABSORBERS

Here the disadvantages of the soda lime canister being so close to the patient are obviated. The patient is connected to the absorber via two corrugated hoses, one inspiratory and the other expiratory, as shown in Fig. 7.17. The one-way or 'circle' flow of gases is determined by two unidirectional valves V_1 and V_2 which are often accommodated in glass domes so that their correct action may be observed. In the simple system shown in Fig. 7.18a these valves have been replaced by an Ambu-E valve, which performs the same function. The dead space is very small, but the long hoses and unidirectional valves cause some resistance. In the case of the 'jumbo' absorber (Fig. 7.18b), the soda lime

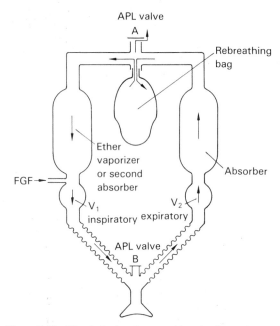

Figure 7.17 The circle closed system. Note the alternative positions for the APL valve. If it is situated at B, less CO_2 will pass through the absorber if there is a relatively high fresh gas flow, thereby affording an economy in soda lime and more efficient CO_2 elimination.

canister may have a capacity of 4 lb ($\sim$2 kg) of soda lime, and since this has a large volume and surface area of granules, the expired air is in contact with the soda lime for a relatively long period of time, so increasing the efficiency of absorption. When a 4 lb canister is employed it usually has two chambers, one above the other, and is reversible. When one half is exhausted it is refilled, and then the canister is inverted so that the previously unused half now bears the brunt of the absorption. Not only is the absorption more efficient in the large absorbers, but also less frequent recharging is necessary. One advantage of the circle system over the 'to-and-fro' system is that in the former the absorber may be switched off without any disconnection of the parts.

Whereas in earlier circle units there was both an absorber and an ether vaporizer, recently the ether vaporizer has been omitted, or replaced by a second absorber. When manual controlled ventilation is being used, the rebreathing bag may be mounted on a length of corrugated hose in order to 'mobilize' the anaesthetist. It is convenient to mount a manually operated 'spill valve' next to the bag so that excess gases may be voided during manual ventilation. This is more efficient than keeping the expiratory valve partially open.

Although there is little dead space, the capacity of the hoses alone is over a litre, and of the whole apparatus considerably more. At the beginning of an administration there should be a high fresh gas flow to purge the system of air and nitrogen evolved from the patient's plasma.

Daily maintenance of circle absorbers

After use the corrugated hose should be washed and hung up to dry. During prolonged administration water vapour condenses in the expiratory hose and this needs to be emptied from time to time. Condensation also occurs in the expiratory unidirectional valve. Not only does this obscure the glass dome so that the correct operation of the valve cannot be observed, but also a drop of water on the cage retaining the valve disc may cause the latter to adhere to it by surface tension, thus holding the valve permanently open. This results in the patient breathing backwards and forwards through the expiratory hose — the dead space being enormous — and could be catastrophic for the patient. The tendency of the valve discs to stick is a result of their being made of increasingly lighter materials in order

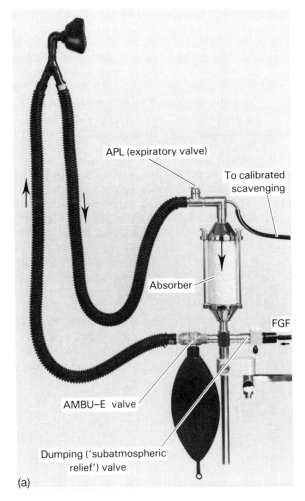

(a)

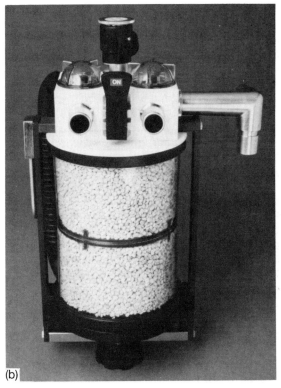

(b)

Figure 7.18 Examples of circle absorbers. (a) A simple circle system employing an absorber and an Ambu-E valve. Note that this is a Hafnia system and that excess gases are removed by an ejector flowmeter. FGF = fresh gas flow. (b) A 'jumbo' absorber (see text).

to reduce the resistance to gas flow. When controlled ventilation is being employed, especially with a negative expiratory phase, the mica disc may need to be replaced by a heavier one or have a small weight placed upon it in order to prevent sticking.

When, after dismantling, the glass domes are screwed back on again, it is important to ensure that the sealing washers are in place, otherwise a serious leak may occur. The drums of the valves controlling the soda lime canister and the ether vaporizer are greased in order to permit free movement but avoid leaks. A special grease is used which is resistant to anaesthetic agents. It requires renewal by the service engineer at regular intervals. Some circle absorbers cannot be autoclaved but may be cleaned by chemical means. More modern ones, especially those connected with ventilators, may be safely autoclaved. It is generally considered that, provided the inspiratory and expiratory hoses are allowed to hang in a loop, droplets precipitate within them and the absorber itself does not become infected. There is little evidence to confirm or deny that this supposition holds good in anaesthetic practice. Certainly it is difficult to obtain positive bacteriological cultures of pathogens from anaesthetic equipment except in those parts very close to the patient. Recently developed respiratory filters may be installed between the expiratory hose and the absorber. There is no doubt that these protect the absorber from infection, and they are constructed of materials that are hydrophobic, i.e. water vapour does not condense upon them, nor do they absorb moisture.

The soda lime container usually has a mark above which it should not be filled. Since it is held in the vertical position, channelling cannot occur as in the Waters' canister. Overfilling may result in granules of soda lime clogging the threads of those canisters that screw into position, or may prevent the correct seating of the sealing washer, thus causing a leak or bypassing of the soda lime.

The use of volatile agents in the circle system
If there is a vaporizer actually within the breathing circuit, it must be of low resistance. Calibrated vaporizers for use in the back bar, such as the Fluotec, are unsuitable. Any vaporizer containing wicks, however low their resistance, is also unsuitable, since water vapour would condense on the wicks. As the same gases are repeatedly passing through the vaporizer, calibration can be misleading. With agents such as halothane, where it would be possible to administer a dangerously high concentration, a vaporizer in circle (VIC) should therefore be used with caution.

Ether has, however, been widely and safely used with a VIC. Adequate vaporization is assisted by baffles within the vaporizer which cause the gases to impinge repeatedly on the surface of the ether, or even by bubbling the fresh gas flow (FGF) through the liquid ether, and to some extent by the heat from the expired gases.

For agents such as halothane, it is more prudent to use a vaporizer out of the circle (VOC) and add the vapour to the fresh gases. When there is a low FGF rate and only a small spill, a relatively high concentration of halothane may be required and a vaporizer such as the MJ version of the *Fluotec*, giving up to 10% halothane, or a 'copper kettle' may be used.

A circular slide rule has been produced which may be used to calculate the halothane concentration in a closed circuit, given data such as the FGF rate, patient's minute volume and concentration of halothane in the FGF.

The use of a closed circuit when the patient is breathing spontaneously has often been advocated for the sake of economy: certainly anaesthetic gases and vapours are costly. Warming and humidification of the inspired gases are also beneficial. It must be remembered, however, that no absorption system is always 100% efficient, and all circle systems offer some resistance. Many an anaesthetist has been surprised when he has been made to try breathing

oxygen through his circle absorber, to find how soon he becomes dyspnoeic! The old adage 'I like to have a bit of soda lime in the circuit' has often covered a multitude of sins. No amount of apparatus will help a patient whose ventilation is spontaneous but inadequate.

Disposable Breathing Tubing

Sets of corrugated hose complete with breathing bag and Y-piece are available for single use after which they may be discarded. The expiratory limb may include a bacterial filter which is intended to prevent contamination of the apparatus. This tubing is lightweight, but being less robust is more prone to kinking or obstruction by being pinched. It is particularly useful in the treatment of patients with a tracheostomy and intermittent positive pressure ventilation (IPPV) since it has less tendency to pull on or dislodge the tracheostomy tube. Although this type of tubing does not stand up to autoclaving, it can often be pasteurised and reused.

Dead Space

Patient dead space

Patient dead space is that part of the respiratory system that is occupied by air that does not come into contact with the respiratory epithelium and does not take part in respiratory exchange. In an adult the volume of this space is ~ 150 ml, but varies with the movements of the lung during breathing. During anaesthesia it may be reduced by endotracheal intubation. Whereas anatomical dead space consists of the air passages from the lips or the nares down to the alveoli, physiological dead space includes in addition that part of the air in an overdilated alveolus that does not take part in respiratory exchange and the air in an unperfused alveolus.

Apparatus dead space

Apparatus dead space is the volume of the part of the anaesthetic equipment that at the end of expiration is filled with exhaled gases, which in a non-

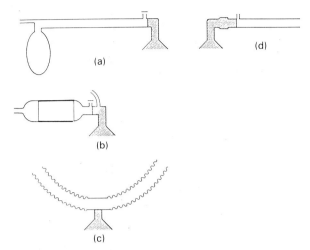

Figure 7.19 Dead space. (a) In the Mapleson-A system. (b) In the 'to-and-fro' system. (c) In the circle system. (d) In the T-piece system. In (a) and (b) an inadequate fresh gas flow rate will lead to rebreathing of gases from an area greater than that shown in the diagram. In (b) the dead space will be extended to the surface of the soda lime if the fresh gas flow rate is very low, and in (c) if the absorber is switched out of circuit or the soda lime is exhausted. The whole circle system acts as a dead space.

rebreathing system are destined to be re-inhaled at the next breath, and in a closed system to be re-inhaled without first passing through the CO_2 absorber (Fig. 7.19). As has already been pointed out in the discussion of the Mapleson-A system, these exhaled gases have not necessarily been subjected to respiratory exchange, since they may have occupied only the anatomical dead space. In this case, their re-inhalation does not constitute functional re-breathing. The dead space of various systems has already been described.

Breathing system volume

Breathing system volume is the volume of the breathing system excluding that of any limb that is occupied by gases that are to be entirely vented. In a circle system, this may be termed 'circuit volume'. Although it is not dead space, it is of significance, since in various systems it may influence:

1. The time taken to alter the constitution of the gases inspired, as, for example, when the concentration of oxygen in the fresh gas flow (FGF) is increased.
2. The time taken and the FGF rate required at the

start of the anaesthetic to purge air from the system and subsequently the nitrogen that is 'washed out' of the patient.
3. In intermittent positive pressure apparatus, the loss of stroke volume by virtue of elongation of the corrugated hoses (of which there may often be four in the circuit).
4. The loss of stroke volume in ventilators by compression of the gases. In a volume of 3 l this may account for a 'loss' of about 25 ml per litre at an inspiratory pressure of 25 cmH$_2$O.

Intentional dead space

Although it is usually desirable to reduce dead space to a minimum, there are occasions when it is augmented intentionally. This is to enable hyperventilation without lowering the patient's PCO_2. It may be done by increasing the volume of the catheter mount or by interposing a length of corrugated hose between the patient and the rest of the breathing attachment.

In the case of paediatric and neonatal anaesthesia, dead space may be created by using a Rees T-tube and connecting it as shown in Fig. 7.20a. Dead

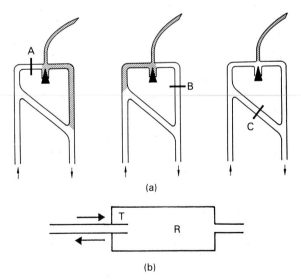

Figure 7.20 The intentional provision of dead space. (a) In a paediatric system using a Jackson Rees T-tube, a cross shunt may be used. If a clamp is applied at A, the dead space is maximal; if at B, it is less; and if at C, it is minimal. (b) The position of the end of the tube T within the reservoir R may be altered in order to vary the effective volume of dead space.

space will be maximal if the circuit is blocked at A and minimal if it is blocked at C. Alternatively it may be increased by an arrangement as shown in Fig. 7.20b. Note that here the volume of dead space may be varied by adjusting the length of the smaller tube within the reservoir.

Modification of Breathing Systems

Some modifications of the above systems aimed at reducing resistance and facilitating scavenging are described at the end of this chapter.

The Components of a Breathing System

Rebreathing and reservoir bags (Fig. 7.21)

These are identical, the distinction being solely in the use to which they are put, as explained previously. The commonly used size in the Magill attachment is 2 *l* (i.e. that which when fully but not

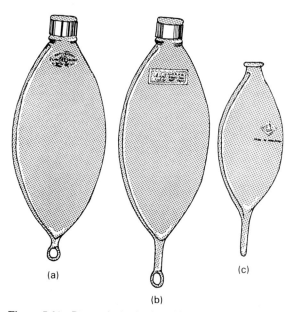

Figure 7.21 Reservoir (and rebreathing) bags. (a) A single-ended, two-litre bag. (b) A two-litre bag in which the extended tail loop may be removed to convert it into a double-ended bag. (c) A half-litre bag with a small neck, which may be converted into a double-ended one, for paediatric use.

forcibly distended has a capacity of 2 *l*; in clinical practice it is seldom filled beyond this capacity). Larger bags are used as reservoir bags in ventilators, and smaller ones in paediatric anaesthesia.

In the Magill attachment and closed-circuit apparatus, the capacity to which the bag may easily be distended must exceed the patient's tidal volume. A larger capacity, though harmless, is unnecessary. Bags are frequently provided with a loop at the bottom end which makes it possible to double the bag back on itself by hanging the loop from a knob on the top of the bag mount. This manoeuvre, or tying the bag around with string, is used when anaesthetizing small children. It does not alter the mechanics of the breathing attachment, and is justified only in that it makes movements of the bag easier to observe. Certainly it should not be used if it makes the bag 'stiffer'.

'Double-ended' bags may be used in two ways. The narrow end may be connected to the fresh gas flow, provided that rebreathing is prevented as in the Digby Leigh paediatric attachment (see Fig. 12.3). In the Rees T-piece paediatric attachment, a double-ended bag is added to the expiratory limb (Fig. 7.14) and the smaller end acts as an expiratory port which can be controlled by the anaesthetist's little finger.

The 'pressure-limiting' bag (Fig. 7.22), seldom used now, was intended for use as a reservoir for ventilators. When it is distended a string within it pulls open the flap of a valve in its wall, allowing the escape of excess gases. It should be noted that it would be dangerous to use such a bag in a Magill attachment, since if the opening pressure of the valve on the bag were less than that of the expiratory valve, the latter would fail to open and so expired gases would not escape through it. Fresh gases would escape from the bag, and the patient would rebreathe the gases in the corrugated hose, the capacity of which would present a dead space of about 500 ml!

The material of which the bag is constructed is important. Where ventilation is spontaneous, the opening pressure of the expiratory valve must exceed that required to prevent the bag from emptying spontaneously due to its weight or resistance to distension. Therefore, to maintain a low expiratory pressure, the bag must be 'soft'.

A stiffer bag with stronger walls is required for use with minute volume divider ventilators such as

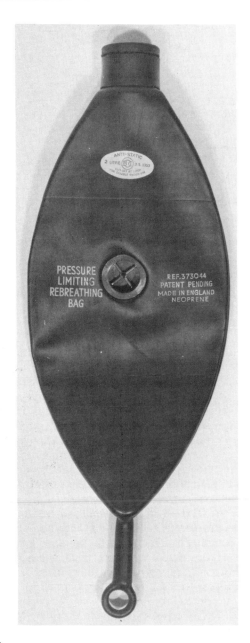

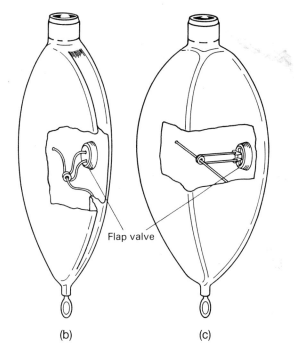

Figure 7.22   (a) The 'pressure-limiting' bag. (b) The bag before it is distended. (c) The bag when full and the flap valve has been opened.

(a)

the East–Freeman Automatic Vent (p. 209), where the back pressure on the bag may rise to 30 mmHg or more, and the elasticity of the bag plays a part in the operation of the valve.

The black antistatic rubber of which it is constructed may make movements of the bag difficult to observe under some conditions. In this case a couple of strips of white adhesive plaster stuck diagonally on the bag may help. The observed movement of the bag depends on several factors, such as its shape, size, degree of filling, the tension of the expiratory valve and the fresh gas flow rate, as well as on the patient's tidal volume. An accurate estimate of the patient's tidal volume cannot be made simply by watching the bag, especially in the case of the Magill and Lack attachments.

When ordering bags, the size of the neck should be specified. Whereas in some bags, including those for the East–Freeman Automatic Vent, etc., the neck is integral with the bag itself and relatively easily stretched, in others the neck includes a stiff moulded rubber fitting which is suitable only for the appropriate size of bag mount.

The bag mount may incorporate a valve that can exclude the bag from the breathing attachment. This is no longer widely employed, but where an intermittent flow machine is used 'on demand', either the valve should be closed or the bag and its mount should be removed from the machine. The bag also needs to be disconnected when minute volume divider ventilators such as the Manley are used.

Expiratory ('pop-off' or adjustable pressure limiting) valves

In the latest British and International Standards this valve is called the *adjustable pressure limiting valve*, or APL valve, but it is felt that for a long time the older terms *expiratory valve* (EXP) or 'pop-off' valve will be used.

The purpose of this valve is to allow the escape of exhaled (expired) and surplus gases from a breathing attachment, but without permitting entry of the outside air, even during a negative phase. Usually it is desirable that the pressure required to open the valve should be as low as possible, in order to minimize resistance to expiration. It must, however, present sufficient resistance to prevent the reservoir bag from emptying spontaneously, particularly when a scavenging system is employed that exerts a subatmospheric pressure upon it.

A commonly used type of expiratory valve is the *Heidbrink* (Fig. 7.23). The valve disc is as light as possible, and rests on a 'knife-edge' seating which presents a small area of contact. This lessens the tendency to adhesion between the disc and seating due to the surface tension of condensed water from the expired air, or after washing or sterilizing. The disc has a stem which is located in a guide, in order to ensure that it is correctly positioned on the seating, and a coiled spring, of light weight, which

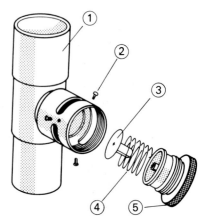

Figure 7.23   The Heidbrink valve. 1, Female taper; 2, retaining screw; 3, disc; 4, spring; 5, valve top.

promotes closure of the valve.

Some people prefer to remove the spring in order to reduce resistance to the opening of the valve. When this is done, if the valve is orientated so that the disc is in a horizontal plane over the seating (i.e. upright), it would seem that gravity would be sufficient to close it, obviating the necessity for the spring. However, as the disc is very light, dampness might lead to surface tension holding it open. Also, if the valve is placed obliquely or sideways, friction between the stem and the guide might prevent it from closing, and if it is upside-down gravity could keep it open. Another problem arising from the absence of the spring is that there may be some delay in the closing of the valve at the start of inspiration, in which case air could be drawn in.

The spring is a delicate coil and is of such dimensions that when the valve top is screwed fully 'open' there is minimal pressure on the disc when seated. However, during the 'blow-off' phase the disc rises and shortens the spring so that the pressure it exerts on the disc is greater and will close it at the appropriate time. Screwing down the valve top produces progressively increasing tension in the spring. When the top is screwed fully down the valve is completely closed. If, due to damage or fatigue, the spring is shortened, the top may have to be screwed down a little in order to assure closure at the start of inspiration. If it has been elongated, the pressure at which it opens may be excessive. Small grub screws in the body of the valve, and a groove in the skirt of the top, prevent it from being unscrewed so far that it falls apart.

(a)

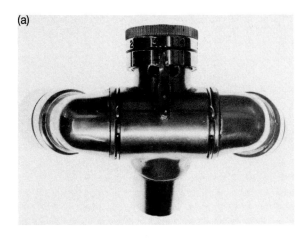

Figure 7.24 The Magill calibrated expiratory valve.

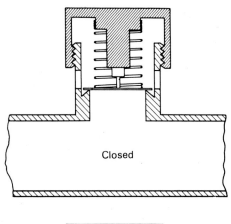

Closed

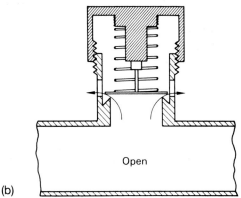

Open

(b)

There are various modifications of the Heidbrink valve and the similar '*Magill spring-loaded*' *valve*, such as the 'calibrated' valve (Fig. 7.24), that offer variable resistance to expiration. Such a valve might be used, for example, when employing a circle absorber with manually controlled or assisted ventilation.

In paediatric anaesthetic equipment it is difficult to produce and maintain in good working order an expiratory valve of suitable size and mass that can be relied on to offer a sufficiently low resistance. This problem can be solved either by using a valveless system such as a 'T-piece' or by using a simple flap valve with a lightweight mica disc, as in the Digby Leigh attachment. These mica discs are prone to damage and it is advisable to have a few spare ones to hand.

Some workers have attempted to modify the ordinary Heidbrink valve for paediatric use by in-serting a safety pin through two of the vent holes so that it is interposed between the disc and the seating. This manoeuvre renders the expiratory valve inefficient and actually resembles a T-piece system. To ensure that no air is drawn in through the valve there must be a relatively high fresh gas flow, and this in itself may cause resistance to expiration.

The *McKesson expiratory valve* (Fig. 7.25) is used on nasal inhalers for dental anaesthesia. It is spring loaded, and the tension on the spring closing the valve may be altered by adjusting the calibrated 'clutch'. This valve was useful when a degree of rebreathing against a spring loaded bag was intended; a technique rarely used now. The disadvantages of the McKesson valve are that the flap is relatively heavy and inclined to stick and that it is often held closed by accidental pressure from the back of the dentist's hand as he works.

The *Salt valve* has no spring, in order to minimize

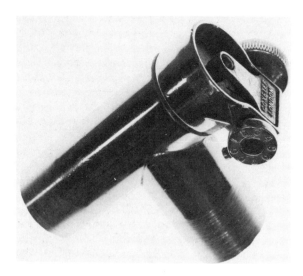

Figure 7.25   The McKesson expiratory valve (Coxeter version).

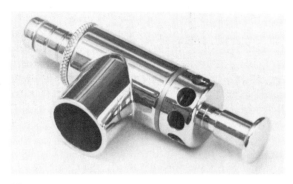

(a)

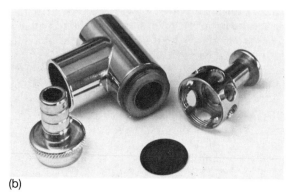

(b)

Figure 7.26   (a) The Salt valve. There is no spring, but the valve may be closed by applying pressure to the plunger at the top. (b) The valve dismantled to show its component parts.

resistance. It has, however, provision for easy and rapid closure for use in controlled ventilation (Fig. 7.26).

In the case of several ventilators there is an expiratory valve whose opening and closing is operated by the force that, intermittently, causes inflation and deflation of the lungs. In some cases the pressure of the gas that inflates the lungs is also applied to a diaphragm or balloon which closes the valve to prevent expiration (Fig. 7.27).

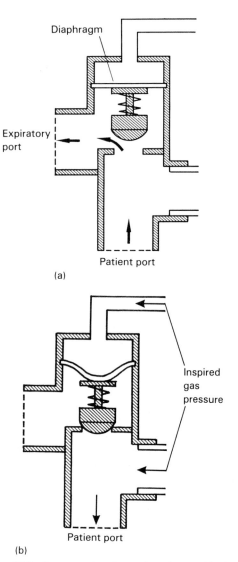

Figure 7.27   A pneumatic valve such as that used in the Bird Mark 7 ventilator (a) during expiration; (b) during inspiration.

Breathing tubes

The tubing connecting the components of a breathing attachment must be of such a diameter as to present a low resistance to gas flow. Its cross section must be uniform, in order to promote laminar flow where possible, and although it should be flexible, kinking should not occur. It should 'drape' easily so that a deep loop may hang between the patient and, say, a circle absorber, since this tends to trap droplets of moisture which could carry infective organisms back to the apparatus.

The most commonly used type of tubing has for a long time been a corrugated hose of rubber or neoprene (Fig. 7.28). The corrugations allow acute angulation of the hose without kinking. Various plastics, both in corrugated and smooth form are now in use and may possibly replace the rubber one in the course of time. The disadvantages of the corrugated rubber or neoprene hose are that its irregular wall must cause turbulence and may harbour dirt and infection, and that it is much heavier than most of the plastic variety. Its advantage is that its ends are more easily stretched, and so will make a better union with other components of different diameters.

There are several standard sizes of corrugated hose (sometimes known as 'elephant tubing'), both ends of which have parallel walls for about 1 in. (2–3 cm). These ends may be fitted with a metal or hard-rubber tapered connector, which fits a component such as an expiratory valve or a bag mount.

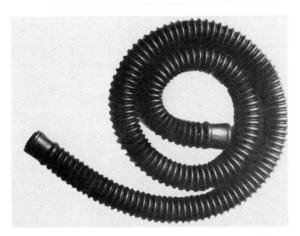

Figure 7.28 A standard length of wide-bore corrugated hose.

(Fig. 7.29). Various sizes of taper have been used for these interconnections in the past, but the British and International Standard 22 mm taper is now virtually universal. Tapered connections are described as having a male half and a female half and in the British Standard these are strictly sequential, i.e. the upstream component end has a male taper and the downstream component end has a female one. (For further details of tapers see p. 170.) There are, however, exceptions to this, such as the expiratory valve shown in Fig. 7.30.

The tapered connectors and other parts of the breathing attachment sometimes present as rather a large mass of 'ironmongery' which can drag on the facepiece or endotracheal tube, particularly when the patient is a child. The dead space may also be greater than necessary. By using the end of the corrugated hose as a simple push-fit much of this trouble can be prevented (as seen in Fig. 7.31).

There is a wide variety of materials for the plastic tubing, some of which may be sterilized by all means including autoclaving. Others, however, will not withstand these temperatures, and are regarded by the manufacturers as disposable. In some centres, however, these are disinfected by pasteurization.

Following the advent of scavenging, some of these plastic hoses are supplied in long coils, the appropriate length of which may be cut off at one of the frequent intervals where the corrugations give way to a shaped connector (Fig. 7.32).

Facepieces

Facepieces are also referred to as face masks. They are designed to fit the patient's face perfectly, without any leaks, and yet to exert the minimum of pressure, which might either depress the jaw and cause respiratory obstruction or cause pressure sores. A snug fit is achieved by anatomical shaping and by the use of an air-filled cuff which has a soft cushioning effect or a flap which takes up the contour of the face. The facepiece (Fig. 7.33) consists of three parts: A, the mount; B, the body; and C, the edge.

The mount may be a 22 mm or other female taper. It is usually constructed of hard rubber but may be plastic or metal. When ordering facepieces it is important to specify the size, as both the new British and other standards still exist.

The body may be of rubber, neoprene or plastic.

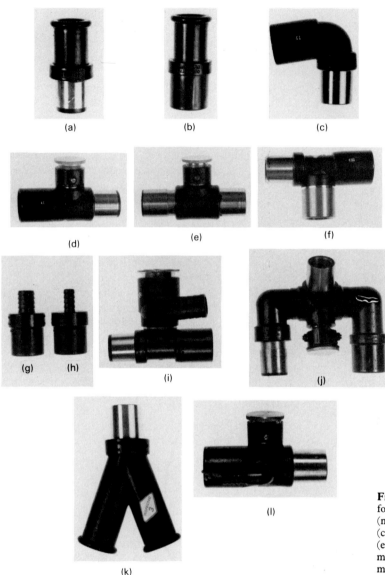

Figure 7.29 Various superlite connections for breathing attachments. (a)Hose adaptor (male). (b) Hose adaptor (female). (c) Facepiece angle mount (elbow). (d) APL (expiratory) valve. (e) APL valve with double male tapers. (f) Bag mount. (g) Catheter mount. (h) Feed mount. (i) Exhaust valve. (j) Swivel Y-piece. (k) Fixed-Y piece. (l) APL (expiratory) valve with side feed.

In some cases a wire stiffener or a wire gauze is incorporated so as to make it malleable in order that its shape might be altered to fit the patient's face. The transparent body of the Ambu and other facepieces is particularly useful in resuscitation. It permits the early detection of vomit.

The edge may be anatomically shaped and fitted with a cuff or a flap. Where there is a possibility of explosive anaesthetic agents being used, the cuff, like the rest of the equipment, must be of antistatic material, but otherwise a soft latex is most satisfactory. There is a small filling tube with a plug to enable the degree of inflation of the cuff to be regulated. It may be blown up by mouth.

It is advisable to stock a variety of types of facepiece since none will fit every type of face well.

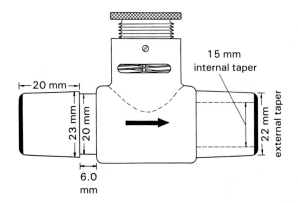

Figure 7.30 An expiratory valve with the British and International Standard 22 mm taper. Note that the proximal taper may be pushed directly into the end of a corrugated hose and the square shoulder will help to secure this joint. The distal 22 mm taper will also accept a 15 mm endotracheal connector.

15 mm internal taper

20 mm

23 mm 20 mm

6.0 mm

22 mm external taper

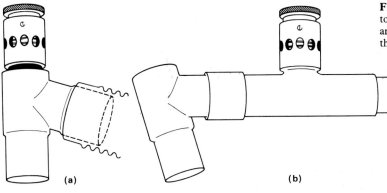

Figure 7.31 (a) A Heidbrink valve attached to an elbow in order to lessen both dead space and the weight of ironmongery hanging on the facepiece, as shown in (b).

(a)   (b)

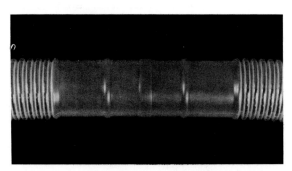

Figure 7.32 Lightweight plastic corrugated hose. There are frequent intervals at which the corrugations give way to a shaped connector, where a long roll of this hose may be cut.

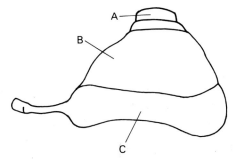

Figure 7.33 The parts of an anaesthetic facepiece. A, the mount; B, the body, C, the edge.

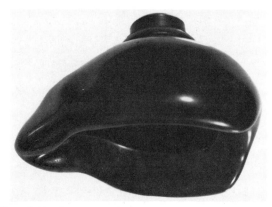

Figure 7.34   The Everseal facepiece (MIE)

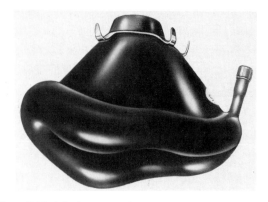

Figure 7.35   The Anatomical facepiece (BOC).

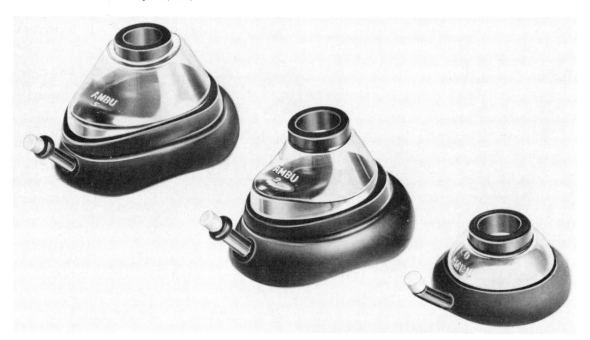

Figure 7.36   Three examples of the Ambu facepiece, which has a transparent body which enables the presence of vomitus to be seen.

Facepieces are made in various sizes and examples of some types are shown in Figs 7.34 to 7.37. Note that the smallest facepiece does not necessarily give the lowest dead space (Fig. 7.38).

Whereas some facepieces withstand the high temperature of autoclaving, others do not. Since these are not easily distinguished, it is advisable to adopt a policy that all facepieces are disinfected by means of low-pressure autoclaving (p. 297), boiling or pasteurizing. Chemical means can also be satis-factory, but there have been cases where agents such as Dettol have been absorbed by the material of the facepiece and later result in injury to the patient's skin.

Endotracheal tubes

There are various situations in which it is not feas-ible to administer anaesthetic gases via a facepiece or

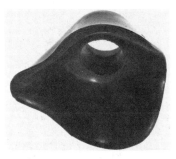

Figure 7.37   The Rendell–Baker paediatric facepiece.

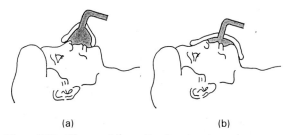

Figure 7.38   The use of the smallest facepiece does not necessarily result in the minimum of dead space. (b) The patient's face may fit into a larger facepiece resulting in less dead space.

nasal inhaler. In these cases an endotracheal, or occasionally a tracheostomy, tube is used. Where positive pressure ventilation is contemplated it is also necessary to make an airtight connection with the trachea.

The majority of endotracheal tubes used are made of red rubber and may be resterilized for repeated use. Armoured tubes made of latex are also used,

but these have the disadvantage that they are expensive and may easily be damaged during autoclaving. Armoured tubes of silicone rubber are less delicate than the latex ones, and their very much greater expense is offset by the fact that they are capable of being used many times provided care is taken in sterilization.

Plain red rubber tubes (Fig. 7.39a) may be used

Table 7.1   Lengths of endotracheal tubes

Internal diameter (mm)		Age (years)	Length (cm)	
Oral	Nasal		Oral	Nasal
2.5	2.5	PREMATURE	10.5	13.0
3.0	3.0		10.5	13.0
3.5	3.5	0–1	11.0	14.0
4.0	4.0		12.0	14.5
4.5	4.5	1–2	13.5	15.0
5.0	5.0	2–4	14.0	16.5
5.5	5.5		14.5	17.0
6.0	6.0	5–12	15.0	17.5
6.5	6.5		16.0	18.5
7.0	7.0	13–16	17.5	19.0
8.0	8.0		18.5	19.5
—	6.0	ADULTS — Small women	—	24.0
—	6.5		—	24.0
7.0	7.0		—	24.0
7.5	7.5		—	25.0
8.0	8.0		23.0	26.0
8.5	—		24.0	—
9.0	—		25.0	—
9.5	—		25.0	—
10.0	—		26.0	—
11.0	—	Large men	26.0	—

A widely used formula for selecting the diameter of an endotracheal tube suitable for children over the age of one year is:

$$\frac{\text{Age in years}}{4} + 4.5 \, mm$$

The exact length to which a new tube should be shortened cannot be categorically specified. In some operations it is necessary to pass the tube further down the trachea than in others. Cuffed tubes are generally trimmed to a centimetre or so longer than plain ones.

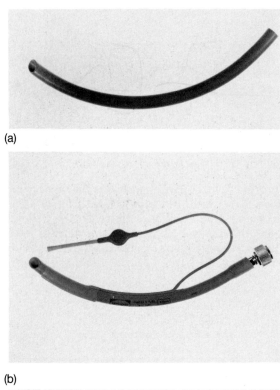

(a)

(b)

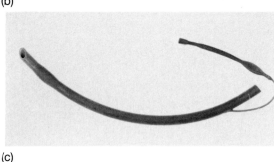

(c)

Figure 7.39 Endotracheal tubes. (a) Plain. (b) Cuffed. (c) Streamlined cuffed nasal.

when the patient is to breathe spontaneously, particularly when passed via the nasal route. Table 7.1 shows the various sizes, with an approximate indication of the age range of patients for whom they are suitable. They are usually supplied longer than necessary and need to be cut to the correct length before use.

Various types of plastic endotracheal tube, some of them disposable, are being increasingly used.

Although some of the earlier ones failed to keep their shape, the modern ones have proved more satisfactory — particularly for long-term cases where they cause less tissue reaction. It must be noted that tubes for nasal intubation need to be longer, and they also have thinner walls, which unfortunately renders them more liable to be obstructed by kinking or compression.

Cuffed red rubber endotracheal tubes (Fig. 7.39b) are usually used for orotracheal intubation only, since the extra external diameter due to the cuff and its pilot tube make it difficult to pass them through the nose without damaging the nasal or nasopharyngeal mucosa, especially on extubation. Cases have been known where epistaxis resulted in considerably greater blood loss than the operation itself! New 'streamlined' cuffed nasal tubes (Fig. 7.39c), which are made of either rubber or plastic, present much less of a problem in this respect.

The small-bore tube leading to the cuff contains a 'pilot' balloon. The inflation of this pilot balloon indicates that the cuff is also inflated. Care must be taken to prevent the accidental kinking of this small tube when the endotracheal tube is being fixed in position with strapping.

The cuff is inflated with air either by a Mitchell's inflator (Fig. 7.40a) or a 10 or 20 ml syringe. An artery forceps is applied to the pilot tube between the syringe and the balloon when the cuff has been inflated just sufficiently to make an airtight fit in the trachea (Fig. 7.40b). Some pilot tubes have a self-sealing valve which prevents air from escaping when the syringe has been removed, in which case the syringe is reinserted to deflate the cuff (Fig. 7.40c).

If these tubes are to be sterilized by autoclaving, care must be taken to completely evacuate the cuff of both air and water, since during sterilization this could expand it to the point of rupture.

Cuffs on tubes should be inflated only just enough to prevent leaks because (1) this limits the pressure on the cilliated columnar epithelium of the trachea, which can cause damage or even necrosis; and (2) if there were over-pressure in the breathing attachment, it would permit leakage around the cuff, thereby (a) allowing excess gases under pressure to escape and (b) giving a warning by the gurgling noise produced.

We must admit that accidents will continue to happen, and over-pressure in breathing attachments is one of them. Any steps that may be taken to minimize the effects of such an event will promote safety.

Red rubber tubes may be sterilized by cold solution or, better, by being pasteurized or autoclaved. In either case, connectors should be removed before treatment. Tubes may be wrapped separately, in which case a transparent packet should be used so that they may be inspected before opening. Alternatively, a day's supply may be kept in a single sterile box or tray. The cuff should be tested before reuse — the technician can do this with all those in the tray or box just before the start of an operating list. When they are packed singly the cuff should be tested before packing.

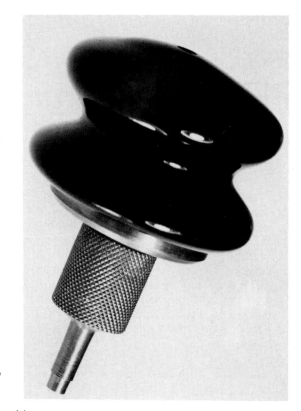

(a)

Figure 7.40 Methods of inflating the cuff. (a) Mitchell's inflator. (b) Syringe and artery forceps. (c) Self-sealing valve, into which a syringe may be re-inserted to deflate the cuff.

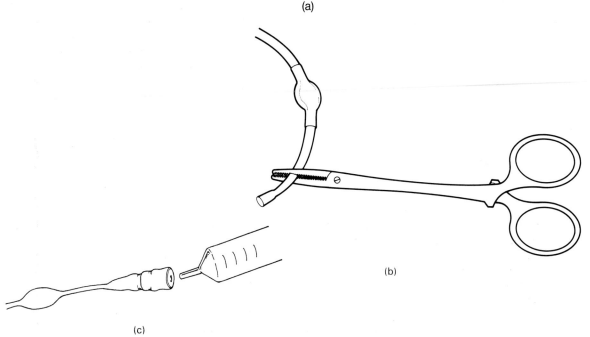

(b)

(c)

The common faults with the use of endotracheal tubes are as follows:

1. A tube may be passed too far down the trachea and enter the right main bronchus. This occurs because the tube selected is too long and it needs shortening.
2. There may be a leak between the cuff and the trachea. This may be either because the cuff has not been sufficiently inflated in the first place, or because it has leaked. The latter may be due to a fault in manufacture, or to over-inflation. The presence of a leak may be demonstrated by immersing the whole tube, pilot and all, in water, inflating the cuff and watching for bubbles. As mentioned above, it is possible to accidentally kink the pilot tube and prevent inflation of the cuff even though the pilot balloon is blown up.

   The cuff may become stretched and baggy after repeated use and autoclaving, and it is possible for it to form a 'diverticulum' which can protrude over the open end of the tube and obstruct it (Fig. 7.41). This is more likely to occur if the tube is withdrawn a little after the cuff has been inflated. For this reason it is a better practice to fix the tube into position before inflating the cuff. With age, the cuff may become wrinkled and prune-like, and this can make extubation difficult.
3. The tube may be obstructed in one or more of

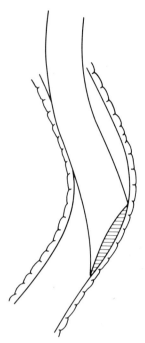

Figure 7.42   If there is marked deviation of the trachea the end of the tube may be obstructed.

several ways. The opening may be occluded if the larynx or trachea is deviated to one side, as seen in Fig. 7.42. This may happen particularly during thyroidectomy, when the gland is being pulled to one side by the surgeon. The 'Murphy eye' (Fig. 7.43) will prevent this hazard. During nasal intubation the tube may be blocked as it harvests a polyp. It may also kink when bent to too small a radius, particularly if soft from frequent use. If it must be acutely bent, an armoured tube or one that is specially shaped should be used (see below). A tube may be compressed by a throat pack that has been inserted too firmly, and it may also be obstructed if

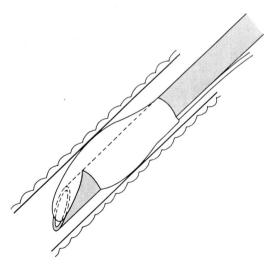

Figure 7.41   A herniation of the cuff which may occlude the distal end of the tube.

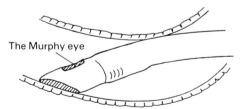

The Murphy eye

Figure 7.43   The distal end of an endotracheal tube with a 'Murphy eye'.

as oesophagoscopy are being performed, or during operations when extreme flexion of the head on the neck is required, as in some neurosurgical procedures.

All sorts of foreign bodies have been found within endotracheal tubes, blocking them, including the tops of ampoules. This emphasizes the fact that tubes, airways, etc. that are to be reused should not be placed in the same 'dirty dish' as discarded syringes, needles, ampoules, etc. A diaphragm of dried mucus or K-Y Jelly has been found blocking a tube, and even if the tube is straightened so that one can look through it to confirm patency, it is almost invisible.

For neurosurgical anaesthesia it may be considered wiser to use an anatomically shaped tube such as the Oxford non-kinking tube (Fig. 7.45) which may be either cuffed or plain. There is a special stylet or 'director' available to assist the insertion of these tubes. Alternatively, armoured tubes may be used. These are made of latex, plastic or red rubber and contain in their wall a spiral of metal wire or tough nylon. The latest models are constructed of silicone rubber and are of considerably superior quality. If they are to withstand repeated use they must be sterilized with care. On autoclaving, the cuff must not be over-distended by steam, and to this end the self-closing valve or the

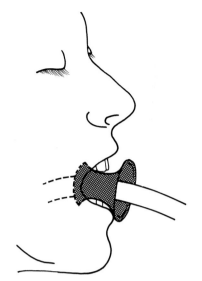

Figure 7.44 The London Hospital airway prop.

the patient is lightly anaesthetized and bites it. This may be prevented either by inserting an airway alongside the tube or by using a 'London Hospital airway prop' (Fig. 7.44).

Endotracheal tubes may be kinked in the mouth or nasopharynx when the patient's neck is flexed, and this is particularly likely when procedures such

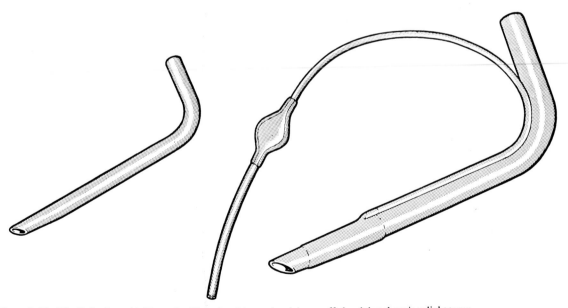

Figure 7.45 The Oxford non-kinking tube. Note that this may be plain or cuffed and that there is a slight taper.

pilot tube should be kept open, if necessary by a dummy syringe (Fig. 7.46). In the resting state they may be either straight or curved. A stylet or 'director' may be needed to introduce them, but care must be taken to avoid injuring the larynx or trachea (see below). Typical armoured tubes are shown in Figs 7.47 and 7.48. They must be handled with care since if the armouring is distorted by handling roughly with forceps, especially while hot, after autoclaving or boiling, there will be a considerable narrowing of the lumen. When an endotracheal connector is

being inserted into an armoured tube it is important to ensure that there is no 'soft spot' between the end of the connector and the start of the spiral reinforcement, since kinking could occur at this point (Fig. 7.49). A little of the unreinforced end of the tube may need trimming off. However, if all the unreinforced end is removed altogether, it is difficult to insert a connector of the appropriate size, since the reinforcement will not stretch to admit it. The use of an unsuitable connector may obstruct the lumen of the tube (Fig. 7.50).

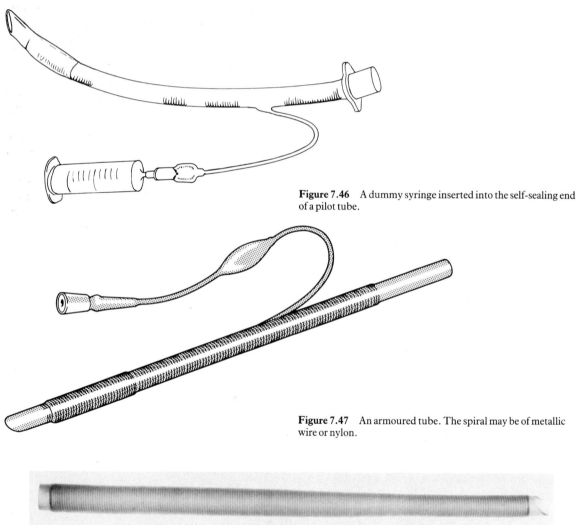

Figure 7.46   A dummy syringe inserted into the self-sealing end of a pilot tube.

Figure 7.47   An armoured tube. The spiral may be of metallic wire or nylon.

Figure 7.48   The Enderby paediatric armoured tube.

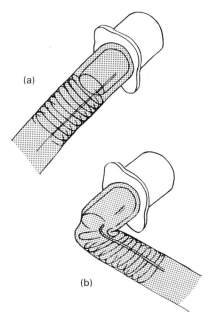

(a)

(b)

Figure 7.49 Obstruction at the 'soft spot' between the connector and the spiral of an armoured tube. (a) With the connector placed correctly. (b) With incorrect placement leaving an unarmoured segment of tube.

With any endotracheal tube it is important that it is cut to the correct length so that the connector is as close as possible to the patient's mouth. If there is an excess of tube sticking out of the mouth, as in Fig. 7.51a, kinking may easily occur. A tube may also be obstructed by being twisted in its long axis if the position of the catheter mount is altered.

Tubes for children, infants and neonates require special consideration. The thickness of the wall is important. Since it must be adequate to prevent kinking, it represents a considerable proportion of the cross-sectional area of a small tube. (It will be seen below that there may also be a similar problem in the case of connectors.) The resistance of such a narrow tube may be decreased by tapering it (Fig. 7.48), the narrow end being just small enough to enter the larynx, but the larger end leading to a less resistive connector. It is true that a tapered tube has a slightly larger dead space, but the disadvantage of this is more than offset by the decrease in resistance.

ENDOTRACHEAL TUBES FOR SPECIAL PURPOSES

Many 'special' tubes have been devised — they are

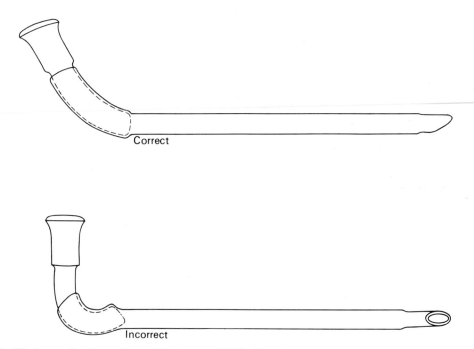

Correct

Incorrect

Figure 7.50 The lumen of a tube may be partially obstructed if a Magill nasal connector has been wrongly fitted.

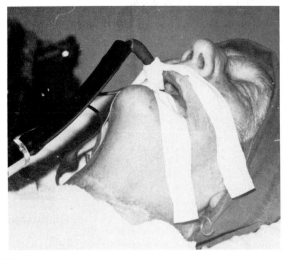

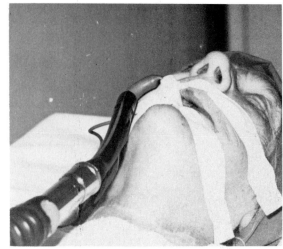

(a)

Figure 7.51 (a) Kinking of an endotracheal tube outside the mouth due to its being too long. (b) Kinking of an endotracheal tube within the mouth which may develop slowly during anaesthesia owing to its becoming warmer and softer, all having seemed to have been well at induction.

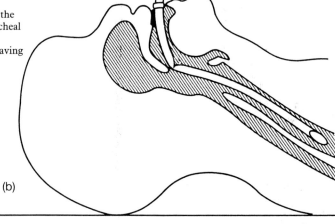

(b)

too numerous to all be described here. A few examples are shown in Figs. 7.52–7.55.

The Carden tube has been developed in order to facilitate microsurgery of the larynx. As will be seen in Fig. 7.52 the part occupying the larynx during surgery is very slender, and can be kept out of the way of the surgeon's manipulations. The tracheal portion has a cuff which when inflated prevents aspiration of blood or debris and may also make artificial ventilation feasible. The tube may be inserted either by grasping it with the Magill's endotracheal forceps, or as follows:

A Carden tube and a plain nasal tube are threaded in series onto a stylet (Fig. 7.53). This assembly is then introduced through the larynx so that the Carden tube and a centimetre or so of the nasal tube pass into the trachea. The stylet is then withdrawn and until all is ready for the laryngoscopy the anaesthetic is maintained through the plain tube. When the laryngoscopy is to be performed the cuff on the Carden tube is inflated and the plain nasal tube is removed. The breathing attachment is then discarded and the anaesthetic gases are delivered directly to the Carden tube through a feed mount. The expired gases escape via the lumen of the Carden tube.

Figure 7.54 shows the Jackson Rees paediatric tube which is especially useful for cases of prolonged intubation, and which incorporates its own T-piece and suction facility.

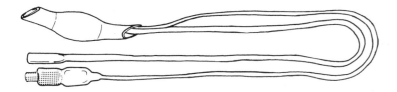

Figure 7.52   A Carden tube.

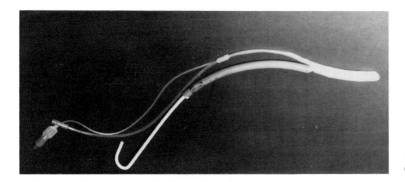

Figure 7.53   A method of inserting the Carden tube.

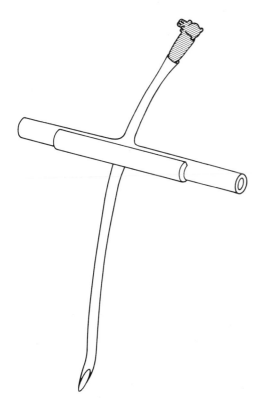

Figure 7.54   The Jackson Rees paediatric T-tube. Note the provision for suction.

There are several special tubes for endobronchial anaesthesia during lung surgery. Examples of these are shown in Fig. 7.55. These enable the anaesthetist to administer the anaesthetic via one lung, the other being 'blocked'. In some cases, suction tubes are also incorporated. Detailed description of these specialized tubes can be obtained from the manufacturers.

There are also many varieties of tracheostomy tube; most of these connect with a catheter mount with a 15 mm female taper. Various swivelling adaptors, some with facilities for suction, are available. Two examples of tubes are shown in Fig. 7.56.

The advantages and disadvantages of the use of various materials for endotracheal tubes are set out in Table 7.2.

Aids to difficult intubation

There are occasions when intubation by the nasal or oral route may be difficult, due to anatomical abnormalities in the patient, or other factors.

In some of these situations intubation may by assisted by prior insertion of a stylet of gum elastic, plastic or wire, into the tube so as to maintain it in a particular shape. This is particularly useful for tubes of silicone rubber, etc., which may be very floppy. When the tube has been inserted into the larynx, the stylet is withdrawn.

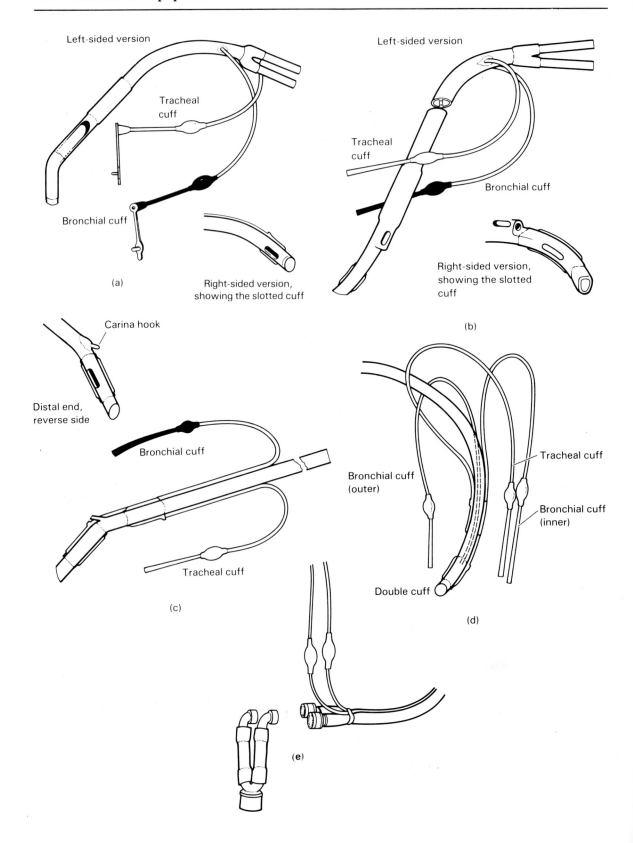

Left-sided version

Tracheal cuff

Bronchial cuff

(a)

Right-sided version, showing the slotted cuff

Left-sided version

Tracheal cuff

Bronchial cuff

Right-sided version, showing the slotted cuff

(b)

Carina hook

Distal end, reverse side

Bronchial cuff

Tracheal cuff

(c)

Bronchial cuff (outer)

Tracheal cuff

Bronchial cuff (inner)

Double cuff

(d)

(e)

	Red rubber	Plastic	Latex	Silicone rubber
Plain oral	Satisfactory and relatively inexpensive · With careful handling may be used many times. Eventually they soften or perish. Not suitable for prolonged use in intensive care	Single use only; therefore expensive. Do not perish like rubber but may harden on storage and become brittle · Hard and therefore traumatic to nasopharyngeal mucosa. Cuff wrinkled during extubation	Particularly useful in intensive care · Perish easily and offer no advantages over red rubber	Floppy but otherwise satisfactory. No real advantage over red rubber for anaesthesia or plastic for intensive care to justify extra expense
Cuffed oral				
Plain nasal				
Cuffed nasal	In some types the cuff becomes wrinkled			
Double lumen	May be found to be perished on prolonged storage	Disposable; therefore expensive. Tendency for bronchial cuff to burst	Not generally available	Not generally available
Armoured	Not generally available	Not generally available	Satisfactory but perish on storage. Cheaper than silicone rubber	Expensive but ideal for operations such as cataracts and thyroids. Extra-long tubes available
Nasopharyngeal airway	Satisfactory	Some have too small a flange	Not generally available	Expensive but atraumatic and does not perish

Table 7.2   A 'best-buy' for endotracheal tubes

Figure 7.55   Various endobronchial tubes. (a) Robertshaw left-sided double-lumen tube. The insert shows the right-sided version, which has a slotted cuff to connect with the right upper lobe bronchus. Note that in each case there are two cuffs, one for the trachea and the other for the bronchus. (b) Brice-Smith double-lumen tube. Note the slot for the right upper lobe bronchus on the right-sided version, shown in the insert. (c) Gordon–Green tube. Note the slot for the right upper lobe bronchus and the hook which is engaged with the carina. (d) Brompton left-sided triple-cuffed tube. If the outer bronchial cuff is damaged during surgery, the inner one may be inflated. (e) Catheter mount for a double-lumen tube. Note that either side may be blocked by a robust pair of artery forceps, if required.

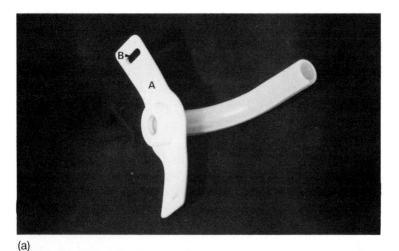

(a)

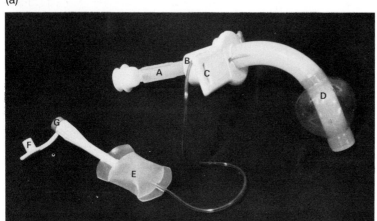

(b)

Figure 7.56   (a) A plain tracheostomy tube (which is supplied by Portex in a variety of sizes). Note that there is a flange A with slots B, to which the securing tape may be tied. Another version has a 15mm male taper for connection to a condenser/humidifier filter. (b) The Portex siliconized PVC cuffed tracheostomy tube with a replaceable internal cannula A, which may be changed with minimal disturbance to the patient. The cuff inflating tube has a self-sealing inlet, but there is also a bung to ensure that the cuff does not accidentally deflate before it is required. This tracheostomy tube has a 15mm male taper which fits the Interantional 15 catheter mount, even when the internal catheter is in place, provided that it is correctly installed. B, 15mm OD connector; C, flange with slot for tape; D, cuff; E, pilot balloon; F, bung; G, one-way valve.

This procedure is not without dangers, especially with wire stylets, which may protrude from the end of the tube and injure, or even perforate, the trachea.

There are plastic stylets available of extra length, such as the so-called 'endotracheal introducer' manufactured by Eschmann (Fig. 7.57). This is of such a length that it may first be passed on its own and then, when the tip has passed through the larynx, there remains outside the mouth a sufficient length on which the tube may be threaded and railroaded through the larynx into the trachea.

In recent years a fibre-optic endoscope (see Chapter 22) has been used in place of a stylet. In skilled hands this may be very useful, but in most instances anaesthetists who are faced with difficult intu-bations will not have familiarized themselves with this type of equipment. One prudent salesman advised his would-be customers that they should practice on at least fifty easy intubations by this means before depending on it in times of difficulty.

A more recently used aid to intubation consists of a disposable electric torch, which has a small bulb at the end of a long, narrow, flexible limb. The endo-tracheal tube is threaded upon this and then in-serted. The light from the bulb may be seen through the skin of the neck and serve as a guide when passing it into the larynx (Fig. 7.58).

There is a variety of other stylets, hooks, etc. designed to facilitate intubation. In the author's view, however, it is prudent to avoid dependence on these potentially dangerous devices, and if assist-

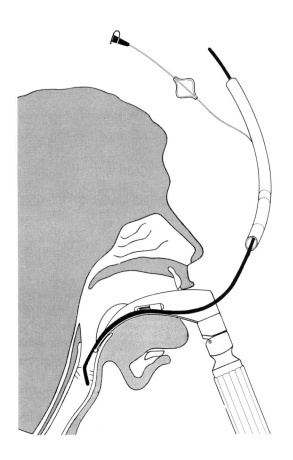

Figure 7.57   The Eschmann endotracheal introducer.

ance is required it is safer to grasp the tube with Magill's endotracheal forceps.

Endotracheal connectors

Endotracheal connectors join the endotracheal tube to the catheter mount. Various types are shown in Figs. 7.59–7.68. Their particular features are:

1. The two-part design of the connectors, which permits rapid disconnection and reconnection.
2. The provision for suction.
3. The incorporation of a special angle, as, for example, for nasal tubes.

When delivered from the suppliers, connectors frequently have a length of wire threaded through them, as seen in Fig. 7.60. This is to demonstrate that the lumen is patent and was introduced following an accident in which one was found to be blocked by a metal diaphragm as a result of faulty manufacture. Obstruction may also result from the improper fitting of a nasal connector, as may be seen in Fig. 7.50. Another cause of obstruction is the use of an unsuitable bung in a Magill suction connector (Fig. 7.69).

In selecting a connector, thought should be given to using one with an adequate internal diameter, which should be no less than that of the endotracheal tube. Any abrupt reduction of bore will result in resistance and this is rendered even greater by turbulence.

Turbulence may also be caused by an acute bend, as in the Rowbotham connector (Fig. 7.60), but is considerably reduced in the Rink connector (Fig. 7.65). The disadvantage of the latter is either that it protrudes a long way from the patient's mouth and the pressure of towels, etc., covering it may cause kinking of the tube, or that the point of attachment of the tube is well within the mouth and accidental disconnection here would be unobserved. It is also difficult to fix the tube and connector securely with adhesive plaster. These dangers are minimized with the Rowbotham connector and it is difficult to recall any harm resulting from turbulence due to the acute bend.

In paediatric anaesthesia connectors of small size are used. When choosing these, one should be careful to avoid those with very thick walls, since their lumen is likely to be smaller than the tubes into which they can be inserted (Fig. 7.70).

If the need for bronchial suction is envisaged, the most convenient type of connector is either one such as the Cobb or Magill suction connector, or a two-piece connector such as the Nosworthy or the Knight's paediatric connector, which may easily be disconnected and reconnected (Figs 7.62 and 7.63).

Metal endotracheal connectors may be autoclaved or cold sterilized. When fitting them to a tube they will be found to slip in very much more easily if they are lubricated by dipping them in ethanol (surgical spirit).

The catheter mount

The term 'catheter mount' does not appear in BS 6015 (ISO 4135), which is the official glossary of terms used in anaesthesiology. Its modern

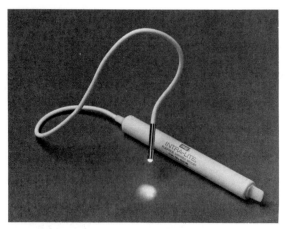

Figure 7.58   A torch on which endotracheal tubes may be 'railroaded'.

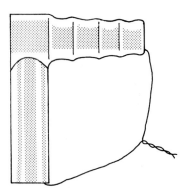

Figure 7.60   Rowbotham connector. Note that there is a piece of wire threaded through this connector when supplied, to demonstrate that the lumen is patent.

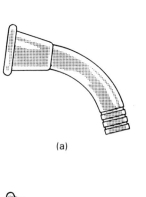

(a)

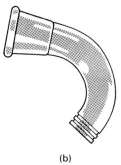

(b)

Figure 7.59   Magill connectors. (a) Oral (b) Nasal.

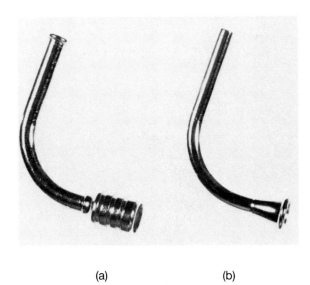

(a)   (b)

Figure 7.61   (a) The Worcester and (b) the Doughty connector.

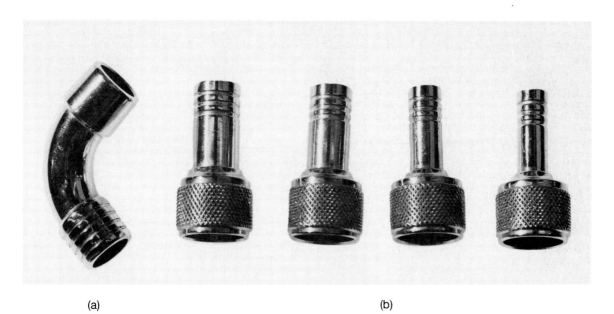

(a)   (b)

Figure 7.62   Nosworthy connectors. (a) To attach to the catheter mount. (b) To be inserted in the endotracheal tube.

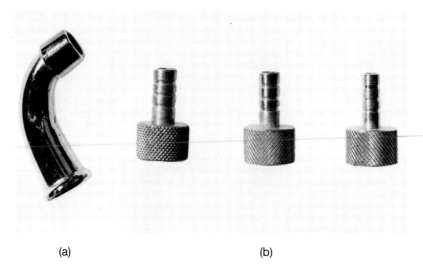

(a)   (b)

Figure 7.63   Knight's paediatric connectors. (a) To attach to the catheter mount. (b) To be inserted in the endotracheal tube.

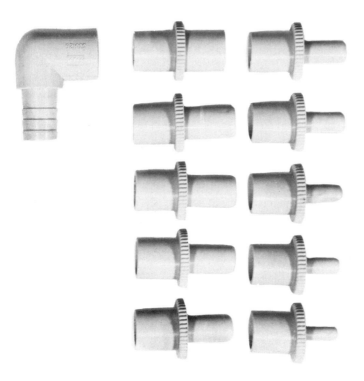

Figure 7.64   'International 15' connectors.

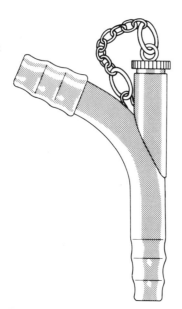

Figure 7.65   Rink connector.

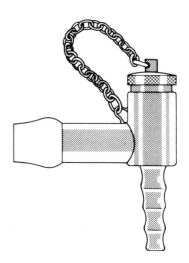

Figure 7.66   The Cobb suction connector.

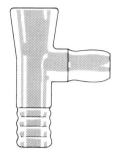

Figure 7.67   The Magill suction connector. Note that a cork is required to occlude the suction limb.

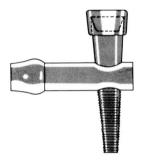

Figure 7.68   The Cardiff paediatric suction connector.

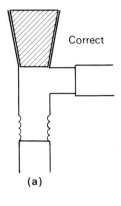

Correct

(a)

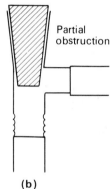

Partial obstruction

(b)

Figure 7.69   The lumen of a Magill suction connector may be obstructed by the use of an inappropriate bung. (a) Correct (b) Too long a cork has been used.

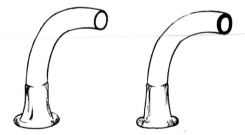

Figure 7.70   Two Magill oral connectors of the same size, but supplied by different manufacturers. Note that due to the thickness of the wall in one of them, the lumen is considerably smaller than that of the other.

equivalent 'tracheal tube adaptor' will probably be slow to replace the older and more familiar term, as will the term 'tracheal tube' rather than the older 'endotracheal tube'. Some explanation of these terms would perhaps be apt.

Before the introduction of the Boyle's machine with the Magill breathing attachment, the mixed gases, with added vapour of volatile agents, were fed via a narrow-bore tube to the patient, with no reservoir bag or expiratory valve in the positions that we now know them. The end of the tube could be attached to a Boyle-Davis gag, a modified open-drop mask such as the Tyrrell, a bag on a Hewitt's stopcock or to a catheter which was passed through the larynx into the trachea. The gases and/or vapours were blown constantly down the catheter and were exhausted to the atmosphere by passing out through the trachea but outside the catheter. Spontaneous ventilation became very shallow, respiratory exchange being mainly by diffusion. A thoracotomy was possible under these conditions. This technique was known as intratracheal insufflation. Thus when the catheter was replaced by a wider bore tube through which the patient could breathe (or be ventilated) in both directions, this was called endotracheal intubation.

Modern techniques with high-frequency jetting seem to hark back to the older technique and the author would therefore have preferred to retain the older terms, 'catheter mount' and 'endotracheal'.

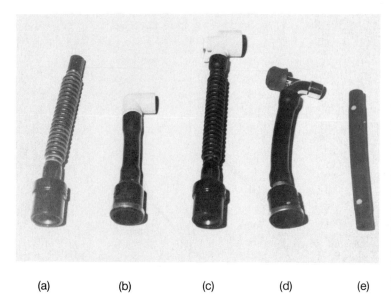

(a)   (b)   (c)   (d)   (e)

Figure 7.71 Catheter mounts (endotracheal adaptors). (a) For use with Magill, Rowbotham or similar connectors. (b) For use with International 15 connectors. (c) For use with International 15 connectors, with a facility for suction. (d) For use with Nosworthy connectors. This fitting has a side branch for suction, which is closed by a rubber bung. (e) With spiral reinforcement to prevent kinking. Note that this mount should not be shortened by cutting, since the part that is reinforced cannot be distended to accommodate the nozzle of a 22 mm tapered fitting catheter mount or a endotracheal connector. N.B. The corrugated tubes also resist kinking when flexed.

The catheter mount acts not only as an adaptor between the breathing attachment and the tracheal tube (or tracheostomy tube), but also to minimize the transmission of accidental movements of the breathing attachment to the endotracheal tube. Repeated movements of the tube within the trachea are undesirable since they can cause injury to the tracheal mucosa. Various types of catheter mount are shown in Fig. 7.71.

Tapered connections

The dimensions of various tapered connections are given on p. 170. Those used by McKesson, MIE and the original 23 mm BOC (cage mount) have to a large extent been replaced by the British and International Standard 22 mm taper. Unlike some of the earlier systems, in the British Standard all the tapers are directed in the same way — i.e. a male taper upstream and a female one downstream. This 'sequential' arrangement was adopted to promote safety — one point being that it should minimize the chance of any one component of the breathing attachment being accidentally omitted. Unfortunately it is not successful in the latter respect.

A further step has been the introduction of the 15 mm taper for items such as endotracheal and tracheostomy connectors. Indeed, the downstream end of the APL (expiratory) valve may have both a 22 mm male and a 15 mm female taper (see Fig. 7.30).

Many accidents have occurred as a result of the accidental and unobserved disconnection of tappered joints, and several systems aimed at preventing this have been described. One consists of a wire clip and another of a screw-threaded cap which engages with a similar thread on the opposite component (Fig. 7.72).

The application of either of these depends on the vigilance of the anaesthetist — but the vigilant anaesthetist will make his connections with care, not only by inserting the taper but also by giving the joint a slight twist to ensure a firm union. He will also observe, with minimal delay, any disconnection. As stated in Chapter 14, if it can be avoided, no part of the breathing attachment should be covered with drapes, as this could hide such a disconnection.

Modifications of Breathing Systems and their Components

It has long been appreciated that part of the energy required to propel the gases along the passages of a

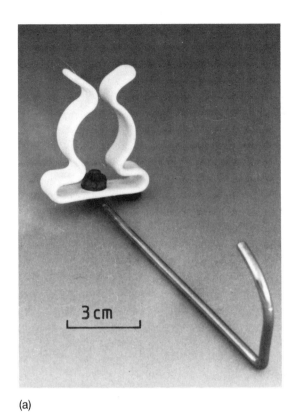

(a)

Figure 7.72   (a) Antidisconnection clip devised by Dr Condon. The hook is placed between the limbs of the 'Y'-piece and the clip attached to the catheter mount. (b) Penlon Safelock tapered connector. An O-ring which retains the nut does not contribute towards the gas tight seal.

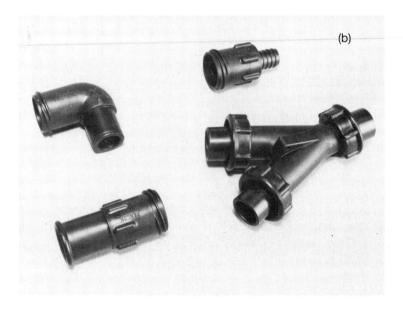

(b)

breathing system must be derived from the patient's respiratory effort. The latter, being prejudiced by the depressant effects of narcosis, becomes inefficient and any form of resistance would further impair respiratory function. On the other hand, any form of assistance to flow or of reduction of resistance would be beneficial. To this end various 'circulators' have been devised and expiratory valves that are not spring loaded have been advocated. Some of these are described below.

Breathing systems with assisted circulation

These attempt to reduce the problems of resistance to flow, the inertia of gases, and dead space.

REVELL'S CIRCULATOR

A small fan helps to assist the circulation of gases in a closed system. It will be noted that this is used in conjunction with a 'chimney' which is part of the facepiece mount or catheter mount. As is shown in Fig. 7.73, this causes a continual flow of fresh gases into the facepiece, thereby reducing the effects of dead space. The Revell's circulator may be incorporated in a circle system and thereby help to overcome the friction of the valves and other parts of the system. The design features are of particular benefit

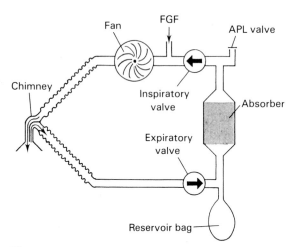

Figure 7.73   The Revell's circulator and chimney. Driven by compressed air or other gas, a fan induces the circulation of anaesthetic gases within a circle breathing system. The 'chimney' directs a flow of fresh gases into the facepiece, thus minimizing the effective dead space. FGF = fresh gas flow. APL valve = adjustable pressure limiting valve.

in paediatric anaesthesia, and enable a circle system designed for adults to be used for small children.

NEFF'S CIRCULATOR

In 1968 a venturi circulator was described by Neff, Simpson, Burke and Thompson. This makes use of the power that is latent in the fresh gas flow at regulated pressure entering the breathing attachment from the back bar (Fig. 7.74).

These circulators enabled the exploitation of the advantages of the circle system, such as the economy in fresh gas flow and the retention of water vapour and heat, but without the disadvantages of resistance, dead space and the inertia of gases in a large apparatus volume.

Further developments

When scavenging systems were devised, this led to the development of the various Hafnia breathing systems (Fig. 7.75). The common feature of these is that there are no valves but simply one port delivering the fresh gas flow and another through which excess gases are removed by the scavenging system, the flow rate of the latter being adjusted so that the reservoir bag is never fully distended, nor completely emptied. One method of controlling the rate at which excess gases are extracted is the use of the ejector flowmeter. In this device a jet of oxygen or compressed air, or any other gas, utilizes the venturi effect to draw the gases through a flowmeter. The rate of extraction may be controlled by a flow control valve so that it balances the combined inflow of the fresh gases (Fig. 7.76).

A more recent embodiment of all these features is to be seen in the system described by Jorgensen (Fig. 7.77), in which the circulation of gases is assisted by a venturi, and the excess gases are removed by an ejector flowmeter. It will be seen that this is a circle closed system with spill which enables the fresh gas inflow to be reduced to well below the minute volume of the patient. This affords economy of gases and also a reduction of the total volume of gases to be scavenged. During the first few minutes of anaesthesia, with a high fresh gas flow, the control may be turned to 'D', whereupon the system will behave as a Mapleson-D system.

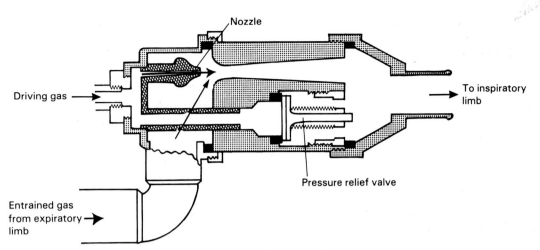

Figure 7.74 Neff's circulator, which is a venturi powered by the fresh gas inflow.

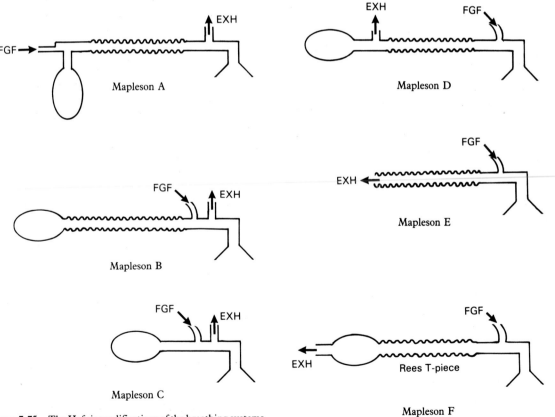

Figure 7.75 The Hafnia modifications of the breathing systems described by Mapleson. Note that in each case the expiratory valve is replaced by a connection to the scavenging system. FGF = fresh gas flow. EXH = exhaust to scavenging system.

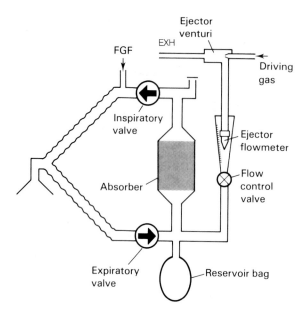

Figure 7.76   The principle of the ejector flowmeter. By means of a flow control valve, the total volume of gases drawn from the breathing system and delivered to the scavenging system is adjusted so as to be equal to the fresh gas flow (FGF) rate.

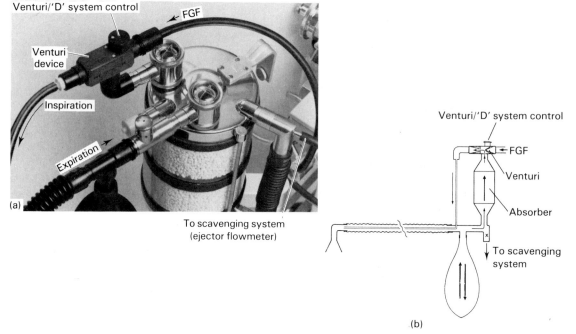

Figure 7.77   (a) Jorgensen's venturi circulator. (b) Diagrammatical representation of its use with a Mapleson-D coaxial breathing system. Note that the control knob maybe turned to 'D' during induction and the first few minutes of the maintenance of anaesthesia, while a high fresh gas flow (FGF) rate is used.

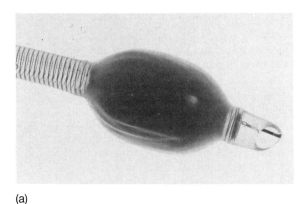

(a)

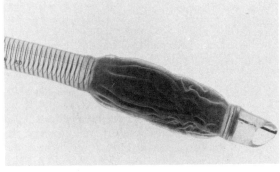

(b)

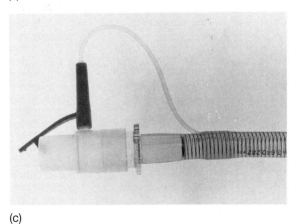

(c)

Figure 7.78   The Fome cuf endotracheal tube. (a) the cuff is filled with foam rubber, which in the resting state keeps it distended. (b) At intubation, a vacuum is applied by means of a syringe to collapse the cuff against the elastic recoil of the foam rubber. When the syringe is removed, the foam expands so that the cuff occupies the whole of the lumen of the trachea. (c) The pilot tube from the cuff is then connected to a side branch of the endotracheal tube connector. This maintains the pressure within the cuff at the same level as that in the airway.

A new concept in cuffs

The risk of damage to the tracheal mucosa caused by over-inflation of the cuff of an endotracheal tube is well known. Recently, however, it has been pointed out that if it is initially inflated with air, and then the patient breathes or is ventilated with a mixture containing nitrous oxide, the latter diffuses into the cuff, thereby increasing the pressure within it. During operations of long duration it is therefore prudent to check the pressure within the cuff from time to time.

The Fome cuf (Fig. 7.78) has recently been developed in order to avoid the risk of overpressure. When in situ, the inflating tube is open to the atmosphere, the cuff being inflated by inclusion within it of a specially shaped piece of foam rubber. When inserting or withdrawing the tube, the cuff is collapsed by applying a vacuum with a syringe to the pilot port. Tracheostomy tubes with the same type of cuff are also available.

Tapered Connections

The British and International Standards provide for a sequential mounting of the fittings in adult breathing systems in such a way that the male taper is always upstream and the female downstream. This necessitates the provision of various adaptors, for example at each end of the corrugated hose. The result is rather an excess of heavy ironmongery, the weight of which can result in kinking of the endotracheal tube or displacement of the facepiece. Hard rubber connectors are lighter, but they tend to fall apart and would be better discarded. They are not a satisfactory substitute for metal connectors, which however, may be distorted by being dropped on the floor or may stick together by the phenomenon of cold welding which occurs particularly with aluminium alloys. Attempts at preventing the latter by coating the surfaces have proved unsatisfactory since the coating can flake off and could be inhaled by the patient. The recently developed fitting known as Superlite is made of plastic with a stainless steel lining on the bearing surfaces; it certainly seems to be an improvement since it is not prone to the defects mentioned above.

However, it would seem that it is simpler to push the corrugated hose over the end of the component concerned, as may be done, for example, in the case of the expiratory valve with two male tapers shown in Figure 7.30.

The sequential arrangement under the 'New British Standard' was intended to prevent accidents arising from misconnections. However, it does not prevent the accidental omission of components such as the reservoir bag or the expiratory valve.

Details of the various tapers are shown in Table 7.3.

Table 7.3   Details of various types of tapered connections

Name or nominal diameter	M → F = male upstream F → M = female upstream	Maximum diameter of spigot or socket (mm)	Purpose	Angle of taper
15 mm	F → M	15.47	Endotracheal connectors Paediatric breathing systems	1 in 40
22 mm British and ISO Standard	M → F	22.37	Adult breathing systems Paediatric facepieces Vaporizers in breathing system	1 in 40
Cagemount 23 mm	F → M	23.75	Back bar fittings including high-resistance vaporizers	1 in 36
30 mm	M → F	30.9	Scavenging	1 in 20
McKesson M + IE	M → F M → F	19.75	McKesson fittings MIE back bar	— —
Nosworthy connectors	M → F	15.4	Endotracheal connectors	—
Knight's connectors	M → F	9.7	Paediatric endotracheal connectors	—

The Boyle's machine, the components of which have been described in previous chapters, is known as a *continuous* flow machine. This means that when the fine-adjustment valves have been set, the various gases flow at a regular, continuous rate to the breathing attachment. The inspiratory effort to the patient, as he inhales, may vary the amount of mixed gases drawn from the reservoir bag, but the fresh gas flow rate remains constant until readjusted by the anaesthetist.

In a *demand* flow apparatus the gases flow only in response to the patient's respiratory effort. Figure 8.1 shows the basic principles upon which such a system operates. In order to fill the reservoir bag R, the gases pass through the valve V_1. As R becomes progressively distended, the plate P is deflected; this operates V_1, which is eventually closed, whereupon the supply of gases ceases. Under static conditions the weight of the disc D in the valve V_2 (assisted by a spring, the tension of which is set in the factory) is just sufficient to prevent gases escaping from R. However, when the patient inhales, V_2 is drawn

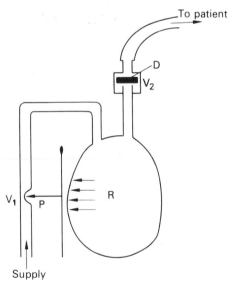

Figure 8.1 Basic principles of demand flow apparatus. The supply gases pass through the valve V_1 and enter the reservoir bag R. The outlet of R is closed by the gravity valve V_2. As R distends it pushes the plate P sideways and this by lever action closes V_1. No more gases enter R and it remains in the filled (ready) position. The weight of the disc D in V_2 is just sufficient to prevent gases flowing to the patient until he makes an inspiratory effort. The latter produces a subatmospheric pressure above D just sufficient to raise it and the gases flow to the patient on demand.

open and the gases flow from R to the patient. When this happens R partially empties, P returns towards its former position and V_1 reopens to admit more gases, refilling R. This is the principle used in the original Minnitt's analgesia apparatus (Fig. 8.2), which is now obsolete. However, Minnitt's apparatus is of considerable historical interest, since it was the first apparatus devised for the self-administration of nitrous oxide and air analgesia during labour.

If we add to the demand flow apparatus a means of applying variable counter-pressure to P, e.g. a screw T and spring S (Fig. 8.3), a greater pressure has to be built up in R in order to close V_1. This pressure is too great to be contained by the weight of D, which is therefore lifted and gases flow from R even when they are not demanded by the patient. Of course, when the patient inhales there is an even greater flow of gases. The 'intermittent' flow machine has now been converted into one which gives an uninterrupted but *varying* flow of gases. The flow rate is not indicated, and the only calibration that is possible is that of the pressure against which the gases are able to flow, this being dependent on the force with which S acts on P. Even when this 'pressure setting' is constant, the flow rate varies with the demand from the patient. This principle is used in the McKesson anaesthetic machine.

The McKesson machine (Fig. 8.4)

Nitrous oxide and oxygen are delivered to their respective reservoirs at a pressure of 60 lb/in^2 ($\sim$ 4 bar)

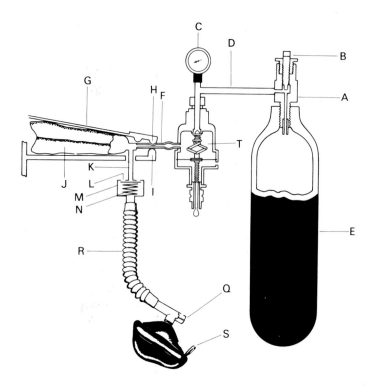

Figure 8.2   The Minnitt nitrous oxide and air analgesia apparatus. A, cylinder valve block; B, valve spindle; C, contents gauge; D, delivery pipe; E, cylinder; F, rubber tube; G, pressure plate; H, I, cut-off valve; J, reservoir; K, delivery tube; L, air inlet; M, valve disc; N, valve spring; Q, expiratory valve; R, wide-bore hose; S, facepiece. In this case the valve spring opposes gravity and is accurately adjusted at the factory to give exactly the correct opening pressure.

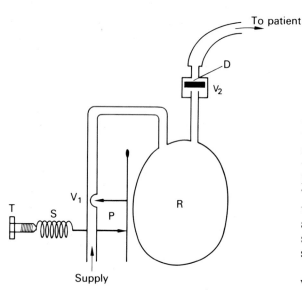

Figure 8.3   This is a similar arrangement to that shown in Fig. 8.1, except that a spring S and screw T are added. The pressure exerted on the plate P by S prevents the reservoir bag R from pushing P sufficiently to close valve V_1. The pressure in R therefore rises enough to overcome the weight of the disc D and gases flow without demand.

either from the pipeline or from cylinders via 60 lb/in² regulators. For each gas there is a pressure gauge which is not as a rule calibrated in units of pressure, but shows a segment of the scale marked 'operating range' to indicate that the pressure is sufficiently close to 60 lb/in² to ensure accuracy of the mixing mechanism. Each gas passes to the appropriate reservoir via a cut-off valve V. This valve is closed by the pivoted lever L, when the latter is pushed by the fully distended reservoir. This cuts off the gas flow. When gas is drawn from the reservoir, L returns towards its former position allowing V to reopen. Up to this point the McKesson resembles the Minnitt's machine, already described.

The outlets of the two reservoirs lead through variable ports to the mixing chamber M. The gravity valve is just heavy enough to prevent the flow of gases during stand-by conditions ('0' on the dial). When the patient inhales, the gravity valve is lifted and the mixed gases pass to the breathing system.

The mixing chamber consists of a drum that

rotates within a cylinder, both being drilled with corresponding ports. By rotating the drum, the relative degree of opening of the ports may be varied, so determining the proportions of the two gases delivered to the outlet. The dial on the mixing chamber is calibrated in percentage of oxygen in the mixture, and there is a fine-adjustment knob calibrated from 0 to 50, which makes two complete revolutions between the positions for pure oxygen and pure nitrous oxide. So, for example, if the latter reads 15, the mixture may contain either 15 or 65% oxygen and reference to the main mixing valve dial will determine which is the case.

Under the conditions so far described, the McKesson delivers gases only when demanded, and it is therefore called a *demand flow* or *intermittent flow* machine. However, it can be made to deliver a continuous flow as follows. The pressure dial, when rotated, actuates a balanced mechanism that presses equally on the oxygen and nitrous oxide levers, pushing them against the reservoirs. This prevents the valves from closing until a higher pressure is reached in the reservoirs. This increase in pressure is sufficient to open the gravity valve, producing a flow of mixed gases even when not demanded by the patient. The pressure control, which is calibrated in mmHg, indicates the pressure at which the gases flow (or alternatively the back pressure required to stop gas flow). With the dial set at '0', flow is on demand only, and when at 'OFF', there is no flow under any circumstances.

There is an oxygen flush control which delivers oxygen directly to the mixing chamber above the gravity valve, so that the latter is closed and the flow of nitrous oxide is stopped when it is operated.

Originally the McKesson was fitted with a rebreathing bellows, the volume and compliance of which could be varied (Fig. 8.4c). Later this was replaced by a simple bag — but in present day models this too has been omitted for reasons that will be explained below — and the connection to it blanked off by a plate and gasket. In Great Britain, at least, there are many of these old Nargraf heads still in existence, though kept with the bellows closed and out of use. Since the latter are made of rubber and prone to perish, the risk of a leak occurring at this point should be prevented by the removal of the Nargraf head, which should be replaced by the blanking plate referred to above.

A vaporizer may be fitted to the outlet of the McKesson. This may be one that is appropriate for halothane, but the older model had as a fixture a vaporizer that was intended for diethyl ether, and if this were used for halothane, it would give a lethally high concentration.

THE PRACTICAL USE OF THE McKESSON
BREATHING SYSTEMS

With demand flow, as seen in Fig. 8.5a, there is no rebreathing bag (if one is fitted it is turned off or the bellows closed). A vaporizer may be included but there is no reservoir bag. There is an expiratory valve at the patient end of the corrugated hose.

The disadvantage of this system is that it depends on a slight subatmospheric pressure in the breathing attachment to produce a supply of gases. If the facepiece is not a perfect fit, air is drawn in and dilutes the gases.

With varying flow and intentional rebreathing, as seen in Fig. 8.5b and c, the pressure control is turned sufficiently to produce a low fresh gas flow rate — less than the patient's minute volume. As rebreathing into the bellows occurs the gases pass backwards and forwards through the vaporizer. This might have been deemed satisfactory when ether was employed, but now that halothane is used it is inadvisable, since a dangerously high vapour concentration would result, owing to the gases passing repeatedly through the vaporizer. Also there would be an undesirable accumulation of carbon dioxide.

With continuous flow and no rebreathing, as seen in Fig. 8.5d, a vaporizer and a Magill's attachment (Mapleson A) have been added. The McKesson is now being used in much the same way as the Boyle's machine — except that there is no precise indication of the mixed gas flow rate, the percentages only of the gases being known. If the flow rate is too low, rebreathing occurs.

It is not easy to determine in practice the exact setting of the pressure control to guarantee an adequate flow rate, and very often an excessive rate is used not only to prevent rebreathing, but also to make sure that the patient does not inhale air. However, it is possible to prevent rebreathing by interposing a check valve between the reservoir bag and the corrugated hose (Fig. 8.5e).

It is most important that, if there is no check valve, the reservoir bag should be fitted on the

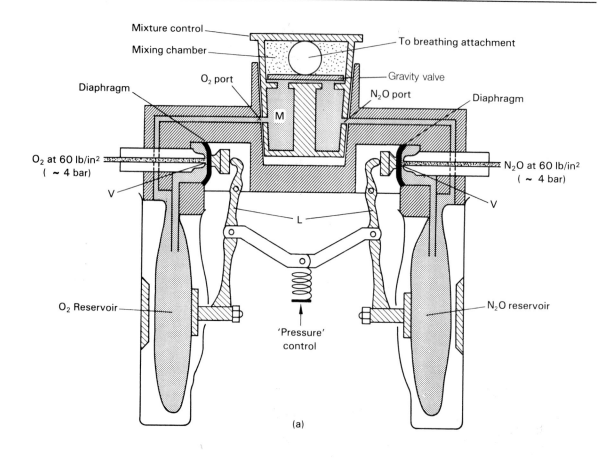

Mixture control

Mixing chamber

O_2 port

To breathing attachment

Gravity valve

N_2O port

Diaphragm

Diaphragm

M

O_2 at 60 lb/in² (~ 4 bar)

V

N_2O at 60 lb/in² (~ 4 bar)

V

L

O_2 Reservoir

N_2O reservoir

'Pressure' control

(a)

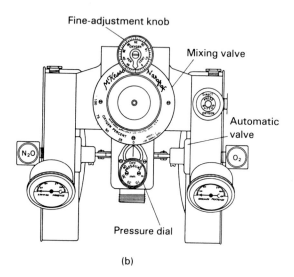

Fine-adjustment knob

Mixing valve

Automatic valve

N_2O

O_2

Pressure dial

(b)

Figure 8.4 McKesson intermittent flow gas and oxygen apparatus. This consists of two demand flow arrangements, one for oxygen and the other for nitrous oxide. The gases are mixed in the mixing chamber and passed through the gravity operated check valve to the patient. (a) A diagrammatic representation showing the principle of operation (see text). (b) The top view showing the dials, pressure gauges and oxygen bypass. (c) The side view, including the Nargraf rebreathing bellows. (d) A recent model incorporating an oxygen-failure safety device.

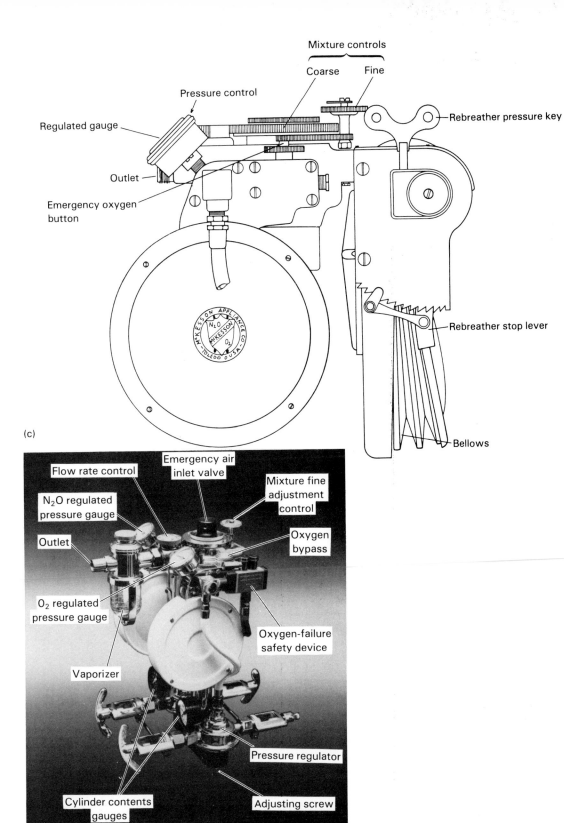

Mixture controls

Coarse   Fine

Pressure control

Regulated gauge

Rebreather pressure key

Outlet

Emergency oxygen
button

Rebreather stop lever

Bellows

(c)

Flow rate control

Emergency air
inlet valve

Mixture fine
adjustment
control

N$_2$O regulated
pressure gauge

Outlet

Oxygen
bypass

O$_2$ regulated
pressure gauge

Oxygen-failure
safety device

Vaporizer

Pressure regulator

Cylinder contents
gauges

Adjusting screw

(d)

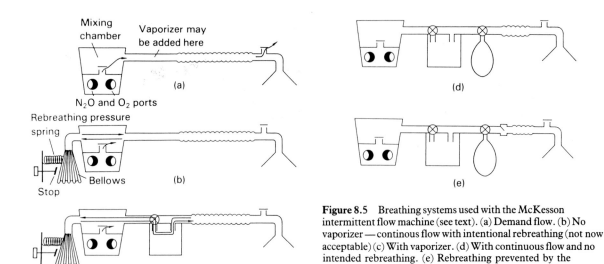

Figure 8.5   Breathing systems used with the McKesson intermittent flow machine (see text). (a) Demand flow. (b) No vaporizer — continous flow with intentional rebreathing (not now acceptable) (c) With vaporizer. (d) With continuous flow and no intended rebreathing. (e) Rebreathing prevented by the interposition of a check valve.

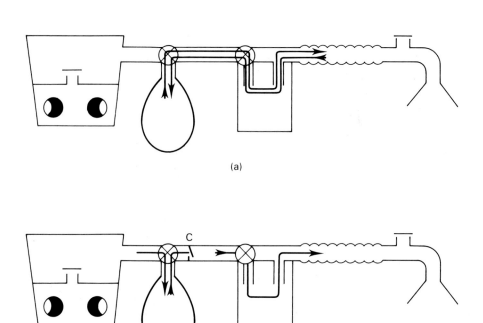

Figure 8.6   (a) The effect of mounting a vaporizer between the reservoir bag and the patient on a varying flow machine. If there is a low fresh gas flow rate, gases pass more than once through the vaporizer, generating an excessive vapour concentration. (b) A check valve C prevents rebreathing and the gases pass once only through the vaporizer.

downstream side of the vaporizer to prevent the gases being exposed more than once to the halothane, which would then produce too high a concentration (Fig. 8.6).

From time to time the regulated pressure should be checked and, if necessary, corrected so that the gauges read 60 lb/in^2 or indicate the middle of the segment marked 'operating range'.

In the author's experience the McKesson Simplor is the most reliable of all anaesthetic machines. Some of those used are over 40 years old and still working satisfactorily, in spite of the fact that the dentists who own them have had them serviced and recalibrated far less often than should have been the case. The accuracy of the percentage of oxygen tends to vary with flow rate, but it is rare for it to be less than that indicated (see Further Reading).

The Walton Five machine (Fig. 8.7)

The Walton Five machine works on a different principle from that of the McKesson. There are two low-pressure regulators to which gas is supplied at about 11 lb/in^2 (~ 0.7 bar). The chambers above the diaphragm of each of these are interconnected by a pressure loading tube, thereby making the oxygen regulator a slave of the nitrous oxide regulator. The latter contains a sensing diaphragm which, when deflected by the inspiratory effort of the patient, causes the valve to open and nitrous oxide to flow to the mixing chamber and the outlet. This nitrous oxide is mixed with oxygen which flows from its regulator at the same time. There is a pressure control knob analagous to that of the McKesson machine. This causes deflection of the diaphragm of the nitrous oxide regulator and a rise of pressure therein. This change is transmitted by the loading tube to the oxygen regulator. The nitrous oxide and oxygen flow to the mixing drum, the percentages being determined by the relative degree of opening of ports X_1 and X_2, which are varied by means of the mixture control lever.

The machine also includes high-pressure regulators for nitrous oxide and oxygen, an emergency oxygen control valve, a pressure relief valve and a cut-out unit which will prevent the flow of nitrous oxide should there be a failure of the oxygen supply. There is also an air inspiratory valve, complete with a whistle, which will act if the supply fails and the patient makes a respiratory effort. Note that this might not operate if the breathing attachment includes a reservoir bag.

As with the McKesson and the AE (see below), if large wall-mounted cylinders or a piped gas supply are used, the high-pressure regulators are mounted on the cylinder so that the tubing carries the gases at the regulated pressure.

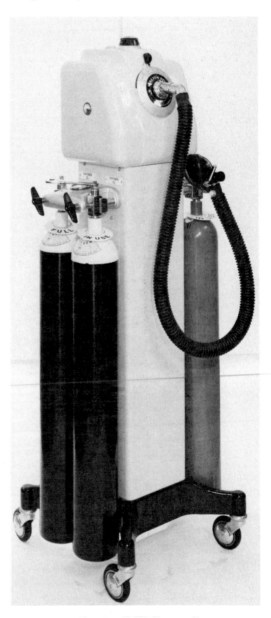

Figure 8.7   (a) The Walton Five machine.

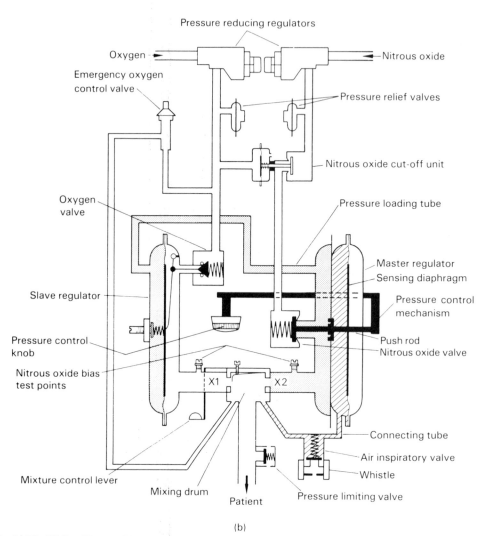

Pressure reducing regulators

Oxygen

Nitrous oxide

Emergency oxygen control valve

Pressure relief valves

Nitrous oxide cut-off unit

Oxygen valve

Pressure loading tube

Master regulator

Sensing diaphragm

Slave regulator

Pressure control mechanism

Pressure control knob

Push rod

Nitrous oxide valve

Nitrous oxide bias test points

X1   X2

Connecting tube

Air inspiratory valve

Whistle

Mixture control lever

Mixing drum

Patient

Pressure limiting valve

(b)

Figure 8.7 (b) The Walton Five machine; working principles.

The Walton Five is accurate, economical and very convenient to operate. Many anaesthetists regret that it has been declared obsolete by the manufacturer.

Although in the illustration it is depicted with neither reservoir bag nor vaporizer, it is most commonly used in the same manner as described above with the McKesson intermittent flow machine, and a non-return valve downstream from the reservoir bag is recommended.

The AE gas–oxygen machine (Fig. 8.8)

The working principles of this machine depend on three stages of pressure regulation. In the first stage there are two high-pressure regulators R_1, one each for nitrous oxide and oxygen. The cylinders or pipelines are attached at HP, and there is a pressure gauge P for each gas. The output pressure from these regulators is $60\,lb/in^2\,(\sim 4\,bar)$, and from them the nitrous oxide and oxygen pass to their appropriate second-stage regulators R_2. These two regulators have a spring S, which is common to both and

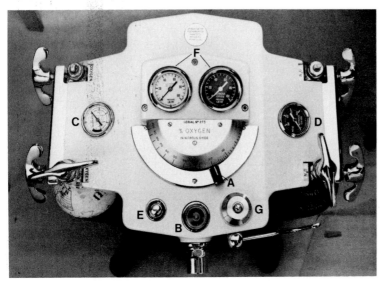

(a)

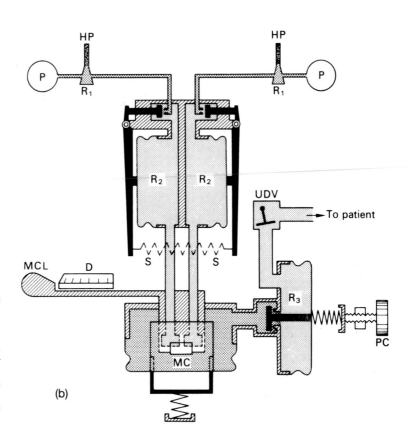

Figure 8.8 (a) The AE intermittent flow anaesthetic machine. A, mixture control lever; B, unidirectional valve; C, oxygen cylinder contents gauge; D, nitrous oxide cylinder contents gauge; E, oxygen flush button; F, first-stage regulated pressure gauges; G, pressure control knob.
(b) Working principles. R_1, R_2 & R_3, first-, second- and third-stage regulators; P, first-stage regulated pressure gauges; S, balancing spring; MC, mixing chamber; MCL, mixture control lever; D, mixture indicating dail- PC, pressure control knob; UDV, inidirectional valve.

(b)

Figure 8.9   (a) The Entonox valve. (b) Working principles (see text).

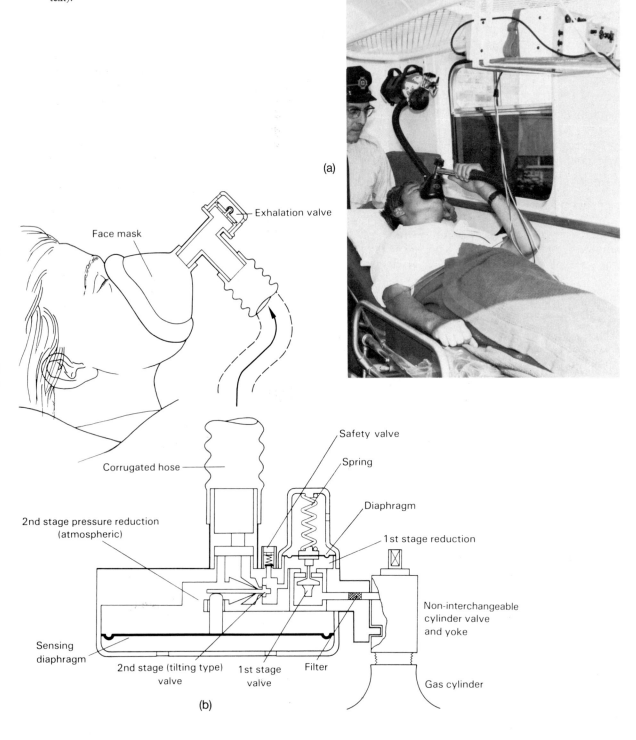

ensures that their output pressures are maintained equal — at about 70 cmH$_2$O (52 mmHg). The gases then pass to the mixing chamber MC, where they are mixed in any proportion required, depending on the position of the mixture control lever and the consequent degree of opening and closing of the ports in the mixing chamber. They then pass to the third stage, which is a simple regulator R$_3$, the output pressure of which can be varied by a spring which is controlled by the pressure control knob PC. The gases then pass via a unidirectional valve UDV to the outlet and breathing attachment. The unidirectional valve has a glass dome so that the anaesthetist can see the disc move as an indication of the fact that the patient is breathing, if he is unable to hear the 'hiss' of the expiratory valve.

Also incorporated in the AE machine is a device that cuts off the nitrous oxide supply if the oxygen fails, an oxygen flush, and gauges showing the pressure at the output of the first stage (4 bar).

'Demand' valves

Demand valves may be used, in the same manner as the now obsolete Minnitt machine, by the patient for self-administration. Suitable instruction and only general supervision, which may be by a nurse or ambulance man, is required. Two valves for the delivery of Entonox — a 50/50 mixture of nitrous oxide and oxygen, supplied in cylinders by BOC — will be described.

THE ENTONOX VALVE

The Entonox apparatus is used to administer 'premixed' nitrous oxide and oxygen (50% of each) to produce analgesia.

The valve (which is shown in Fig. 8.9) clamps directly onto a pin-index cylinder. It contains a first-stage regulator and a second-stage demand valve. A sensitive diaphragm, which is deflected by the patient's inspiratory effort, operates a push rod which tilts the valve lever, opening the valve and letting the gases flow. Very little inspiratory effort is required to achieve a high gas flow rate, making this a most efficient demand valve.

Since the nitrous oxide is in the gaseous state in the cylinder of premixed gases, the pressure gauge gives a direct indication of the cylinder contents. When small cylinders are used they may be placed in any position, but large ones should be maintained upright.

THE PNEUPAC ANALGESIA VALVE (Fig. 8.10)

Although this valve also uses Entonox and may be used on demand by the patient, it embraces some additional features to those mentioned above.

A pressure regulator is attached to the cylinder yoke and clamps directly onto the cylinder. A narrow-bore delivery tube connects this to the demand valve which is mounted directly onto the facepiece. Two versions of the demand valve are available, one having a push-button by which the attendant can inflate the lungs of a patient in respiratory failure.

The delivery tube between the regulator and demand valve may be several metres long and this may facilitate its use in the roadside treatment of accident cases and also allows the cylinder to be kept inside the ambulance so that during cold weather it will not become too cold. The joints at either end of the tube are secure, and disconnection is therefore rendered less likely.

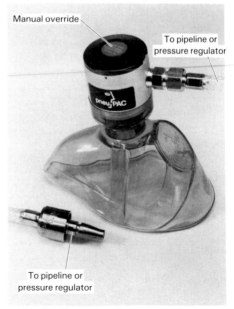

Figure 8.10   The Pneupac analgesia valve.

For the purposes of this chapter, dental anaesthesia is defined as general anaesthesia for the removal or conservation of teeth, in the dental operatory (surgery) and exclusively for outpatients. Whereas it is possible to intubate inpatients undergoing oral surgery in hospital, to pack the pharynx completely and afterwards to let the patient remain in a recovery ward for a prolonged period, this is often impracticable in dental anaesthesia.

In the dental operatory rather different circumstances appertain, namely:

1. The patient is required to be fit to leave for home within a short period of time.
2. The induction of anaesthesia is often by inhalation, and
3. During the operation the anaesthetist must allow the dentist access to the open mouth, thereby sharing the air passages with him, usually without the advantage of endotracheal intubation.

These seemingly impossible requirements are met by the use of a nasal inhaler. For inhalational induction the patient is instructed to keep his mouth closed so that he breathes through the nose. When anaesthesia is established the mouth is opened and a pack inserted to prevent mouth-breathing and the inhalation of blood or dental debris during the operation.

The patient may be sitting upright, though in some cases the lying position is preferred. It is not always possible to obtain a good fit between the inhaler and the face at the start of induction, so a high flow rate of gases must be available to prevent the inhalation of air rather than the anaesthetic mixture. It is desirable to be able to make changes of flow rate and of the percentage of nitrous oxide and oxygen independently of each other, on a 'breath to breath basis' and with minimal manual manipulation.

Therefore a so-called intermittent flow machine with an N_2O/O_2 percentage control is preferable to a continuous flow machine. It is, however, usually used with the pressure control turned somewhat 'up' so that there is always some flow of mixed gases. This somewhat resembles 'continuous flow', but since the rate is dependent on the patient's demand, which is continually altering, it may conveniently be called 'varying flow'.

9
Equipment for Dental Chair Anaesthesia

Continuous flow machines for dental anaesthesia

An ordinary Boyle's machine can be used, but it may present difficulties. The maximum flow rate of nitrous oxide may be lower than is convenient and the manipulation of the flow control valves may require more movements of the hand than are desirable.

The recently developed Quantiflex RA dental machine (Fig. 9.1) does have flowmeters — but they are capable of a greater flow rate than those on the average Boyle's machine. Note that the Quantiflex RA always gives at least a minimum flow rate of oxygen, usually preset at 3 l/min.

The McKesson 883 RA and 882 RA/GA machines (Fig. 9.2) both have flow control valves for oxygen and nitrous oxide and an on/off switch. The regulated pressure is 60 lb/in^2 ($\sim$ 4 bar) and they both have not only an emergency oxygen flush button but also an arrangement whereby a fall in the oxygen regulated pressure is automatically accompanied by a fall in nitrous oxide pressure so that the percentages of the gases remain the same. If the oxygen pressure falls below 10 lb/in^2 ($\sim$ 0.7 bar), the nitrous oxide is cut off altogether. In the 883 RA there is a minimum flow rate of oxygen of 3l/min but in the 882 RA/GA this operates only when the switch on the side is turned to RA. The 882 also carries a halothane vaporizer. Both machines have a valve that admits air if the oxygen and nitrous oxide supply fails and the reservoir bag is mounted on the machine itself with a one-way valve in the mount for the corrugated tube.

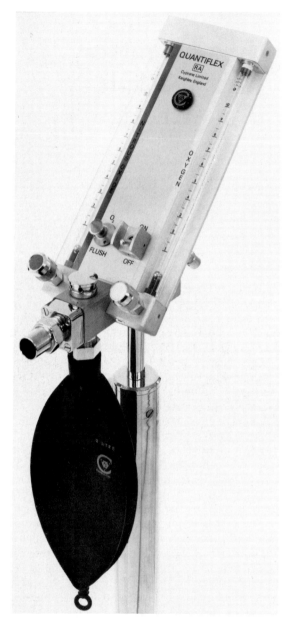

Figure 9.1   The Quantiflex RA machine. Note that in this range of machines there are many models in which the control and flowmeter for oxygen is on the right-hand side, as opposed to the left-hand side, which in the United Kingdom and many other countries, is the traditional position.

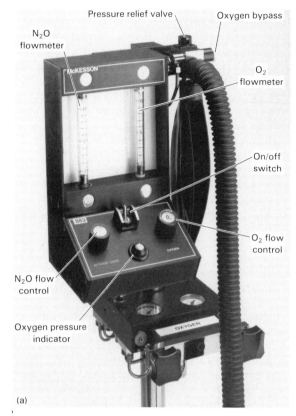

(a)

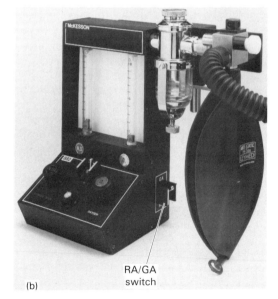

(b)

Figure 9.2   (a) The McKesson 883 RA machine. (b) The 882 RA/GA machine.

Intermittent (varying) flow machines

Intermittent flow machines were described in Chapter 8. They may be used for demand flow or a modified Magill attachment (Mapleson A) may be employed with the 'pressure' control turned up. The modified Magill attachment differs from the traditional one in that a non-return (check) valve downstream from the reservoir bag prevents rebreathing. This modification is made because there is no indication of flow *rate*, and therefore there would be no indication if there were an inadequate fresh gas flow rate resulting in rebreathing. Where true demand flow is required, the reservoir bag may be omitted, but theoretically this is not necessary if there is a non-return valve.

Vaporizers for dental anaesthesia

The halothane vaporizer is often detachable. It must be mounted upstream of the reservoir bag — otherwise gases might flow repeatedly backwards and forwards through the vaporizer as the patient breathes and would contain a higher concentration of halothane than intended. The check valve mentioned above would also prevent this (see Fig. 8.6).

CHOICE OF VAPORIZERS FOR DENTAL
ANAESTHESIA

Although other volatile agents are used, halothane is at present the most popular, and will be considered here. When selecting a vaporizer, distinction should be made between static apparatus, as kept in a hospital or group dental practice, where bulky or heavy apparatus may be used, and the type of vaporizer that may be conveniently carried by the itinerant dental anaesthetist in his case.

With a continuous flow machine, such as the Boyle's, the usual temperature and level compensated vaporizer, such as the Fluotec, may be used, but with the so-called 'intermittent flow' machines, such as the McKesson, Walton Five or AE, vaporizers of low resistance are required, since they are within the low-pressure breathing system and would better be described as VIBS (vaporizer in breathing system). The patient draws gases through them on demand. Vaporizers containing wicks may be used, since the moist exhaled gases do not pass through them. A most satisfactory type is the AE halothane

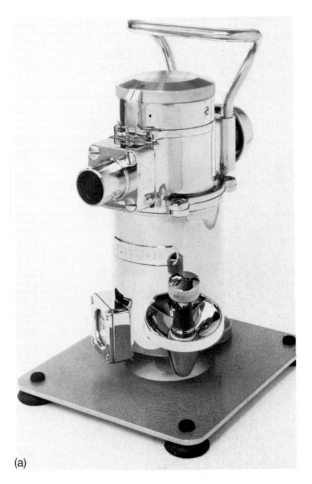

(a)

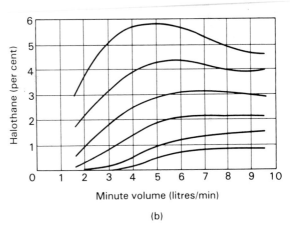

(b)

Figure 9.3   (a) The AE draw-over halothane vaporizer.
(b) Performance characteristics.

vaporizer by Cyprane (Fig. 9.3). This is suitable more for static apparatus, since it is rather bulky and needs to be drained before transportation. It is a calibrated compensated vaporizer of satisfactory accuracy.

Most of the suitable portable vaporizers are neither calibrated nor compensated for temperature or level, but tables giving typical performance characteristics are available. Provided that the vaporizers are used correctly they do not give a dangerously high concentration of halothane.

It must be emphasized that only a vaporizer designed for halothane should be used for this agent, since those designed for other volatile anaesthetics might give a dangerously high concentration of halothane.

Examples of portable vaporizers are shown in Figs. 5.25–5.27. As stated in Chapter 5, agitation or tilting of such vaporizers increases the vapour concentration. If the vaporizer is accidentally overturned and then used soon afterwards, liquid halothane in the bypass or tubing could give rise to a lethally high concentration of vapour.

Nasal inhalers

There are two traditional types of nasal inhaler (or hood) — the McKesson and the Goldman, and from these numerous modifications have been made.

The *McKesson inhaler* (Fig. 9.4) is constructed of rubber and fits over the nose. It is quite flexible and can be widened or narrowed. The gas enters through two narrow tubes, one on each side of the inhaler. These tubes pass round each side of the patient's head and are held together by means of a sliding clamp behind the head. Thus, when properly applied, the inhaler stays in place on its own, thereby freeing the anaesthetist's hands for other manipulations. It may be fitted with either a Heidbrink expiratory valve (Fig. 9.5) or a McKesson lever-action valve (Fig. 7.25) the former being the more satisfactory. The latter has the disadvantage that it may be closed by accidental pressure from the dentist's hand as he works.

The McKesson inhaler may be augmented by a mouth cover, as shown in Fig. 9.6. This is used if the patient persists in mouth breathing, particularly before the pack is inserted. When the mouth cover is out of use it falls downwards, automatically turning off the supply of gas to it. Mouth covers are rather

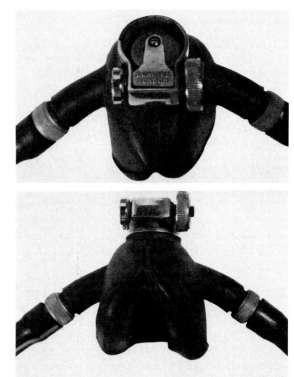

Figure 9.4 The McKesson nasal inhaler. Note that the lever-action valve manufactured by Coxeter was used at one time.

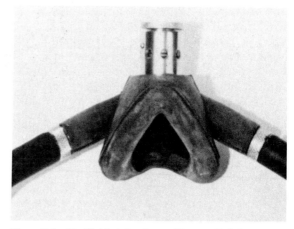

Figure 9.5 The Heidbrink valve used in a nasal inhaler.

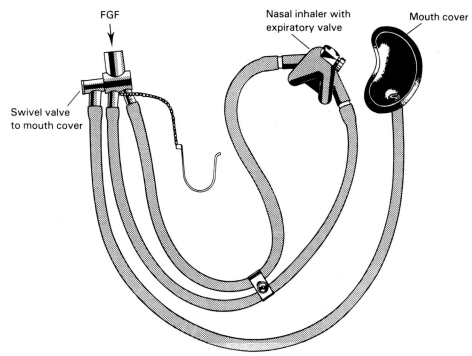

FGF

Nasal inhaler with
expiratory valve

Mouth cover

Swivel valve
to mouth cover

Figure 9.6 The McKesson nasal inhaler
complete with a mouth cover.

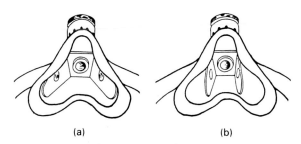

(a)

(b)

Figure 9.7 (a) The Braun nasal inhaler. Note the metal
stiffener. (b) An inhaler with a stiffener made of too flimsy a
material which has become bent.

objectionable to the patient, and most experienced
dental anaesthetists manage without them.

The *Braun modification* of the McKesson inhaler
(Fig. 9.7) has a metal stiffener inside to spread it
open and prevent it from pinching the nose. This
makes it much more acceptable to the patient. It
may also be used to cover both the mouth and nose
of an infant during induction. The stiffener should
be made of strong metal, since otherwise the two
sides may be pressed together and become impaled
on the patient's nose, so defeating the object of the
exercise.

The *Goldman inhaler* (Fig. 9.8) is rigid and has a
rather larger capacity than that of the McKesson.
The pad, which is moulded to fit the face, can be
replaced when damaged or perished. Gases enter via
a wide-bore hose, which passes over the top of the
patient's head, and escape through a Heidbrink

expiratory valve. The inhaler can be held in place by a harness of the Connell type (see Fig. 22.21b).

The advent of the vogue for scavenging exhaled anaesthetic vapours and the partial relaxation of regulations concerning the employment of electrically conductive materials (containing black carbon) have led to the diminution of the use of the 'black mask over the face', the insensitive and unsympathetic use of which has, in the past, kindled such fear in the patients on whom it was imposed.

Figure 9.9 shows a prototype nasal inhaler produced by Cyprane several years ago. It has been successfully used by the author in about 15 000 cases (repairs and replacements excepted). The Frazer–Sweatman hood is better accepted by nervous patients and the whistle either reassures the dentist that all is well or the lack of its intermittent sound warns him that he may be obstructing the airway. When the author has occasionally disconnected the whistle as an experiment, the educated dentist has complained of its absence! It should be noticed that even if it is not connected to a

scavenging system, the expiratory limb directs the expired gases to the floor and the extract fan rather than towards the operator, nurse and anaesthetist.

Another dental nasal inhaler is the Brown scavenging mask, manufactured by Narco-McKesson (Fig. 9.10), in which the fresh gases are delivered through an internal nasal hood and the expired gases pass via an external hood to the disposal system.

The author has no experience in the practical use of this inhaler, but found on examining it that the various components were easily disconnected, which may prove unsatisfactory during a 'lively' induction!

Further information on scavenging will be found in Chapter 15.

Nasal inhalers may be sterilized by cold methods such as immersion in chlorhexidine solution, but not all can be autoclaved. Usually, however, they are simply washed in hot running water after use on each patient and may then be dipped into a sterilizing solution. In busy dental practices it is rather expensive to provide a fresh inhaler for each patient.

An anaesthetist who has to resort to the use of the 'full facepiece' for a difficult patient more than *very* infrequently must admit that he is deficient in technique.

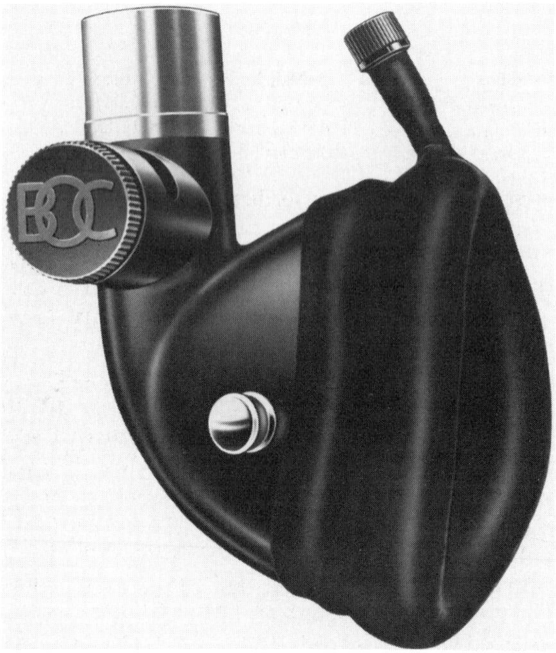

Figure 9.8   The Goldman nasal inhaler. Note the studs for the attachment of a head harness.

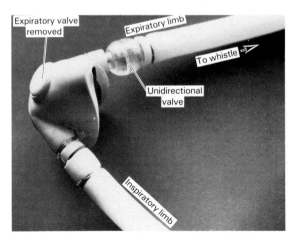

Figure 9.9   A protoype nasal inhaler manufactured by Cyprane.

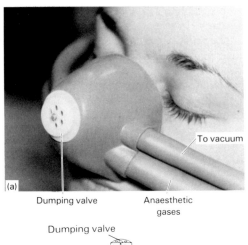

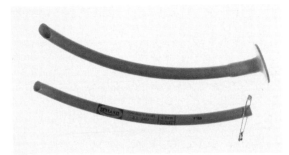

Figure 9.11 Nasopharyngeal airways. (a) Purpose-made with a flange. (b) The improvised version.

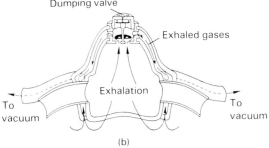

(b)

Figure 9.10 (a) The Brown scavenging nasal inhaler (manufactured by Narco-McKesson). The anaesthetic gases are delivered through the wider bore tubes and the vacuum for scavenging is connected to the narrower pair. The dumping valve admits air only if the reservoir bag has been emptied. The inhaler has a double skin, as shown in (b), the anaesthetic gases being delivered to the interior and the vacuum to the gap between the two layers.

Endotracheal tubes used in dental anaesthesia are described in Chapter 7. Nasopharyngeal tubes (or airways) may be purpose-made, with a flange to prevent their slipping out of reach from the nostril, or may be improvised by inserting a safety pin through an old nasotracheal tube cut short (Fig. 9.11). A no. 7 tube, 7 in. (17 cm) long, or a no. 6 tube, 6 in. (15 cm) long should suit most adults.

Gags and props

Mason's and Ferguson's gags are described in Chapter 22. The blades should be covered with plastic or rubber tubing to protect the patient's teeth from damage. As shown in Fig. 9.12, the pieces of tubing should not be so short that they might fall off and be inhaled by the patient. Plastic tubing is more easily threaded onto the blade of the gag if it is first

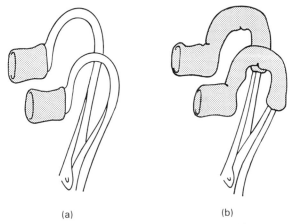

(a)   (b)

Figure 9.12 Mouth gags. (a) With the blades covered by inadequate lengths of tubing which might easily become dislodged and be inhaled by the patient (b) With the blades covered by longer lengths of tubing.

softened by immersion in boiling water.

When the gag is being inserted into the patient's mouth it should be held by the blades, as shown in Fig. 9.13a, and not by the handles, since the latter causes the gag to open before it is inserted (Fig. 9.13b).

Instead of a gag, a prop may be used to keep the patient's mouth open. Since the days of Hewitt (1857–1916) the prop has been re-invented many times and a typical set is shown in Fig. 9.14. A prop should be attached to a length of cord or chain to facilitate its retrieval if it slips into the patient's mouth. Conveniently, three or four props of different sizes may be linked together by their chains.

Various forms of throat pack have been produced, including those consisting of absorbent tampons and preformed foam-rubber. Strips of gamgee about 2 in. (5 cm) wide remain the most popular and

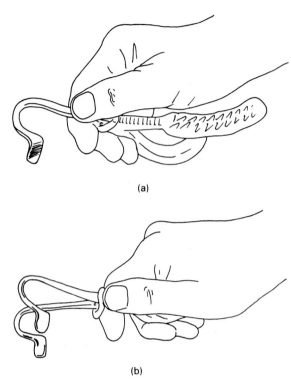

(a)

(b)

Figure 9.13   A mouth gag held (a) correctly; (b) incorrectly.

adaptable. This material comes in rolls, in various thicknesses. It may be precut into lengths which should be not less than 12 in. (30 cm) long. When in use the end of the pack should always remain outside the mouth to facilitate its removal. If one pack is inadequate, a second should be used and the ends of both should be kept outside the mouth.

Suction equipment

In the dental operatory this should be of the high displacement type (see Chapter 16). The high-pressure, low-displacement type, such as that produced by a hospital piped medical vacuum or a good quality portable electrically operated suction pump, may be satisfactory, but low-displacement types such as the foot-operated suction pump or the venturi type working off the water tap give far less than the desirable performance.

The sucker is used most commonly to remove blood and debris from the site of operation, and only seldom to remove regurgitated or vomited stomach contents, or secretions, from the respiratory tract.

It should be remembered, however, that with the low-pressure, high-displacement type of suction equipment, the nozzle should be of wide diameter, between 0.5 and 2 cm and as short as possible. Long, narrow-bore suction catheters are inappropriate.

The dental chair

The chair itself is justifiably included in this chapter since the ease with which the posture of the patient may be altered and, equally important, the security with which he, and his head in particular, may be maintained in the desired position are of paramount importance in the pursuit of safety during dental anaesthesia.

Whether the patient is anaesthetized and subjected to operation in the sitting, semirecumbent or horizontal position is a matter for individual choice. Whichever is preferred there is no argument that the patient who collapses must be placed, quickly, in the horizontal position — preferably with the legs raised. The anaesthetist should, therefore, be familiar with the workings of the chair and also check, before use, that any electric controls are turned on and functioning correctly.

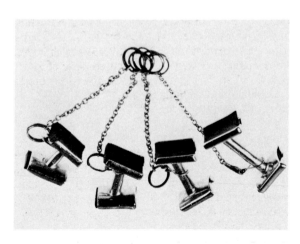

Figure 9.14   A set of mouth props.

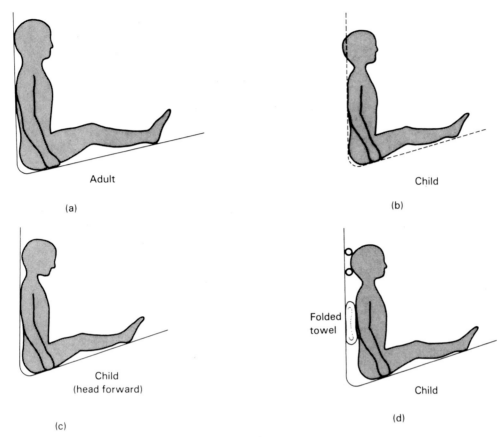

Figure 9.15 (a) When an adult sits in the dental chair, his occiput is roughly in line with his back. (b) Children tend to have slender necks and prominent occiputs, (c) causing flexion of the neck. (d) A folded towel behind the back and the 'ring of confidence' may help to maintain the head in the correct position.

One of the problems of the modern electrically operated dental chair is that it may be slow to operate when the horizontal position is required urgently and, in most types, if the electric supply is not energized, there is no manual override to lower the back of the chair speedily.

The other disadvantage of modern chairs is that the old 'doughnut' type of headrest which maintained the position of the patient's head so positively has been replaced by the flat rest which permits the head of the anaesthetized patient to wobble about. In the case of children this is of even greater importace, since their necks are even more slender, and the occiput more prominent, making the maintenance of a suitable position more difficult (Fig. 9.15).

Makeshift additions to the headrest include a home-made 'bean bag', consisting of a 3 *l* infusion bag filled with rice, designed by J. V. I. Young (personal communication) (Fig. 9.16) and the 'ring of confidence' (Fig. 9.17), which consists of a circular head-rest constructed from a discarded length of corrugated breathing tubing.

Piped medical gases

The decision as to whether to install a piped gas system in the dental operatory must be influenced by the frequency of use of general anaesthesia and relative analgesia and on the aesthetic aspect of the design of the establishment. Piped gas systems are described in Chapter 4.

Considerable economy of running expenses and time may be achieved by installing large cylinders of

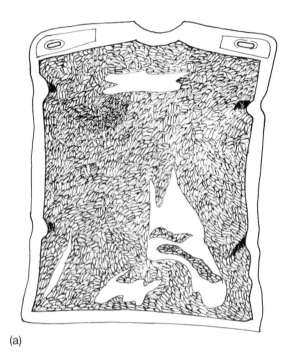

(a)

Figure 9.16 (a) The 3 *l* infusion bag ('bean bag') filled with rice. (b) The 'bean bag' used to hold the patient's head steady during dental chair anaesthesia.

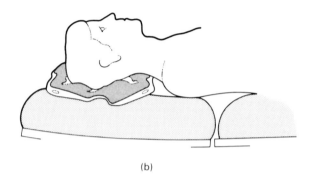

(b)

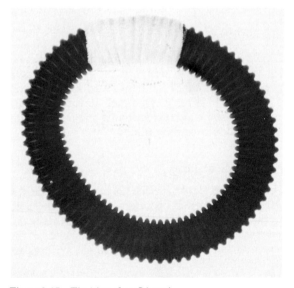

Figure 9.17 The 'ring of confidence'.

nitrous oxide and oxygen instead of small ones mounted on the anaesthetic machine itself. This may be done in several ways:

1. A single trolley may carry two large cylinders *and* an anaesthetic machine. This is rather cumbersome, but portable, and may be wheeled, with some effort, from operatory to operatory. The longevity of the cylinder contents is a distinct advantage.
2. Two cylinders at the wall of the operatory with regulators and contents gauges attached. These may be secured by a chain or special rings into brackets screwed to the wall. Rubber tubing delivers gases to the anaesthetic machine — and may be detached if non-interchangeable connectors similar to those on the pipeline are used.

**The itinerant dental anaesthetist's case —
a suggested list of contents**

The instrument case has four drawers, the top ones
shallow and the lower ones deep.

Top drawer

Endotracheal tubes, with connectors
Nasopharyngeal tubes
Bronchoscope blade (to fit laryngoscope handle)
Spare washers for cylinders, vaporizers, etc.
Spare O-rings for bullnose cylinder fittings
Adhesive plaster
Specimen bottles for blood samples
Safety pins

2nd drawer

Drugs, including those for resuscitation, and
    isoprenaline spray
Ampoule files
Sickledex kit
Hawksley haemoglobin scale
Scissors
Airways
Tongue-and-towel forceps
Spencer Wells forceps

3rd drawer

Syringes, 5 and 10 ml
Selection of needles
Methohexitone, thiopentone and sterile water
Ampoules of atropine or glycopyrronnium bromide
    (glycopyrrolate)
Miniswabs or cotton wool

4th drawer

Nasal inhaler(s)
Vaporizer

Reservoir bag on mount
Check valve (for use in Mapleson A)
Adaptors, McKesson to BOC and New BS, etc.
Bottles of halothane and 70% alcohol skin
    preparation
Funnel
Cylinder key (ratchet)
Laryngoscope (with batteries removed from handle)
Mouth gag
Straight and angled expiratory valves
Facepiece
Catheter mount
Spare laryngoscope batteries and bulb
Spare reservoir bag
Stethoscope
Sphygmomanometer

Equipment to be kept at the dental operatory

Anaesthetic machine, complete with breathing
    attachment and preferably a compensated
    vaporizer
Cylinder key
Throat packs
Mouth gag or props
Suitable headrest
Spare cylinders
Resuscitation equipment (independent of
    anaesthetic machine and oxygen cylinder)

**Equipment that may be kept in the anaesthetist's
car when parked nearby**

Manual resuscitator (such as Ambu or Air Viva)
Spare tracheal tubes and laryngoscope
Cardioscope
Defibrillator   at his
Pulse monitor   discretion
Portable suction
(standby)

10

Draw-over and Air-driven Apparatus

Draw-over Apparatus

The main object of this type of equipment is to enable a volatile anaesthetic agent to be vaporized in air with complete independence from supplies of nitrous oxide and oxygen, or any other motive force other than that of the patient's breathing. Its main use is for emergency work in the field and in remote areas where the supply of compressed gases is restricted or impossible. There are several sophisticated draw-over machines, some of which are described later in this chapter, but the principles can best be understood if the more primitive methods are described first.

Figure 10.1 shows the 'open-drop' administration of ether or chloroform. The Schimmelbusch mask consists of a simple wire frame over which is stretched layers of gauze or lint. As the patient breathes, air is drawn backwards and forwards through the mask and vaporizes the volatile anaesthetic agent which has been dropped onto it from a suitable drop bottle. This apparatus is extremely cheap and portable, but has several disadvantages:

1. It requires considerable skill to make the administration pleasant for the patient. Induction may be time consuming.
2. It is a wasteful method which may greatly add to the expense of administering costly anaesthetic agents.
3. The lint or gauze quickly becomes sodden with

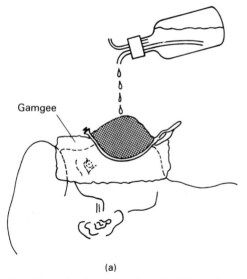
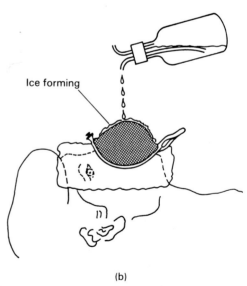

(a) (b)

Figure 10.1 'Open drop' administration. The Schimmelbusch mask is covered with 16 layers of gauze in the case of ether; and 12 layers of gauze or one layer of lint for chloroform. (a) The patient breathes backwards and forwards through the gauze onto which drops of the anaesthetic agent are poured from a drop bottle. (b) As liquid ether vapourizes, the gauze is cooled to such an extent that the water vapour in the expired air both condenses and freezes on the surface of the gauze.

Whereas ether is poured relatively rapidly over the whole area of the gauze, chloroform is poured very slowly over only one half of its area. In this diagram the patient's eyes are shown to be open in order to stress the risk of conjunctivitis from absorption of the anaesthetic agent, even though they are covered by the layer of gamgee.

water which has condensed from the patient's exhaled breath. This increases the resistance to air flow of the mask. If ether is being used, this water may freeze and form crystals of ice on the mask.

4. There is no calibration or control of the vapour concentration other than by the skill of the anaesthetist.

5. There is no means of applying artificial ventilation should the patient become apnoeic.

Modifications of the original Schimmelbusch mask have been made from time to time. The most important is the addition of a tube through which oxygen or even an N_2O/O_2 mixture can be fed in such a way that it is supplied to the patient from within the mask (see Figs. 5.1–5.4). It should be noted that the Schimmelbusch mask and nearly all its modifications have been purposely designed so that they do not closely fit the contours of the patient's face, in order to provide a channel through which the patient can breathe some fresh air. This is particularly important in the case of the administration of chloroform and ethyl chloride, where it may help to prevent the inhalation of too high a concentration of the vapour, which would result in an overdose.

Figure 10.2 shows Clover's inhaler. There are several modifications of this, but the working prin-

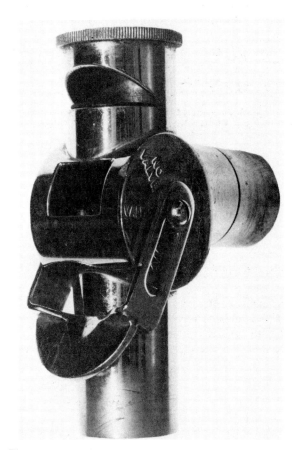

Figure 10.3 The Barth three-way stopcock. Note the three positions for 'air', 'valves' (i.e. with valves allowing the ingress and egress of air) and 'no valves' (i.e. with complete rebreathing).

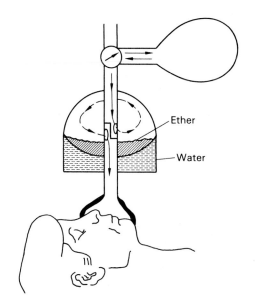

Figure 10.2 Clover's inhaler (see text).

ciples are much the same. A roughly spherical chamber contains ether. Through this chamber there passes a tube which connects the facepiece to a control valve. The valve may be turned either so that the patient breathes fresh air or so that he breathes in and out of the rebreathing bag. By moving the control lever, the patient's breath is made to pass through the ether chamber, picking up ether vapour as it does so. The water chamber provides a reservoir of heat to prevent the ether from cooling to the point where vaporization is significantly reduced. Heat is also derived from the patient's breath and the anaesthetist's hand as he holds the vaporizer.

The Barth valve (Fig. 10.3) and other elaborations on the same principle consisted of a three-way stop-cock to replace the valve. It contained rubber flaps which formed a one-way breathing system.

This type of vaporizer is now, of course, obsolete. The disadvantages included the large dead space. The build-up of carbon dioxide was taken to be an advantage by anaesthetists in years gone by, in spite of the fall in oxygen concentration. This is not acceptable to anaesthetists of the present day.

Figure 10.4 shows the principle of the 'draw-over' anaesthetic apparatus. When the patient inhales, air is drawn through the vaporizer (or its bypass if the vaporizer is turned off) and then through a one-way valve V_1. As the patient exhales it is impossible for him to breathe back through V_1 and the exhaled gases are vented to the atmosphere through the expiratory valve. The vaporizer must be a low-resistance type such as the AE Fluothane vaporizer, the Oxford Miniature vaporizer or the EMO ether

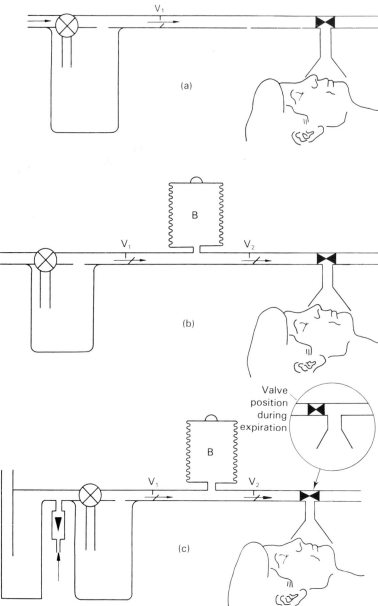

Figure 10.4   The draw-over anaesthetic system. The vaporizer must be of low resistance and valve V_1 prevents reverse flow during expiration. A non-rebreathing valve such as the Ruben valve is used. (b) The addition of a bellows B and a second unidirectional valve V_2 facilitates controlled ventilation. (c) An oxygen flowmeter has been added. During expiration the continuing supply of oxygen flows into the reservoir.

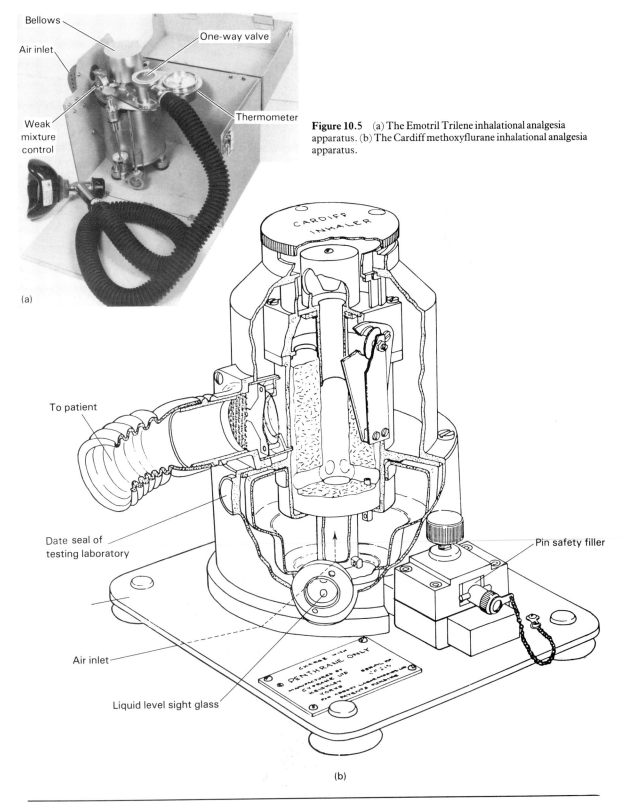

Bellows

Air inlet

One-way valve

Weak mixture control

Thermometer

(a)

Figure 10.5 (a) The Emotril Trilene inhalational analgesia apparatus. (b) The Cardiff methoxyflurane inhalational analgesia apparatus.

CARDIFF INHALER

To patient

Date seal of testing laboratory

Pin safety filler

Air inlet

Liquid level sight glass

CHARGE WITH PENTHRANE ONLY

(b)

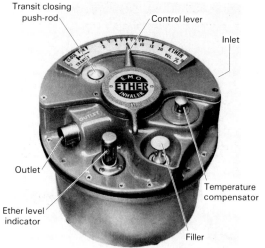

Figure 10.6 (a) The EMO ether inhaler. This is a low-resistance vaporizer which is both temperature and level compensated. (b) Working principles. Note that there is a mass of water, which provides a heat sink. When the control lever is put to the 'close for transit' position, the ether chamber is sealed off to prevent spillage.

(a)

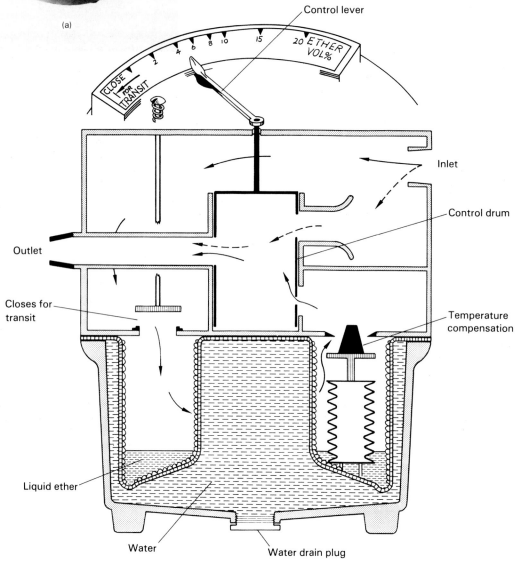

(b)

vaporizer. This scheme has been elaborated in various portable draw-over anaesthetic systems, but in its basic form it is used for inhalation analgesia as employed in obstetrics. Figures 10.5 and 10.6 show the temperature compensated vaporizers for obstetric analgesia. These vaporizers are designed for use with Trilene and methoxyflurane (Penthrane) respectively. In Britain the Emotril is no longer approved by the Central Midwives' Board for unsupervised administration by midwives, mainly because the use of Entonox has almost universally superseded Trilene in obstetrical analgesia.

Figure 10.6 shows the EMO ether inhaler, which is usually used as a draw-over vaporizer with spontaneous ventilation. It may, however, be used in conjunction with the Oxford bellows for anaesthetic techniques employing IPPV.

Figure 10.4b shows a modification of the basic draw-over apparatus. A bellows B and a second unidirectional valve V_2 have been added so that artificial ventilation may be performed should the patient stop breathing. Note that the expiratory valve is of the Ruben or Ambu-E type to facilitate this.

In Fig. 10.4c a supply of oxygen and a reservoir have been added. During inspiration oxygen is drawn through the apparatus with the air. During expiration oxygen flows backwards into the reservoir so as to enrich the air drawn in at the next breath. If required, nitrous oxide may also be added to the system at the same point.

Figure 10.7 shows one of several models of the Portablease machine. Nitrous oxide and oxygen are provided and there is also a bellows for artificial ventilation. The first unidirectional valve is situated between the flowmeters and the universal vaporizer, and at this point there is an air-inlet valve. There are unidirectional valves on both sides of the inflating bellows, and there is a Ruben valve.

The Triservice apparatus is described on p. 350. It is not only versatile but also extremely portable and is therefore particularly suitable for use in major accidents and in the battlefield.

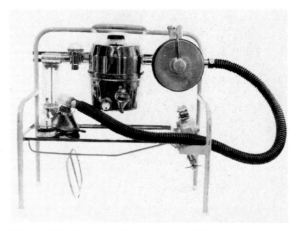

Figure 10.7   The Portablease apparatus. This is another elaboration of the draw-over principle. Note that there are flowmeters for both oxygen and nitrous oxide, but there is no reservoir. The vaporizer is a Blease Universal vaporizer, which may be used for different volatile anaesthetic agents by using the suitably calibrated control knobs.

Draw-over anaesthetic apparatus of the type described above is by no means inexpensive and is not, in practice, a convenient substitute for the Boyle's machine. However, it is indispensable in situations where the latter cannot be employed owing to factors such as a shortage of compressed gases.

Air-driven Apparatus

Interest has recently been taken in a Boyle's type of anaesthetic machine being driven by air rather than nitrous oxide and oxygen. This is partly because some anaesthetists prefer to use air rather than nitrous oxide and oxygen, but mainly because, as mentioned above in connection with draw-over apparatus, in some situations there may be difficulty in obtaining supplies of nitrous oxide and oxygen. Compressed air may be obtained from an electric compressor, a cylinder or some other mechanical device.

11

Resuscitators and Automatic Ventilators

There are three different groups of devices that can be used to produce artificial ventilation of the lungs:

1. Manual resuscitators such as the Air-viva, Ambu, Samson and Oxford bellows.
2. Mechanical ventilators into which the patient is placed in order to stimulate the negative intra-thoracic pressure which occurs in spontaneous respiration. This group includes the cabinet type of ventilator such as the Drinker (Both 'iron lung') and the cuirass. These inflate the lungs by indirect action.
3. Mechanical devices that rhythmically inflate the lungs by means of applying intermittent positive pressure to the air passages (IPPV — intermittent positive pressure ventilation).

Manual Resuscitators

There are several manual resuscitators, and some will be described here.

The Air-viva, Ambu and Laerdal resuscitators

These resuscitators consist of a bag, a valve and a facepiece (Figs 11.1–11.3). The bag is so constructed that in the resting state it is inflated. When it is squeezed a valve closes the expiratory port and the air passes to the facepiece and inflates the patient's lungs. When pressure is released, the bag automatically refills with fresh air and since at the same time the valve moves back to its resting position, the

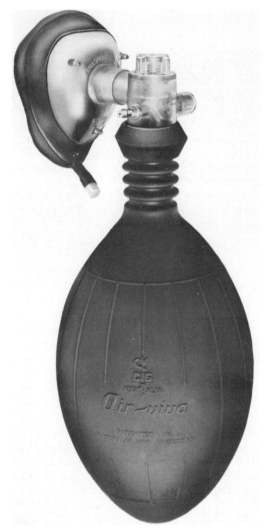

Figure 11.1 The Air-viva resuscitator.

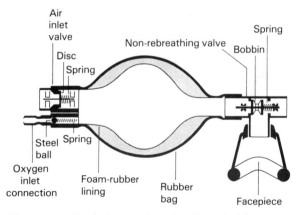

Figure 11.2 The Ambu resuscitator (working principles).

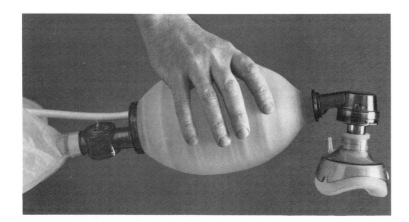

Figure 11.3   The Laerdal silicone resuscitator. Note the optional reservoir bag for supplementary oxygen.

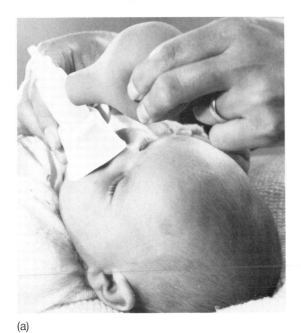

(a)

patient's expired air passes passively to the atmosphere. There is provision for a supply of oxygen to the bag via a tube of small diameter. The nozzle for attaching the oxygen tube is of such small diameter that if the oxygen tube is not connected, very little air is lost through it during the inspiratory phase. In manual resuscitators such as the Ambu, air is drawn into one end of a self-inflating bag and blown out of the other.

The facepieces provided with this type of resuscitator are often constructed of transparent plastic so that if the patient has vomited, this may be more quickly observed. Like most similar devices, the Air-viva is constructed of a material that will not perish, although in some cases the cuff on the facepiece is of latex and requires periodic inspection and massage under warm water to keep them from perishing.

Figure 11.4   (a) The Samson–Blease infant resuscitator. (b) Working principles. A, rubber bulb; B, body; C, facepiece; D, oxygen inlet tube; F, air inlet holes; G, non-return valve; H, side limb for bulb; I, pressure-regulating holes; J, taper for facepiece; K, taper for endotracheal tube connector; L, endotracheal tube connector.

(b)

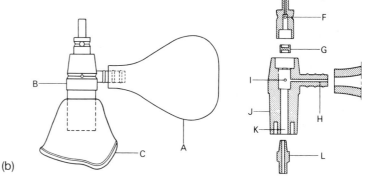

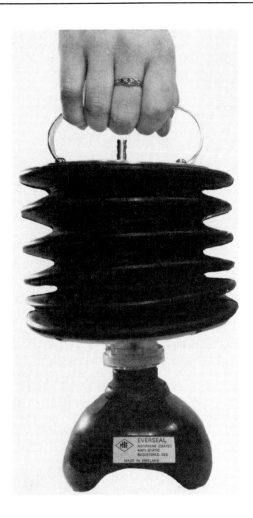

(a)

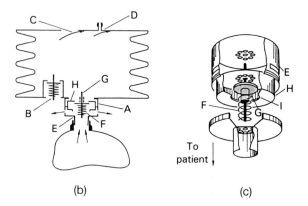

(b)   (c)

Figure 11.5   (a) The Cardiff inflating bellows. (b) Working principles. A, expiratory valve assembly; B, safety valve; C, intake valve; D, oxygen inlet valve; E, valve housing (with expiratory ports); F, spring; G, non-return valve; H, piston; I, valve-seating on piston. E, F, G, H and I constitute the Cardiff inflating valve, which is shown in greater detail in (c).

The Samson-Blease infant resuscitator

The Samson-Blease infant resuscitator works on a similar principle to the above. There are 'pressure-regulating' holes to prevent over-distension of the patient's lungs (Fig. 11.4).

The Cardiff inflating bellows

The Cardiff inflating bellows (Fig. 11.5) employs a concertina bellows and a Cardiff inflating valve (Fig. 11.5b). During inspiration, when the operator compresses the bellows, the valve occupies the inspiratory position and air inflates the patient's lungs. During expiration, as the bellows is drawn open again, the valve returns to the expiratory position, the exhaled air escapes to the atmosphere through expiratory ports and fresh air is drawn into the other end of the bellows through a one-way flap valve C.

The inflating valve has two moving parts, a piston which closes the expiratory ports during inflation and a spring-loaded disc valve G. The latter not only returns the piston H to its former position during expiration, it also prevents the return of expired air to the bellows by closing the holes in the base of the piston. If the valve is dismantled for any reason it is essential to ensure that the parts are replaced in the correct manner.

There is provision for supplying oxygen to the bellows, and a safety valve which opens at 50 cmH2O pressure.

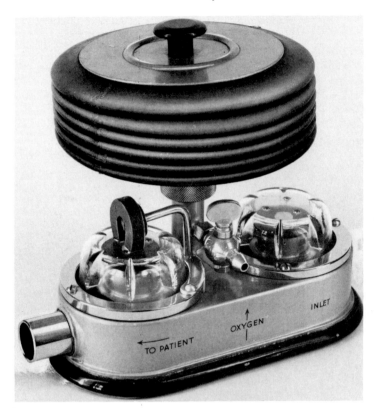

(a)

Figure 11.6   (a) The Oxford inflating bellows. (b) Working principles. Insert shows gas flow with downstream valve V_2 held open by magnet. (See text.)

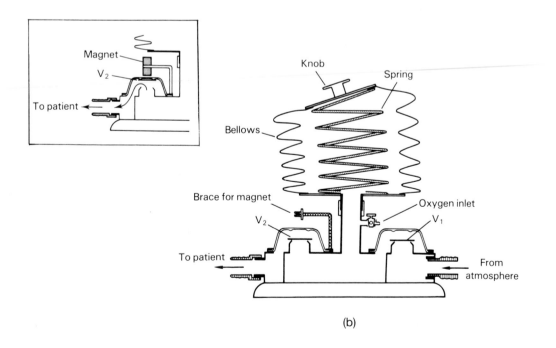

(b)

The Oxford inflating bellows

The Oxford inflating bellows (Fig. 11.6) is most useful in conjunction with draw-over anaesthetic apparatus. It is surmounted by a knob, for easy manual operation, and contains a spring which, when unopposed, opens the bellows, drawing in atmospheric air. The inlet and outlet are guarded by one-way disc valves V_1 and V_2 so that air is drawn in from the atmosphere and blown into the patient when the bellows is depressed. Additional oxygen may be added via a tap in the bellows mount. When the patient breathes spontaneously, air may be drawn through without movement of the bellows, and the resistance is therefore low. Resistance may be lowered even further by placing a magnet on the bracket in such a way that it attracts the disc and by holding it up keeps the downstream valve V_2 open. The disc of V_2 should always be either held up or removed altogether when an inflating valve, such as the Ruben or Ambu E, is employed.

Since the unidirectional valves are of the gravity type, the apparatus must be kept upright when in use.

When the Oxford bellows is connected directly to an apnoeic patient, a non-rebreathing expiratory valve is required, such as the Ruben, which permits expiration but which closes during inflation. Alternatively, a facepiece (when used) can be lifted from the patient's face during expiration.

Mechnical Ventilators that Act Externally on the Chest

These act by applying external pressure to the patient's chest so as to simulate normal respiratory movements.

Cabinet-type ventilators

Figure 11.7 shows a cabinet ventilator. The whole patient, with the exception of his head and neck, is placed in the cabinet, which is connected to a large air pump. The pump blows air alternately into and out of the cabinet, causing an alternating rise and fall of the pressure within it. The patient's chest, being

paralysed, moves in accordance with this rise and fall of pressure, and air is drawn into and out of his lungs. A competent seal around the patient's neck is required in order to prevent leakage at this point. This type of ventilator is seldom used now for the following reasons:

1. It is cumbersome and the patient is difficult to nurse within the cabinet.
2. Air may be drawn into the patient's stomach, rather than into his lungs.
3. It is relatively inefficient.
4. The care of a patient with a tracheostomy is difficult.

The cuirass ventilator

The rigid cuirass ventilator (Fig. 11.8) depends on the same principles as the cabinet ventilator, but consists of a rigid dome which fits over the patient's chest and part of his abdomen. In a manner similar to that of the cabinet ventilator, air is drawn into and out of the dome, producing intermittent positive and negative pressure on the chest and abdomen, thus deflating and inflating the lungs. This ventilator has proved useful in difficult situations such as the transport in aircraft of patients suffering from poliomyelitis, but it is not in general use.

THE PINKERTON INFLATABLE CUIRASS

The Pinkerton inflatable cuirass consists of a rubber bag which is strapped around the patient's chest (Fig. 11.9). It is connected via a tube to another bag and the system is filled with air or any other gas. When the second bag is squeezed manually, the cuirass is inflated and squeezes the chest, providing a measure of artificial ventilation. Note, however, that expansion of the patient's chest is entirely by elastic recoil. The Pinkerton inflatable cuirass was used in anaesthesia for procedures such as bronchoscopy (where short periods of artificial ventilation are required without direct control of the patient's air passages), but has now been replaced by methods such as jetting (see below). However, it is included here for the sake of completeness, and because it is believed that, as in so many other instances, it may be reborn in another guise.

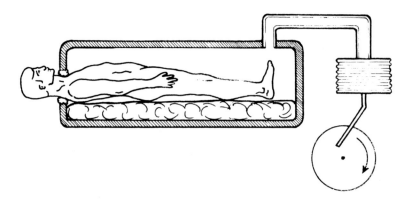

Figure 11.7   The principle of the cabinet ventilator.

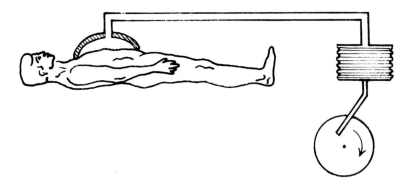

Figure 11.8   The principle of the cuirass ventilator.

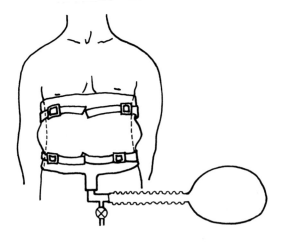

Figure 11.9   The Pinkerton inflatable cuirass.

Automatic Intermittent Positive Pressure Ventilators

Most of the ventilators used for anaesthetic techniques and intensive care procedures fall into this group. They intermittently inflate the patient's lungs by positive pressure applied via a cuffed endotracheal or tracheostomy tube. Deflation of the lungs may be either passive or assisted. The power by which these ventilators are operated may come from an electric motor, or a supply of compressed gases or air. The frequency and pattern of respiration may be varied.

The operation of ventilators may be divided into four phases:
1. Inspiratory.
2. Changeover to expiratory.
3. Expiratory.
4. Changeover to inspiratory.

The repeated change from one phase to the next is called *cycling*, and the functions upon which the changes are dependent may be considered when classifying ventilators. These functions are:
1. The *volume* of gases supplied to the patient in each breath.
2. The *pressure* of gases in the airway.
3. *Time*, which may be determined by means of an electric, mechanical or pneumatic timer, or the speed of a motor and a gear box.
4. *Flow*, as the flow rate during inspiration falls below a predetermined level.
5. *Patient triggering*, i.e. the onset of the inspiratory phase may be initiated by the inspiratory attempt of the patient himself.

Two or more of these functions may be combined in one ventilator. It is also possible to set *limits* to any of these functions, e.g. a high limit for pressure, which if it is reached, will cause the ventilator to cycle. A time-limit may also be set to initiate cycling at a minimum frequency if, when it is on 'patient triggering', the patient fails to attempt to breathe.

At this juncture it would be prudent to distinguish between the terms 'stroke volume' and 'tidal volume'. The *stroke volume* is the volume delivered at each 'breath' by the ventilator. Some of this volume may be lost, as will be described later. The *tidal volume* is the volume by which the patient is actually ventilated.

As explained in Chapter 7, spontaneous respiration is divided into three *phases*:
1. Inspiration, when air is drawn into the lungs.
2. Expiration, when air is either actively forced out of the lungs or simply expelled by the passive recoil of the chest wall.
3. The expiratory pause, which lasts from the end of one expiration until the start of the next inspiration.

In the case of intermittent positive pressure ventilators, during the inspiratory phase air is driven into the lungs by positive pressure (the patient is often paralysed and can neither resist nor assist the ventilator). The expiratory phase may be passive or the machine may assist by applying 'negative' (or subatmospheric) pressure throughout all or part of it.

Not only may the frequency be varied, but the pattern of respiration may also be altered. The duration of the inspiratory phase divided by the duration of the expiratory + expiratory pause phases is known as the inspiratory/expiratory ratio.

Many different ventilators are in current use. A detailed description of these may be found elsewhere (Mushin et al., 1980). However, improvements and innovations are being produced so frequently that in this chapter it must be sufficient to describe the general principles by which ventilators operate, using as illustrations some of the more popular ones.

To demonstrate the different modes of operation of various ventilators, and the uses to which they may be put, they may be classified in a number of different ways. It is hoped that the following description of these classifications will assist in the selection of a ventilator for a specific purpose.

CLASSIFICATION OF VENTILATORS

Ventilators may be classified as: (a) those employed only for anaesthesia, (b) those employed for artificial ventilation of paralysed or apnoeic patients but which are unsuitable for anaesthesia, and (c) those that may be used equally conveniently for both anaesthetic techniques and the long-term ventilation of patients in the intensive care ward.

In an 'open-system' ventilator, fresh gases are delivered to the patient with each inspiration. The expired gases may pass back through the ventilator so that their escape to the atmosphere can be con-

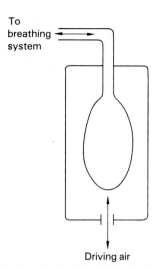

Figure 11.10 The 'bag in a bottle' principle. As the driving air is driven into and out of the bottle, the bag, which is connected to the breathing system and contains patient gases, is pheumatically compressed and re-expanded. By this method the patient gases are isolated from the ventilator, which may be powered by and deliver other gases such as compressed air. The 'bag' is often in the form of a bellows, in which case the stroke volume may be indicated.

trolled by an expiratory valve, so that PEEP or 'negative' pressure can be applied during the expiratory phase, or so that the expired tidal volume can be measured on a spirometer. However, they are always discarded, and none return to the inspiratory side of the ventilator.

A 'closed-circuit' ventilator takes the place of the anaesthetist's manual squeezing of the rebreathing bag of a 'circle' or 'to-and-fro' closed-circuit anaesthetic system. Provision is made for the absorption of carbon dioxide; also, the fresh gas flow may be very much smaller than the patient's minute volume. Most closed-circuit ventilators have provision for the automatic 'spilling' of excess gases.

An open-system ventilator may be converted to the closed-circuit type by interposing a 'bag in a bottle' (Fig. 11.10).

The four principal types of ventilators are as follows:
1. 'Mechanical thumbs'.
2. Minute volume dividers.
3. Bag squeezers.
4. Intermittent blowers.

'Mechanical thumbs'

Figure. 11.11a shows a simple T-piece system for spontaneous respiration (see p. 130). In Fig. 11.11b the anaesthetist has occluded the open end of the T-piece with his thumb. The force of the fresh gas flow inflates the patient's lungs until the anaesthetist removes his thumb from the open end, which allows expiration to occur (Fig. 11.11c). By rhythmical application of the thumb to occlude the T-piece, intermittent positive pressure ventilation (IPPV) is achieved. This is, therefore, an 'open-system' ventilator, which operates on the 'mechanical thumb' principle. In ventilators such as the *Sheffield* (Fig. 11.12) and *Amsterdam* (Fig. 11.13) the anaesthetist's thumb is replaced by an electrical solenoid valve, the cycling of which is achieved by an electronic circuit (Fig. 11.11d). A slide-rule or graph is supplied, from which one can calculate the relationships between tidal volume, inspiratory time, expiratory time and fresh gas flow. In the past decade great advances have been made in fluidics that make use of the Coanda phenomenon (p. 25). Fluidic timing devices have been devised which, requiring the minimum of maintenance, are very reliable and occupy little space. They are ideal for controlling this type of ventilator.

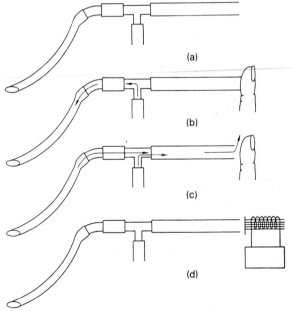

Figure 11.11 The T-piece principle and the 'mechanical thumb' (see text).

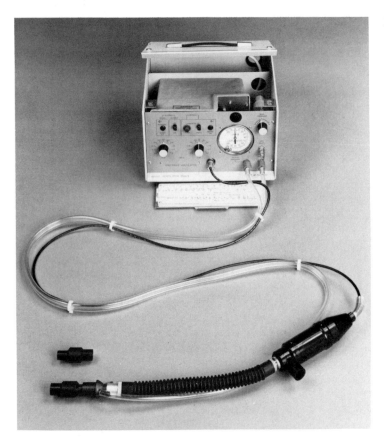

Figure 11.12   The Sheffield infant ventilator.

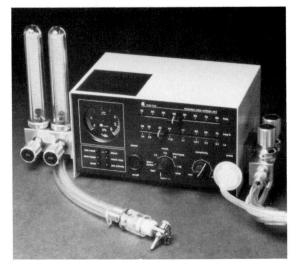

Figure 11.13   The Amsterdam paediatric ventilator.

Minute volume dividers

These ventilators derive their power from the pressure of gases from the outlet of an anaesthetic machine or a similar source. The whole of the driving gas is delivered to the patient and there is no rebreathing. If, for example, the fresh gas flow is 10 l/min, they deliver the 10 l to the patient, but it is divided into 'breaths' or doses of varying volume and frequency — e.g. 10 breaths of 1 l, 20 of 0.5 l, or 25 of 0.4 l.

The principle behind these ventilators is as follows:

A reservoir R, which is continually pressurized by a spring, a weight or its own elastic recoil (Fig. 11.14), is continually being filled by the fresh gas flow (FGF). Two valves, V_1 and V_2, are linked together and operated by a bistable mechanism. When V_1 is open and V_2 closed, the reservoir discharges gas to the patient, i.e. this is the inspiratory

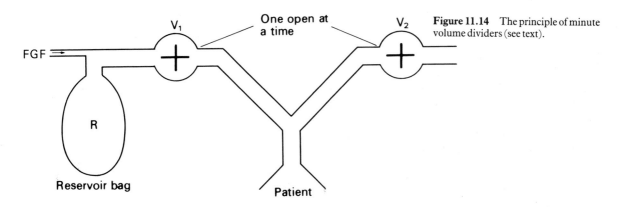

Figure 11.14   The principle of minute volume dividers (see text).

phase. When V_1 is closed and V_2 open, expiration is permitted and at the same time the reservoir bag is refilled.

Minute volume dividers are simple compared with many other types of ventilator and this makes them attractive to the trainee or non-mechanically minded anaesthetist. They are also relatively in-

expensive to purchase and maintain. Some examples of minute volume dividers are described below.

THE EAST–FREEMAN AUTOMATIC VENT (Fig. 11.15)

This replaces the APL (expiratory) valve in the Mapleson A (Magill attachment). The reservoir bag is best replaced by one of a heavy-duty material, since it is distended by a considerably greater pressure than occurs in spontaneous breathing. The valve body has three ports. The upstream one I is connected via a corrugated hose to the reservoir bag. Its aperture is occluded by the seating S on the closed end of the bobbin B, which also carries at its centre a small magnet M_1. The latter is attracted by

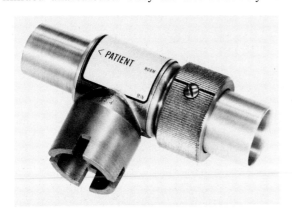

(a)

Figure 11.15   (a) The East-Freeman Automatic Vent. (b) and (c) Working principles. I, upstream port; P, patient port; E, expiratory port; B, bobbin; S, seating; M_1, M_2, magnets; G, gap that allows the exhaled gases to escape via the expiratory port. (See text.)

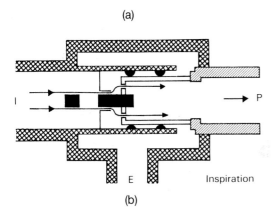

(b)

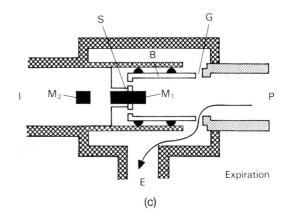

(c)

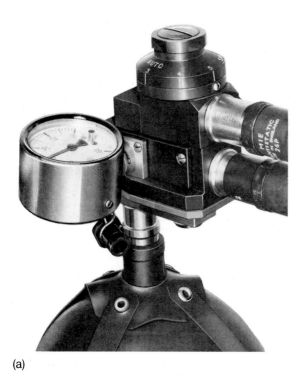

(a)

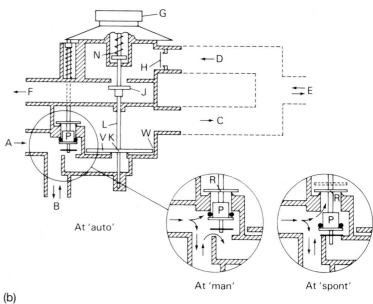

(b)

Figure 11.16   (a) The Flomasta ventilator. (b) Working principles. A, fresh gas inlet; B, reservior bag; C, inspiratory limb;
E, patient; D, expiratory limb; F, expired gas outlet; G, control knob. *For automatic and manual/assisted ventilation*: K, inspiratory
valve; V, disc of inspiratory valve; L, valve spindle; J, expiratory valve; N, spring; W, narrow orifice. *For spontaneous ventialation*:
P, inspiratory/expiratory valve; R, H, non-return valves. (See text.)

another magnet M_2, so that in the resting state the port is closed. Note that there is a gap G between the open end of the bobbin and the patient port P, so that the patient may exhale via the expiratory port E.

The FGF fills the reservoir bag and distends it until the pressure within it is sufficient to overcome the attraction between M_1 and M_2 and force B off S. B then moves downstream until it closes G. At the same time gases pass from the pressurized reservoir via the hose through holes in the periphery of the closed end of B and thus to the patient. (G being closed, they cannot escape via the expiratory port.)

As the reservoir empties the pressure falls and the mutual attraction of M_1 and M_2 returns B to its closed (resting) position. The expiratory phase then starts.

The only adjustments that can be made are to the FGF rate, and the separation of the magnets, which can be altered by twisting a ring on the valve body.

The Automatic Vent may be sterilized by cold methods, but care must be taken to avoid the ingress of grit, which could cause it to jam. A smaller reservoir bag should be used when treating children.

THE FLOMASTA (Fig.11.16)

The Flomasta is a considerably more sophisticated, yet very compact minute volume divider, which is mounted directly on the outlet of the continuous flow anaesthetic machine. A driving gas pressure of $10 - 60$ lb/in^2 (70–420 kPa) is required. The single control knob G has a number of settings: the function of the valve in each mode will be described separately. The reservoir bag is enclosed in a net, partly to avoid over-distension and partly to achieve the appropriate volume/pressure characteristics.

During *automatic ventilation* the fresh gases enter via the inlet A and pass into the reservoir bag B. The pressure within this part of the system rises until it is able to open the inspiratory valve K against the resistance of the spring N. When K opens the gases pass via the inspiratory limb C to the patient, but their escape via the expiratory limb D is prevented by the expiratory valve J (which is connected by the spindle L to the disc V of K), which is closed. The gases therefore pass around V, through a narrow orifice W, and this maintains a relatively high pressure under V until the end of inspiration. As the patient's lungs become distended and the flow through W diminishes, so the pressure difference

across V is reduced, and N successfully opposes the upward movement of V. K then closes and J opens, allowing the expired gases to pass to the atmosphere through the outlet F. From here they may be metered by a spirometer or led to a scavenging system. The point at which inspiration ends depends on the tension in N, which in turn is controlled by setting the control knob to one of the 'auto' positions 1, 2, 3, 4 or 5.

During *manual or assisted ventilation* the inspired gases pass through K, raising V and thus closing J. When manual pressure on the reservoir bag is relinquished, K closes and J opens, allowing the expired gases to escape.

During *spontaneous ventilation* gases are drawn by the patient through valve P, past the non-return valve R. At this stage he cannot inhale via D because the non-return valve H prevents this. During expiration valve P closes, H opens, and the patient may exhale through the expiratory port.

As optional extras, an airway manometer may be inserted into a small socket which is otherwise occupied by a blanking plug, and a Wright respirometer may be directly attached to the exhaust outlet which has a cage-mount (23 mm) taper. The Flomasta may be autoclaved, provided that the respirometer and manometer are first removed. The manometer is not likely to become contaminated when in use, since it is in the inspiratory port.

THE MANLEY MP2, MN2 AND MP3

The *Manley MP2* is a minute volume divider ventilator, in which the bistable system operates by a spring and lever and the inspiratory bellows are pressurized by an adjustable weight. There are several improvements of this simple arrangement, as shown in Fig. 11.17.

The main reservoir is a bellows B_2. During inspiration the fresh gas flow (FGF) is accommodated in a second bellows B_1, which when filled to a predetermined and variable volume trips the bistable system and initiates the expiratory phase. B_1 is loaded with a powerful spring so that during the expiratory phase it discharges into B_2 the gases that entered it during the inspiratory phase, to which is added the continuing FGF. When B_2 has filled to a predetermined volume the bistable mechanism is tripped in the other direction and inspiration starts again.

Inspiratory phase

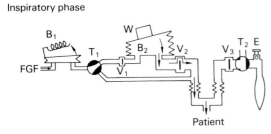

Expiratory phase: atmospheric

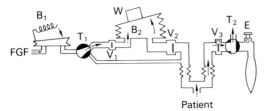

Manual or spontaneous

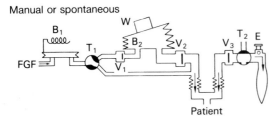

Figure 11.17   Working principles of the Manley MP2 ventilator. B_1, B_2 bellows; W, weight; V_1, V_2, V_3, valves; T_1, T_2, taps; E, expiratory valve. FGF = fresh gas flow. (See text.)

Valves V_1, V_2 and V_3 are linked together pneumatically so as to operate as shown below:

Phase	V_1	V_2	V_3
Inspiration	Closed	Open	Closed
Expiration	Open	Closed	Open

The degree to which B_1 fills before tripping, and therefore the inspiratory time, is determined by the setting of the 'inspiratory phase control'. The 'tidal volume control' may be set to regulate the degree to which B_1 is filled before the bistable mechanism is tripped to initiate inspiration. When the ventilator is used in the mode for spontaneous breathing, fresh gases pass directly to the patient, and the expired gases pass through tap T_2 to the reservoir bag and finally escape via the expiratory valve E. The inspiratory pressure is dependent on the distance

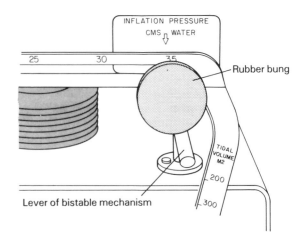

Figure 11.18   A rubber bung used to limit the length of the inspiratory phase.

between the weight W and the hinge (or fulcrum).

By adjusting the position of W to that giving maximum pressure, and by placing the rubber bung of an infusion bottle on the knob that secures it, the bistable mechanism may be made to trip as soon as B_2 has fully emptied, even if the inspiratory phase control had been set to give an inspiratory plateau (Fig. 11.18). Taps T_1 and T_2 change the mode of the ventilator between that for automatic ventilation and that for spontaneous or manual ventilation.

The *Manley MN2* (Fig. 11.19a) has a facility for a 'negative' (subatmospheric) expiratory phase, as shown in Fig. 11.19b. An additional bellows B_3 is mechanically linked to B_2 in such a way that it opens during expiration, drawing air from the patient. An air-inlet valve V_5 also allows the ingress of air once the subatmospheric pressure within B_3 has exceeded a level determined by the position of the weight on the control bar. During inspiration, when the bellows closes, the gases within it may escape via a flap valve V_6. The negative phase may be isolated by turning tap T_2 to an intermediate position. It is only in the latter mode that an expired air spirometer may be attached or scavenging effectively performed. V_4 is an expiratory valve through which those gases that do not pass to B_3 escape to the atmosphere.

To change the mode between automatic and spontaneous ventilation both taps T_1 and T_2 must be operated. This is a potential hazard since if they are turned in opposite directions, neither mode is achieved.

Another problem is that this ventilator may not be

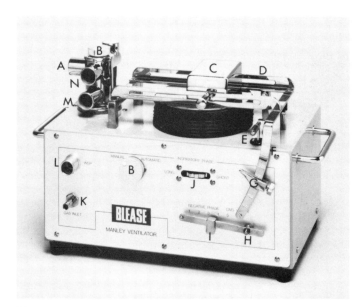

(a)

Expiratory phase: negative

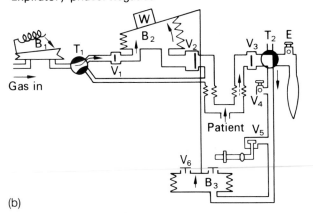

Gas in

Patient V$_5$

(b)

Figure 11.19 (a) The Manley MN2 ventilator. A, to spirometer (not with negative phase); B, control taps; C, sliding weight; D, slide; E, part of bistable mechanism; F, stroke volume selector; G, catch; H, negative pressure control; I, sliding weight; J, inspiratory time control; K, fresh gas inflow; L, to patient; M, from patient; N, to manual bag. (b) Working principles. A 'negative' phase has been added (compared with that shown in Figure 11.17). B$_1$–B$_3$, bellows; W, weight; V$_1$–V$_6$, valves; T$_1$, T$_2$, taps; E, expiratory valve. (See text.)

sterilized easily and quickly. The latter problem has been overcome in its successor, the *Manley MP3* (Fig. 11.20), in which the expiratory unit, complete with a condensation trap, may be detached very easily and autoclaved. This model also has facilities for a higher inspiratory pressure and stroke volume and incorporates an airway manometer. (The *Manley MN3* has a facility for a negative phase.)

THE MANLEY PULMOVENT (Fig.11.21)

The Manley Pulmovent is another minute volume divider ventilator, but its resemblance to the MN2, MP2 or MP3 is superficial only. The driving gases

pass directly to the main bellows B$_1$, which is housed within the cabinet. Cycling is achieved by the stroke volume, which may be varied by the tidal volume control. This ventilator is, therefore, a constant volume generator. The main bellows is closed by a powerful spring rather than by an adjustable weight as in previous models, and there is no provision for the adjustment of pressure. There is an inspiratory flow rate control and again (as in the MN2, MP2 and MP3) there are two controls that need to be adjusted in order to change from the automatic to the manual mode. The bellows B$_2$ surmounted on the top of the cabinet is the expiratory bellows, which may be used to produce a negative expiratory phase, though

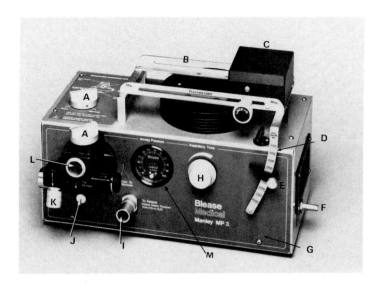

Figure 11.20 The Manley MP3 ventilator. A, control taps; B, slide; C, sliding weight; D, stroke volume selector; E, catch; F, gas inlet; G, alternative position of gas inlet; H, inspiratory time control; I, to patient; J, tap release knob; K, to bag; L, from patient; M, airway manometer.

positive end-expiratory pressure (PEEP) is also available by adjusting the valve NP. Some of the expired gases pass into a small reservoir bag R_1, from which they later enter B_2 during the early part of the expiratory phase. It is therefore not until the expiratory pause, when R_1 has completely emptied, that negative pressure is applied to the patient. The whole of the expiratory system may be removed for autoclaving.

THE BLEASE BM2 BROMPTON MANLEY
VENTILATOR (Fig.11.22)

The Blease BM2 Brompton Manley ventilator is another minute volume divider ventilator resembling the MN2, but it is intended primarily for intensive care, though it may be used equally well for anaesthesia. It may be stood on a flat surface or mounted on a wall-rail system. There is a primary reservoir bellows B_1, from which gases pass to the main bellows B_2, the pressure within which is determined by the position of the weight W. The whole of the expiratory system may be detached, including the negative pressure bellows B_3, which, although housed within the cabinet, may be withdrawn from below. Attached to the expiratory system is a water trap, which should be used if humidification of the inspired gases is employed. On the stroke volume arm there is a small metal block that can be adjusted in such a way that the bistable mechanism is tripped

as soon as B_2 is completely emptied. If it has not been adjusted accordingly, and does not strike the tripping mechanism, the inspiratory time is determined by the opening of B_1 and may be regulated by adjusting the inspiratory time control. There is also an inspiratory flow control and a manometer. In addition to a negative expiratory phase, there is provision for PEEP. This ventilator may, therefore, be used as a constant pressure or a constant volume generator and it may be either volume or time cycled.

THE PHILLIPS AV1 VENTILATOR (Fig.11.23)

This is a time-cycled minute volume divider ventilator. It is intended for both adult and paediatric anaesthesia and intensive care. The cycling is controlled by an electronic circuit and the length of the two phases can be independently varied, except that the inspiratory time cannot exceed the expiratory time.

The inspiratory and expiratory valves (cf. V_1 and V_2 in Fig.11.14) are each controlled by a solenoid (electromagnetic actuator), which in turn is activated by the timing circuit.

During inspiration (inspiratory valve open, expiratory valve closed) the patient's lungs are inflated by the fresh gas flow plus gas driven out of the bellows by the force of the spring. A cam is included in the linkage between the spring and the

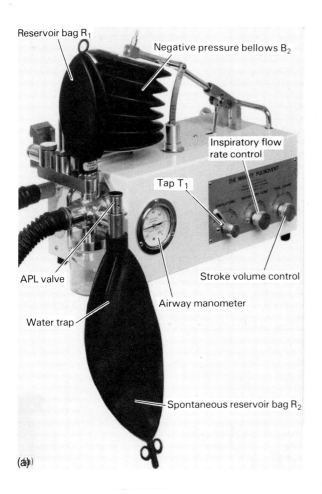

Reservoir bag R$_1$

Negative pressure bellows B$_2$

Inspiratory flow rate control

Tap T$_1$

APL valve

Water trap

Airway manometer

Stroke volume control

Spontaneous reservoir bag R$_2$

(a)

Figure 11.21 (a) The Manley Pulmovent ventilator. Superficially this resembles the Manley MN2, MP2 and MP3, but as will be seen in (b) the mechanism is quite different. The first bellows has been omitted and the fresh gas flow enters the main bellows B$_1$ directly. Whereas the MP2 is a constant pressure generator, in which the stroke volume may be influenced by the patient's compliance, the Pulmovent is a constant volume generator, in which it is the total closure of B$_1$ that leads to the cycling of the ventilator. B$_1$ is closed by a spring, for which there is no adjustment, rather than by an adjustable weight. A negative phase may be added, and is achieved (as in the MN2) by the addition of an extra bellows B$_2$ linked to B$_1$. However, the negative pressure is satisfied during the first part of expiration by the contents of the small reservoir bag R$_1$. Negative pressure is therefore applied only during the expiratory pause. A positive end-expiratory pressure may be achieved by the adjustment of the positive pressure valve NP. Valves V$_1$, V$_3$ and V$_5$ are linked so that when V$_1$ and V$_5$ are open, V$_3$ is closed and vice versa. Taps T$_1$ and T$_2$ must both be turned to change from automatic to spontaneous ventilation, and, in addition, T$_2$ may be turned further to include the negative phase. IF, inspiratory flow rate control; P, airway manometer; VC, stroke volume control; S, overpressure relief valve; C, D, corrugated hose; R$_2$, F and V$_6$, spontaneous breathing system; TV, expiratory tidal volume indicator; E, expirator port; W, trap for condensed water vapour.

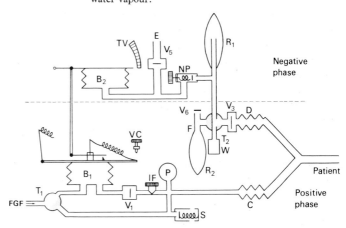

(b)

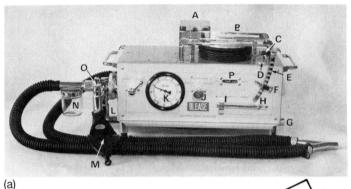

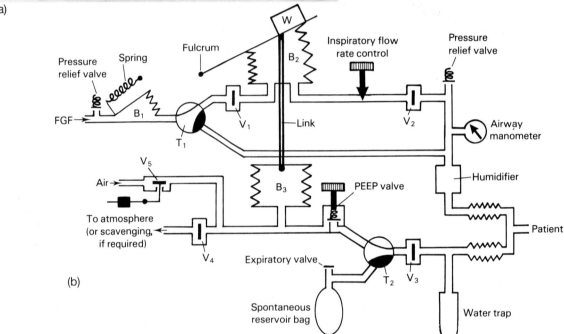

Figure 11.22   (a) The Blease BM2 Brompton Manley ventilator. A, sliding weight; B, slide; C, block; D, trip arm; E, stroke volume selector; F, catch; G, outlet to atmosphere (or scavenging, if required); H, negative pressure control; I, sliding weight; J, inspiratory flow rate control; K, airway manometer; L, PEEP valve; M, spontaneous reservoir bag; N, water trap; O, expiratory valve.
(b) Working principles. During automatic ventilation taps T_1 and T_2 are turned in the direction shown in the diagram. *During the inspiratory phase* the fresh gas flow (FGF) enters the reservoir bellows B_1, which is protected by a pressure relief valve. Valves V_1 and V_3 are closed and V_2 is open. The main bellows B_2 is closed by the weight W, and the gases in it pass to the patient via an inspiratory flow rate valve, valve V_2 and humidifier (if fitted). In this part of the system there is an airway manometer and a second pressure relief valve to protect the patient.

During the expiratory phase V_2 is closed and V_1 and V_3 are open. The fresh gases that had been stored in B_1 now pass to B_2 via V_1, being driven out of B_1 by the force of the spring. These gases and the continuing FGF refill B_2 to an extent determined by the setting of the catch on the stroke volume selector. The expired gases pass via V_3, the PEEP valve and the expiratory valve V_4 to the atmosphere or the scavenging system. The negative pressure bellows B_3, which is mechanically linked to B_2, may draw expired gases from the patient, but this depends on the setting of the negative pressure control V_5. If the weight on the latter is set so that there is no resistance, the ingress of atmospheric air will satisfy the filling of B_3 and no negative pressure will be applied to the patient. As the weight on V_5 is moved so as to cause loading of V_5, negative pressure is generated. Atmospheric air cannot enter via the expiratory valve V_4.

A bistable cycling mechanism consisting of a spring and levers opens and closes V_1, V_2 and V_3. As B_2 refills during the expiratory phase, the catch on the stroke volume selector impinges on the trip arm, pushing it upwards, causes the cycling mechanism to trip and the inspiratory phase to begin. The next change, from inspiration to expiration, is initiated in *volume cycling* by the catch on the stroke volume selector being positioned so that as B_2 reaches the 'empty' position it forces the trip arm down, so tripping the bistable mechanism. Alternatively, in *time cycling*, a lever attached to B_1 trips the mechanism when B_1 has filled to an extent determined by the setting of the inspiratory time control.

For spontaneous or manual ventilation, T_1 and T_2 are turned so that the FGF passes, via the humidifier, if fitted, directly to the patient, and expired air passes via V_3, which is held open, to the spontanous reservoir bag and escapes via the expiratory valve.

On account of the negative pressure system, accurate measurements with an expired spirometer cannot be made at the outlet.

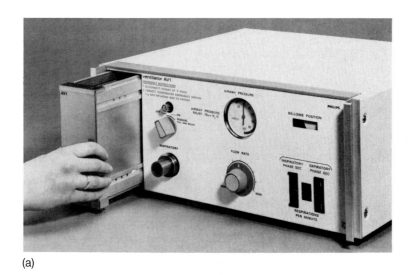

(a)

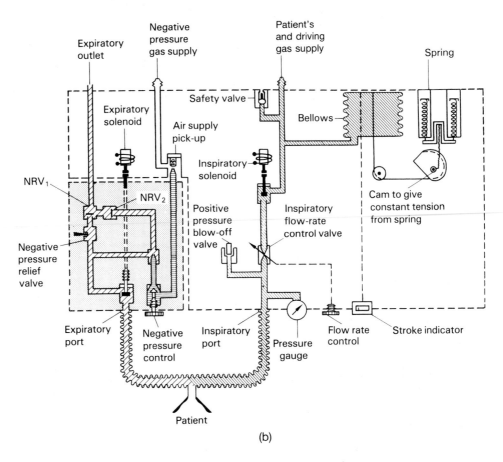

(b)

Figure 11.23 (a) The Phillips AV1 ventilator. (b) Working principles (see text).

bellows in such a way that the closing force acting on the bellows is constant, and therefore this is a constant pressure generator. There is a pressure limiting blow-off valve.

At changeover to expiration, the expiratory valve opens and the inspiratory valve closes. Expiration may be assisted by the application of negative pressure, which is achieved by the passage through a venturi of gas (not patient gas) from another supply. The amount of negative pressure applied is limited by the negative pressure relief valve. NRV1 and NRV2 are non-return valves in the negative pressure system.

During expiration the fresh gas flow refills the bellows.

The inspiratory flow rate can be controlled by a flow restrictor, and the airway pressure is indicated on a pressure gauge.

The expiratory part of the system (shaded in the diagram) can be removed from the ventilator for autoclaving, and a second one may be obtained in order to avoid delay between its use on one patient and the next.

Bag squeezers

This type of ventilator is usually used in conjunction with closed-circuit anaesthesia. It relieves the anaesthetist of having to squeeze the breathing bag and, apart from freeing him to do other things, offers the advantages of producing more regular ventilation, with controllable tidal volume and pressure, as well as the application of a negative phase.

The bag or bellows may be squeezed *mechanically* by means of a motor and suitable gears and levers, by a spring, or by a weight which may be adjusted to vary the pressure produced.

In the East Radcliffe ventilator, for example, the bellows is opened by an electric motor operating through a cam, and closed (during the inspiratory phase) by a weight.

In these mechanically driven ventilators it is often impossible to alter the relative lengths of the inspiratory and expiratory phases, and the inspiratory/expiratory ratio is usually somewhere between 1 : 1 and 1 : 2.

However, when the bellows is squeezed *pneumatically* the respiratory pattern can be varied. This is illustrated in the Blease (Deansway) Pulmoflator.

FUNCTION

If the bellows is compressed during inspiration by a weight, the pressure applied to the patient is limited by the mass of the weight. This type of ventilator is, therefore, called a *constant pressure generator*. It is important to note that the bellows may not be completely emptied if the weight is insufficient to overcome airway resistance or a poor compliance. The tidal volume delivered to the patient may therefore vary.

If the bellows is compressed mechanically by, say, a motor driving a series of gears and a crankshaft, it is emptied at every stroke. (The degree to which it is filled may, of course, be preset). The pressure developed depends on the resistance of the patient and the breathing system. A relief or 'spill' valve may be incorporated to allow the escape of gases at a preset pressure, thereby protecting the patient from over inflation. This type of ventilator is known as a *constant volume generator*.

Other ventilators act as constant flow generators, the pressure within the patient's airway and the tidal volume being determined by his compliance.

In pneumatically operated ventilators, such as the Blease Pulmoflators, one of which is shown in Fig.11.24, *limits* may be set to both volume and pressure, and these may be used in conjunction with time to control cycling.

THE BLEASE CYCLING BOX MECHANISM (Fig.11.25)

A knowledge of the working principles of the 'Blease box' is essential to the user of Blease or Deansway ventilators. The traditional model will be described here. Although it has been replaced over the years by improved versions, it is the easiest to describe and understand, and the principles remain the same. The large 'box' is divided into two compartments by a diaphragm A. On the left-hand side of the box there is a bistable tripping mechanism B which opens and closes an escape valve C. The rubber bellows D is suspended in a glass jar E, which is pneumatically continuous with the left-hand side of the box. Thus the air pressurizing the box also pressurizes E and acts upon D, though it does not mix with the anaesthetic gases contained in the latter.

Starting with C closed, air is delivered by an electric pump to the box via a delivery tube F. (For

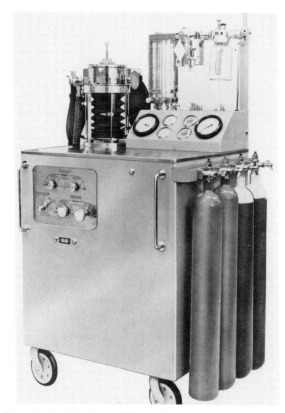

Figure 11.24 The Blease 5050 ventilator, showing the breathing system (top left) which may be detached for autoclaving.

If a second needle valve J is opened, some of the compressed air leaks through it so that A moves less quickly to the right during inspiration. This, therefore, determines the length of time of the inspiratory phase. The tension in H may be varied by the 'inspiratory pressure control'. The greater the pressure required to move A against its own elasticity plus the resistance of H, the greater is the pressure exerted in the box and therefore on D.

The excess gases from the breathing system are not expelled directly to the atmosphere but are fed to the left-hand side of the box during expiration via a tube K, in which a one-way valve L prevents them being driven back during inspiration. Within the box, K ends in a double venturi P, driven by the compressed air supply via F. The two nozzles N and O oppose each other and the compressed air is directed to one or both by the expiratory pressure control valve M. If one nozzle (N) is blowing, the escape of excess gases is assisted; therefore there is a negative expiratory pressure. Conversely, if the other nozzle (O) is blowing, the escape of excess gases is impeded, causing a positive expiratory pressure. A balance

the moment disregard M, N, O and P.) The pressure in the box rises, pushing A to the right and expelling air from the right-hand side of the box via a one-way valve G. At the same time the pressure in E rises, squeezing D (inspiration). As A moves progressively to the right it eventually trips B, and C is opened, allowing the air to escape. The pressure in the box and in E is now relieved, and D re-expands (expiration), this being assisted by a weight within it. The recoil of A, assisted by a spring H, would return it to its resting position, but since G will not allow air to re-enter, it is held to the right by 'negative' pressure. This, however, is relieved by admitting air through the expiratory time control needle valve I, the adjustment of which determines the length of time that A takes to return sufficiently far to the left to trip B, closing C and restarting the cycle.

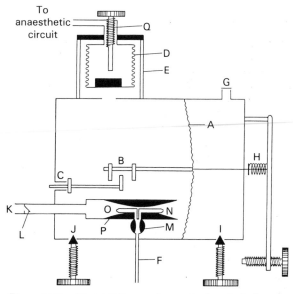

Figure 11.25 The 'old' Blease cycling mechanism. A, diaphragm; B, bistable tripping mechanism; C, escape valve; D, bellows; E, glass jar; F, delivery tube; G, one-way valve; H, spring; I, expiratory time control needle valve; J, inspiry time needle valve; K, tube along which excess gases are fed back to the box; L, one-way valve; M, expiratory pressure control valve; N, O, nozzles; P, double venturi; Q, stroke volume control screw. (See text.)

between these can be achieved. Note that during the early part of expiration the weight in D creates a negative pressure, but once D has fully descended the weight no longer operates and it is solely M that determines the expiratory pressure.

The excursion of D, and therefore the stroke volume of the ventilator, may be limited by a screw Q which projects into D and determines the distance by which its base is able to rise. It is secured by a lock-nut.

A relief valve prevents an excessive pressure developing in the box. This would happen only as a result of malfunction, but it could be relayed to the breathing system.

From the above it will be seen that the following functions may be adjusted:

$\left.\begin{array}{l}\text{Inspiratory time}\\ \text{Expiratory time}\end{array}\right\}$ and therefore $\left\{\begin{array}{l}\text{Inspiratory/expiratory ratio}\\ \text{Respiratory rate per minute}\end{array}\right.$

$\left.\begin{array}{l}\text{Inspiratory pressure}\\ \text{Expiratory pressure}\\ \text{Stroke volume}\end{array}\right\}$ to which limits may be set

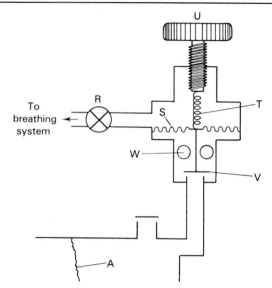

Figure 11.26   The patient triggering mechanism of the Blease cycling box. A, diaphragm; R, on/off tap; S, sensing diaphragm; T, spring; U, screw for adjusting force exerted by T; V, inlet valve; W, air inlet ports. (See text.)

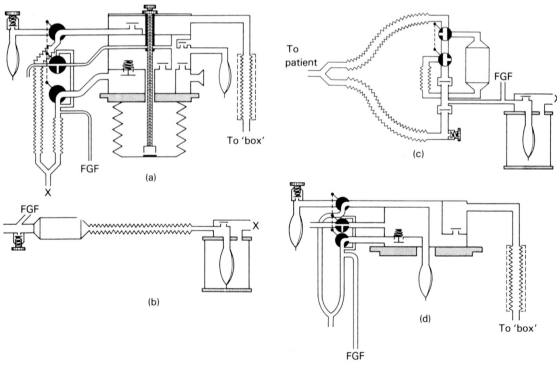

Figure 11.27   The breathing systems available for Blease Pulmoflaters (series 5000). (a) Non-rebreathing system. Note the connecting point X, for use with closed systems. The broken line indicates the position for fitting a bacterial filter, if required. (b) Closed 'to-and-fro' system, with connecting point X to the open system. (c) Closed-circle system, with connecting point X to the open system. (d) The paediatric system, in which a small bag replaces the bellows.

Patient triggering may also be achieved by the mechanism shown in Fig.11.26, as follows. The length of the expiratory phase depends on the rate at which air can re-enter the right-hand side of the box. If the patient's inspiratory effort could be made to affect this, A would be made to move more quickly to the left and the inspiration would begin sooner. This is achieved by the pressure in the breathing system being applied to S when the tap R is turned on. If the patient attempts to breathe, the slight negative pressure in the breathing system lifts S, thereby opening the inlet valve V, admitting air via the inlet ports W to the right-hand side of the box. By loading S with a spring T, the force of which is determined by the setting of the screw U, the additional negative pressure produced by P in the box may be balanced, so that any degree of negative phase may be employed with triggering (which is impossible with many patient-triggered ventilators).

The Blease series 5000 ventilators employ a 'box' working on similar principles. The breathing system can be removed and sterilized by autoclaving, and a filter may be inserted to prevent contamination by expired gases. The breathing systems available are shown in Fig.11.27.

The Blease Pulmoflators are heavy, bulky and expensive, but in the author's opinion they offer a fine control of respiratory pattern which commends them for use in general anaesthesia, rather than intensive therapy, and in particular for open chest operations. A thorough understanding of their mechanism is a prerequisite for their use.

THE CAPE VENTILATOR (Fig. 11.28)

The Cape ventilator is easily understood by nursing staff and is used in intensive therapy. For anaesthesia, it is surmounted by an anaesthetic head, with flowmeters and vaporizers, when it is known as the Cape Waine ventilator. The working principles of the latter are as follows:

A flame-proof electric motor drives a crankshaft 1 through a variable speed gear box. This, in turn, operates two cranks, 4 and 5, two cams, 2 and 3, and a tachometer. The rotation of the first crank 4 operates a lever 7 which opens and closes the main (inspiratory) bellows PPB. The extent to which PPB opens depends on the position at which the fulcrum

6 has been set. This is adjusted by the 'volume' control knob. The nearer the fulcrum is to the crank, the greater is the stroke volume. The first cam, 2, operates the inspiratory valve PV1, which permits gases flowing from PPB to pass to the breathing system and the patient. It opens a short while after PPB starts to close, thus causing a temporary rise of pressure, which serves to accelerate the gases and overcome their inertia. The expiratory valve PV2 remains closed during the inspiratory phase. Any excess pressure is relieved by an over-pressure valve SV2, the opening pressure of which may be pre-set up to 80 cmH2O. There is a manometer indicating the airway pressure.

During the expiratory phase PV1 closes and PV2 opens, PPB is reopened by 4 and fresh gases are drawn in through a unidirectional valve V1 from the reservoir bag SB1 and the flowmeters. The expired gases pass through the soda-lime canister and via PV2 and a unidirectional valve V6 to the first reser-

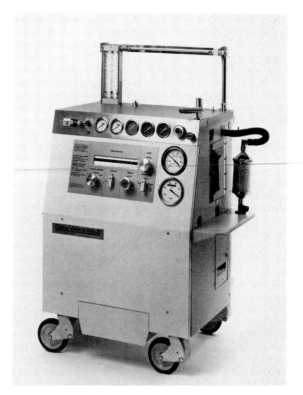

(a)

Figure 11.28 (a) The Cape Waine (anaesthetic) ventilator.

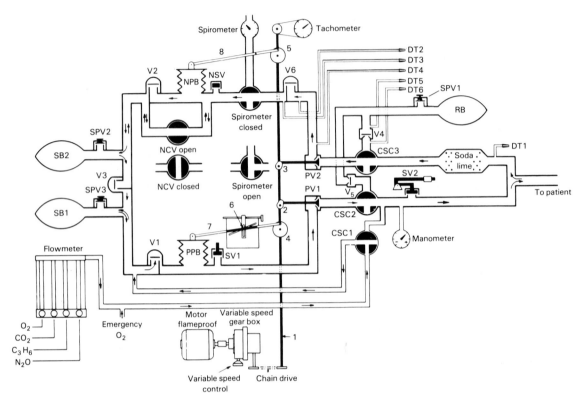

Figure 11.28   (b) Working principles. 1, crankshaft; 2, 3, cams; 4, 5, cranks; 6, fulcrum; 7, 8, levers; PPB, inspiratory bellows; NPB, negative pressure bellows; SB1, SB2, reservoir bags; RB, rebreathing bag; PV1, inspiratory valve; PV2, expiratory valve; SV1, SV2, overpressure valves; V1–V6, unidirectional valves; SPV1, SPV2, SPV3, APL valves; NCV, negative pressure valve; NSV, relief valve; CSC1, CSC2, CSC3, taps. (See text.)

voir bag SB2. At the same time the rotation of the second crank 5 operates a lever 8 which opens the negative pressure bellows NPB, but if the negative pressure valve NCV is open, this will draw in gases from SB2 rather than apply negative pressure to the patient. If NCV is closed, negative pressure is applied to the patient, and if this is excessive, air is drawn in through the relief valve NSV. When SB2 is full, gases pass from it through a unidirectional valve V3 to SB1 and will eventually pass again to

PPB. The two reservoir bags are surmounted with APL valves SPV2 and SPV3, which allow the escape of excess gases. There is also a valve that may divert the expired gases to a spirometer so that they may be measured. This valve is spring loaded so that it returns to its normal position when it is no longer held open by the anaesthetist. If either SB1 or SB2 is removed and its port left open, air may be drawn in. As the ventilator is intended for long-term use in the intensive care ward, a filter can be installed within the cabinet of the machine to prevent the ingress of infection or particles from the ambient air.

The rate per minute is indicated by the tachometer, which is also driven by the crankshaft.

Taps CSC1, CSC2 and CSC3 are mechanically linked to operate together. When the control is turned from 'Mech.' to 'Manual', these three taps are turned through 90° counter-clockwise from the configuration shown in Fig. 11.28b. The fresh gases then flow directly to the inspiratory limb of the breathing attachment and the expired gases to a bag RB from which they may be rebreathed, passing through valves V4 and V5. There is an APL valve SPV1 on the mount of RB to allow the escape of excess gases. The soda-lime canister may be removed, as desired, by the anaesthetist. Water may condense in various parts of the ventilator, particularly when a humidifier is installed, and is drained away by opening the small taps DT1 to DT6, which are located in the cabinet, below the soda-lime canister.

On the latest version, the control taps (CSC1, CSC2 and CSC3) may be depressed and turned to a third position, in which the fresh gases are diverted from the ventilator and pass directly to a Cardiff swivel outlet and a Magill attachment. Older models have a separate tap, but may be converted to provide the same facility

THE EAST RADCLIFFE VENTILATOR (Fig. 11.29)

The East Radcliffe ventilator is used for both anaesthesia and intensive care. It is driven by an electric motor which runs off the mains supply, but there is a second motor which operates from a 12 volts DC battery and may be used in an emergency. If all else fails, there is a handle by which the ventilator can be operated manually. As in the Cape Waine, the motor drives a crankshaft via a gearbox, in this case the Sturmey–Archer gear, which is commonly used in the pedal bicycle. There are two ranges of speed, high and low, of which that required may be selected by the insertion of the appropriate one of two locking plugs which are provided.

The inspiratory (positive pressure) bellows is surmounted by, and fixed to, a metal slide, which is hinged at one end and carries a series of adjustable weights. A large plastic snail cam is driven by the crankshaft; this raises the slide, complete with the weights, and because of their attachment to it, the bellows opens, drawing in air or anaesthetic gases, as the case may be. When the maximum diameter of the cam has passed, the slide is free to fall and this compresses the bellows. The gases from the bellows are unable to pass back through the pathway from whence they came, on account of a unidirectional valve, and pass via the humidifier (if fitted) to an inspiratory valve which is driven by another cam on the crankshaft. When the inspiratory valve is open, the expiratory valve, driven by yet another cam, is closed. The gases therefore pass to the patient. (Note that whereas in the Cape Waine the bellows opens and closes totally come what may, in the East Radcliffe, which is a constant pressure generator, the bellows closes only in accordance with the compliance of the patient, which is matched by the position of the weights on the slide.)

During the expiratory phase the inspiratory valve closes, the expiratory valve opens and the positive pressure bellows is refilled. The expired gases pass either to the atmosphere or are collected, to be returned to the patient, having passed, if required, through a carbon dioxide absorber.

The ventilator incorporates a spirometer, the control of which is spring-loaded so that it operates only as long as it is held in the 'On' position. There is also a negative pressure bellows which is closed by a cam and opened by a spring, the tension of which may be adjusted in order to regulate the degree of negative pressure applied.

Provision is made for the connection of a humidifier, and, in order to remove water resulting from condensation, there are water traps at the inspiratory and expiratory ports.

THE MANLEY SERVOVENT (Fig. 11.30)

Although the Manley Servovent bears a superficial resemblance to some of the minute volume dividers described above, it does, in fact, operate on an entirely different principle and is a bag squeezer. The driving gas, which may be compressed air or oxygen at a pressure of 45–60 lb/in^2 ($\sim$ 3–4 bar), does not reach the patient. Cycling is by a pneumatic logic device with controls for On/Off, expiratory time and inspiratory flow rate. There is also a stroke volume control which permits a maximum of 1300 ml. During the expiratory phase, the piston P of a pneumatic cylinder is driven by the driving gas and opens the bellows B. During the inspiratory phase,

P is returned by a pair of springs S, and B closes, driving the gas to the patient. The inspiratory flow rate control operates by varying a flow restrictor which 'strangles' the exhaust from the cylinder.

Within the breathing attachment there is a diaphragm-operated valve V_1, which is closed during inspiration by pressure from the control unit. Thus during the inspiratory phase the gases from the bellows can pass only to the patient (or to atmosphere via the safety valve). The airway pressure is shown on a manometer G. During expiration, V_1 opens and the exhaled gases from the patient can pass into the reservoir R. They may be augmented by the fresh gas flow (FGF). As B opens, gases are drawn from R and from the FGF. If there is insufficient volume, air may be drawn in through a non-return valve V_3. An excess of pressure in the reservoir is emptied by a relief valve V_2. It will be seen, therefore, that during the expiratory phase, and also when the control unit is turned off, the patient is able to breathe backwards and forwards into the reservoir, the gases being augmented by the FGF and excess gases being voided through V_2, which must *always* be kept open.

The whole of the breathing attachment, including the bellows, may be detached and sterilized by autoclaving. G is isolated by a bacterial filter, since it is not suitable for this treatment.

The driving gas requirement is fairly heavy (the manufacturers claim an average of 12 *l*/min). However, this ventilator may be used in conjunction with a circle absorption system and so the anaesthetic gas flow rate may be low.

THE OXFORD VENTILATOR (Fig. 11.31)

The Oxford ventilator may be used for both anaesthesia and intensive care. It is powered by compressed air and controlled by a pneumatic system (see p. 23). A bellows B containing the anaesthetic gases is operated by a pneumatic cylinder C. The direction of movement of the cylinder is controlled by a spool valve S_1. A second spool valve S_2 controls a smaller cylinder V which operates the expiratory valve of the breathing system. There is a lever on the piston of C which operates a trip valve, T_1 or T_2, at each end of its movement. The lengths of the inspiratory and expiratory excursion are thereby variable, altering the stroke volume of the ventilator. The inspiratory and expiratory flow rates

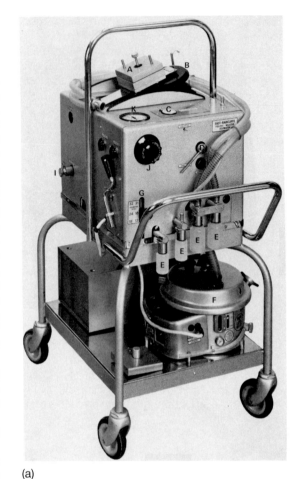

(a)

Figure 11.29 (a) The East Radcliffe ventilator. A, weights; B, bellows; C, spirometer; D, spirometer control; E, water traps; F, humidifier; G, changeover and rate lever; H, handle for manual operation; I, locking plug; J, negative pressure control; K, airway pressure gauge. (b) Working principles (see text.)

are adjusted by needle valves which 'strangle' the exhaust from the cylinder, thereby slowing its movement. The entire patient gas system may be removed from the ventilator for sterilization and the junction between the expiratory valve and the actuator is magnetic.

THE CAMPBELL VENTILATOR (Fig. 11.32)

The Campbell ventilator is a versatile ventilator which is controlled by a fluidic device and may be

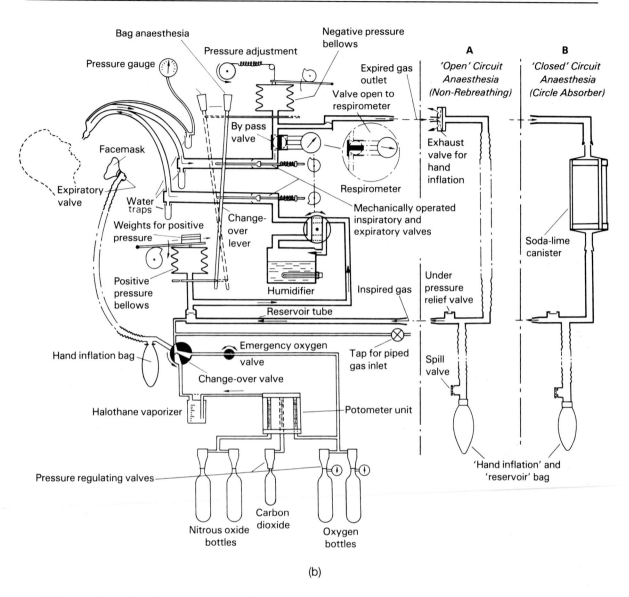

(b)

used in a number of modes, most commonly as a bag squeezer. The cycling system consists of a flip-flop fluidic element (see p. 26), which is controlled by monostable fluidic elements that are in turn controlled by timers, one for inspiration and another for expiration. The manufacturers advise that the driving gas be at a pressure of 50–70 lb/in² (~ 350–450 kPa) and claim that the consumption rate is 11 *l*/min during normal use. In the author's experience the driving gas consumption was considerably higher when a negative expiratory phase was used. The

ventilator is also rather noisy in operation. However, since there are no mechanically reciprocating moving parts, service maintenance is minimal and it is most reliable.

The basic mechanism, which is shown in Fig. 2.34 consists of a fluidic timer (the basic principles of which are described on p. 28), the output from the inspiratory side of which passes to a relay which injects a high-pressure jet into a venturi. The duration and frequency of this is determined by the setting of the controls in the timer system. The

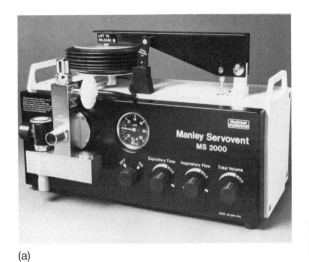

(a)

Figure 11.30 (a) The Manley Servovent ventilator. (b) Working principles (see text). The shaded portion is detachable for sterilization.

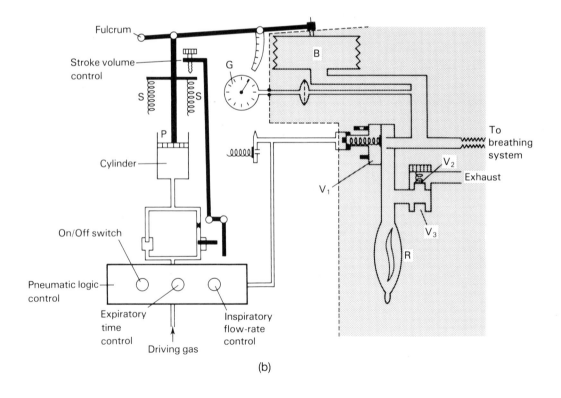

(b)

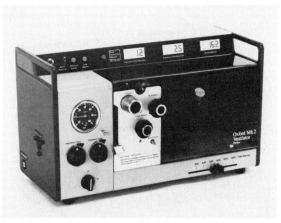

Figure 11.31   (a) The Oxford Mark 2 Ventilator. Note the electronic digital readout of functions, including inspiratory and expiratory times and respiratory rate. (b) Working principles. B, bellows; C, power cylinder; S_1, main spool valve; S_2, second spool valve; T_1, T_2, trip valves; V, cylinder controlling expiratory valve. A third spool valve, connected in parallel with the other two, controls the electronic readout facility but has been omitted from the diagram for the sake of clarity. The portion to the right of the diagonal line is detachable for sterilization.

(a)

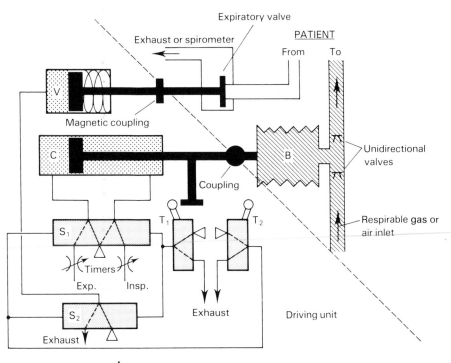

(b)

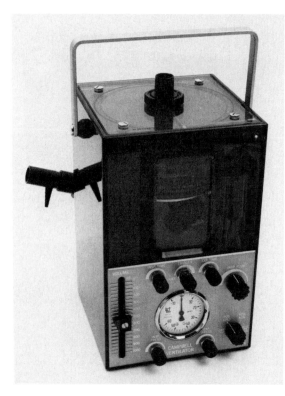

Figure 11.32   The Campbell ventilator. (The working principles are shown in Fig. 2.34.)

venturi may, if desired, entrain air or other gases, and its output may be attached to a variety of breathing systems. Positive and negative end-expiratory phases are available.

Intermittent blowers

These ventilators are driven by a continuous flow of gases or air, a pressure of 45–60 lb/in^2 ($\sim$ 3–4 bar) usually being required. Part only of the driving gas may be delivered to the patient, but by means of an injector air, oxygen or anaesthetic gases may be added to it.

THE BIRD MARK 7 VENTILATOR (Fig. 11.33)

The Bird Mark 7 ventilator is given as an example of an intermittent blower ventilator. It is not suitable for anaesthesia unless it is used in conjunction with a special anaesthesia assistor controller attachment, which is essentially a 'bag in a bottle' device. It is

more useful for the long-term ventilation of patients on oxygen, air or air–oxygen mixtures, and for respiratory therapy. It is driven by medical compressed air or oxygen.

The transparent plastic case C is divided into two compartments by the diaphragm D. Attached to D is a shuttle valve S, at either end of which are soft-iron plates P_1 and P_2. By virtue of the attraction of each of these plates to magnets, a bistable mechanism is created. The distance between each magnet and the adjacent plate (and hence the force of attraction between them) can be adjusted by the control knobs M_1 and M_2 at either end of the case.

During inspiration air passes from the inlet through S not only towards the patient through a wide-bore tube (which has been omitted in Fig. 11.33 for the sake of simplicity) but also to a second tube by which it closes the pneumatic expiratory valve E. The latter tube may also supply air to a nebulizer in order to humidify the inspiratory gases.

If required, air may be entrained by the venturi V to provide an air/oxygen mixture. It is drawn from the left-hand side of the case, which it enters through the filter F.

As the airway pressure increases during inspiration, the pressure within the right-hand side of the case rises until its influence upon D produces a force sufficient to overcome the magnetic attraction between P_2 and M_2. S, being bistable, moves rapidly to the left, P_1 being attracted by M_1.

Omitted from the diagram, for the sake of simplicity, is a smaller chamber bounded by a diaphragm which is reinforced by a spring. This chamber is pressurized during the inspiratory phase, thus moving the diaphragm against the tension in the spring. During the expiratory phase the driving gas is discontinued and the spring drives the diaphragm back to its resting position, at a rate determined by the setting of an expiratory time control needle valve, which allows air to escape from the smaller chamber.

To return to the shuttle valve S, when it moves to the left it interrupts the driving gas supply, the pressure in the right-hand side of the box falls to atmospheric, E opens and the expired gases escape to the atmosphere. As the gas slowly escapes from the smaller chamber, its diaphragm is returned to its resting position and a lever linked to it impinges upon P_1. When it does so with sufficient force to distract P_1 from M_1, the shuttle moves to the right and the cycle recommences.

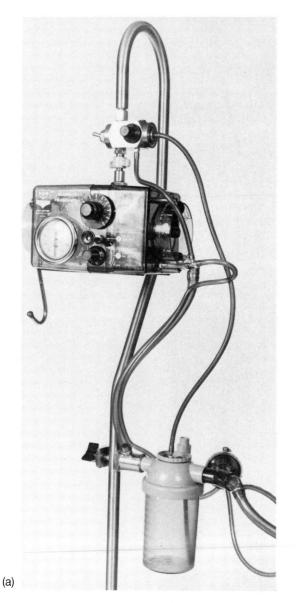

(a)

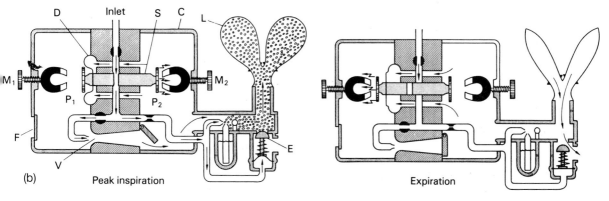

(b)

Figure 11.33 (a) The Bird Mark 7 ventilator. (b) Working principles. C, transparent plastic case; D, diaphragm; S, shuttle valve; P_1, P_2, soft-iron plates; M_1, M_2, magnets; E, pneumatic expiratory valve; L, lungs, V, venturi; F, air inlet filter. (See text.)

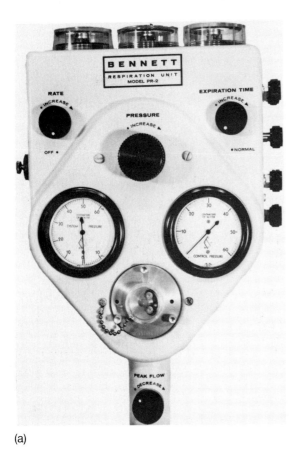

(a)

Figure 11.34 (a) and (b) The Bennett PR-2 ventilator.
(c) Working principles (to demonstrate the principle of a flow-
cycled ventilator). Many parts have been omitted from the
diagram for the sake of clarity. Insert shows the position of the
valve during expiration.

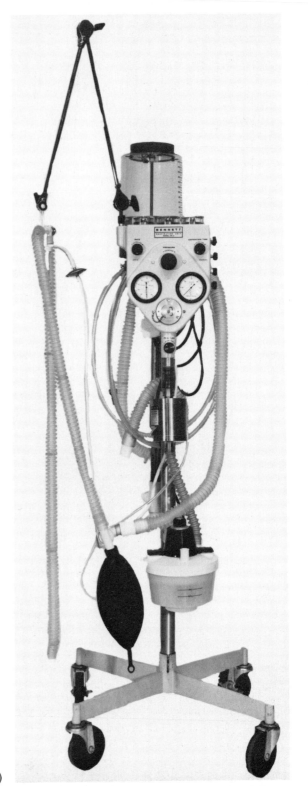

(b)

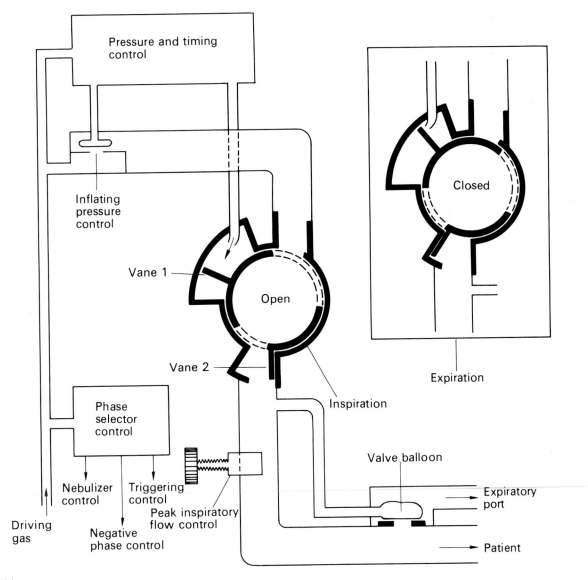

(c)

THE BENNETT PR-2 VENTILATOR (Fig. 11.34)

The Bennett PR-2 ventilator is used for intensive care and is not suitable for anaesthesia. It may be driven by compressed air or oxygen, and in the latter case air entrainment may be employed.

The Bennett valve consists of a cylindrical casing in which there is a rotating cylinder to which two vanes are attached. Pressure of gas acting on vane 1 opens the valve and, so long as the flow rate through the valve exceeds a predetermined level, the valve continues to be held in the 'open' position by pressure on vane 2 even when that on vane 1 ceases. When the flow rate falls below the predetermined level, owing to the resistance of the patient to further inflation, the valve closes. This is therefore a *flow-cycled* ventilator, although pressure and time limits, as well as patient triggering, can be applied. The system consists of three major parts, which we shall consider in turn:

1. The driving gas supply enters the 'inflating pressure control' and from there passes to the Bennett valve and to the patient. The pressure in the breathing system, which is indicated on a gauge, inflates the balloon in the expiratory valve, thereby closing the expiratory port. Another gauge shows the pressure at the output of the inflating pressure control.
2. The driving gas supplies the pressure and timing controls which initiate inflation and can also curtail it by closing the inflating pressure control.
3. The driving gas supplies the phase selector control which regulates humidification, negative phase and patient triggering.

There is a flow restrictor in the outlet of the ventilator which can restrict the peak inspiratory flow rate. There is also an expiratory spirometer available.

THE PNEUPAC AND PENLON A-P VENTILATORS (Figs 11.35–11.39)

These range from a small portable resuscitator to an anaesthetic ventilator, but since they all have the same working principle they will be described together. Each consists of a 'control module'* and a 'patient valve', and the difference between them lies in the extent to which their inspiratory and expiratory timers can be altered. For instance, the two Pneupac models for infants and children each have a single knob for tidal volume, which is actually the variable restrictor in the inspiratory timer. (Since the flow rate is constant, the stroke volume varies directly with time.) The Pneupac adult ventilator has no variables. In the Penlon A-P the inspiratory and expiratory times may be altered and there is also an inspiratory flow rate control.

The patient valve (Fig. 11.37) may be connected to the control module by a long narrow-bore tube, as in the Pneupac ventilator, or it may be attached directly to the control module, as in the Penlon A-P. It contains a piston P which in the resting state, under the control of the spring S, closes the inspiratory port and opens the expiratory port to permit exhalation.

During inspiration the pressure of gas from the control module acts on P with sufficient force to overcome S and so close the expiratory port and open the inspiratory port to the patient.

The Pneupac patient valve, in a special metal form, may be autoclaved, but the more commonly supplied plastic version should not be subjected to temperatures above 90 °C. It may be sterilized by any cold chemical agent.

---

* The term 'module' is, strictly speaking, an arbitrary unit of measurement used in the building and other industries to describe and standardize the sizes of the various units used. Recently the term has been wrongly employed to describe any units that may be connected together regardless of their size and shape.

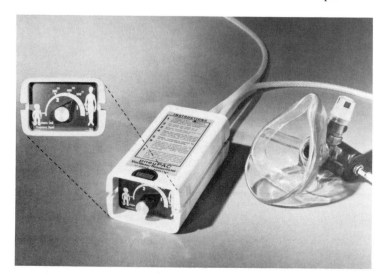

Figure 11.35 The Pneupac child/adult ventilator.

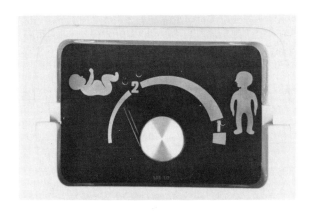

Figure 11.36   The Pneupac child ventilator.

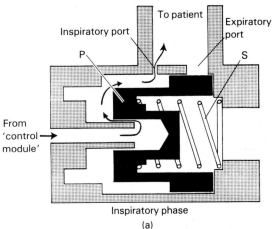

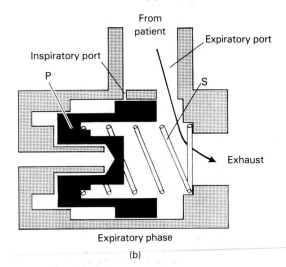

Figure 11.37   Working principles of the Pneupac patient valve. (a) Inspiratory phase. (b) Expiratory. P, piston; S, spring. (See text.)

The Pneupac ventilator

The control module (Fig. 11.38) consists essentially of a spool valve B and two timers, one for the inspiratory phase and the other for the expiratory phase. The spool valve has five ports and there is a pneumatic actuator at each end. Each timer contains a piston which is driven by gas that is metered by a flow restrictor and stored in a capacitator till the pressure is high enough to actuate the piston. When this happens, driving gas is delivered to the end of the spool valve, driving the spool to the opposite end.

The driving gas, which may be oxygen, a nitrous oxide/oxygen mixture or compressed air at a pressure of 35–90 lb/in^2 ($\sim$ 2.5–6 bar), enters the control module at A, passes through a filter F, a pressure regulator R and then to port 1 of B. When the spool is to the left-hand side of the control module, the gas passes from port 1 to port 2 and then on via a flow controller C to the patient valve. This is the inspiratory phase. From port 2 the gas also passes to the inspiratory timer I, where it is metered by the flow restrictor 8, which on the inspiratory side is variable. As the inspiratory flow rate is constant, this control determines the stroke volume. At the end of the time determined by the setting of 8, the timer operates and the gas passes via port 6 to the actuator at the left-hand end of B, driving the spool to the right-hand side of the control module. This is the end of the inspiratory phase. The driving gas entering B at port 1 now leaves by port 3 and passes to the expiratory timer E. The sequence of events now repeats itself, except that there is a fixed restrictor 9 in the expiratory timer and therefore a constant expiratory time. When the expiratory timer operates, the gas passes to B by port 7, driving the spool back to the right-hand side of the control module, initiating the next inspiratory phase. Trapped signals (see p. 24) are vented at ports 4 and 5.

In some versions of the control module both timers are variable, and in others both are fixed.

The Nuffield anaesthesia ventilator, series 200 (Fig. 11.39)

This is an elaboration of the Pneupac ventilator. Here, the patient valve is connected directly on to the control module and there are variable inspira-

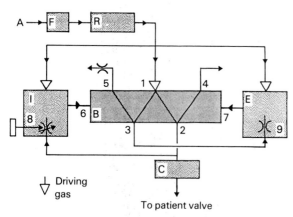

Figure 11.38 The Pneupac control module. A, point of entry of driving gas; F, filter, R, pressure regulator; B, spool valve, with ports 1–5; I, inspiratory timer; 8, 9, flow restrictors; E, expiratory timer; C, flow controller. (See text.)

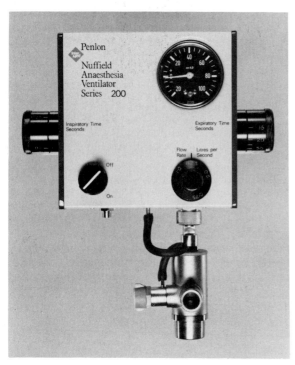

Figure 11.39 The Penlon Nuffield anaesthetic ventilator. The mechanism of this is similar to that of the Pneupac (p. 232). There are both inspiratory and expiratory timers, an airway manometer and a flow restrictor which controls the inspiratory flow rate.

tory and expiratory timers and a variable inspiratory flow rate control. There is also an airway manometer and an on/off switch.

Jet ventilators

There are two ways in which a high-pressure jet may be used to ventilate a patient.

1. SIMPLE JETTING — SHORT TERM

For short procedures such as bronchoscopy, a patient may be paralysed and then ventilated by applying an intermittent jet via the bronchoscope (Fig. 11.40). By the venturi effect, air is entrained by the driving gas, which is usually oxygen, at a pressure of up to 60 lb/in^2 ($\sim$ 4 bar). The jetting may be regulated by hand. Anaesthesia is maintained intravenously.

Alternatively, for procedures such as microlaryngeal surgery, oxygen or a gaseous mixture may be delivered via a Carden tube (see Fig. 7.52) which is inserted into the trachea entirely below the larynx. With only the narrow bore catheter passing through the larynx, the vocal cords may be easily seen and operated on by the surgeon. Exhaled gases pass to the atmosphere by the natural air passages.

The Carden jetting device (Fig. 11.41) may be run from a 60 lb/in^2 ($\sim$ 4 bar) pipeline outlet, from a cylinder with an appropriate pressure regulator, or from a blender for oxygen and air or oxygen and nitrous oxide. It includes a variable pressure regulator and a pressure gauge. It is intended for short-term application only.

2. HIGH-FREQUENCY JET VENTILATION

This technique, which is now in its infancy, has so far been used mainly in the intensive care ward, but some workers consider that it will also replace, in many instances, IPPV at the customary rate of 10–

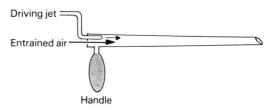

Figure 11.40 A simple jetting device attached to a bronchoscope (see text).

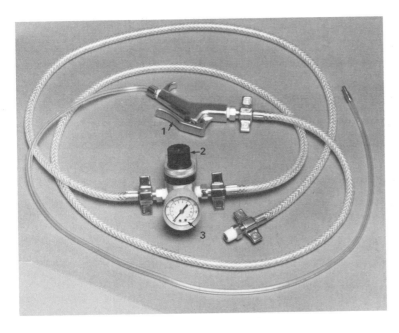

Figure 11.41   The Carden jetting device.
1, trigger; 2, pressure regulator;
3, pressure gauge.

20 breaths per minute in anaesthetic techniques. Its claimed advantages are that it has a less undesirable effect on the cardiovascular system, that the apparatus is relatively simple and that it is effective when there is a leak in the system, such as a bronchopleural fistula, or when suction is being applied to the trachea for the removal of secretions. To many experienced anaesthetists a comparison will be drawn with insufflation anaesthesia, dating back to the year 1910. In the latter a constant blast of air or oxygen with ether or chloroform was blown down the catheter. (Hence the term catheter mount!) Although the patient remained reasonably oxygenated, the PCO_2 (then not measured) rose considerably.

With high-frequency jet ventilation, the patient is well oxygenated and the clearance of CO_2 is efficient. Some of the clinical problems of a raised mean intrathoracic pressure, especially when PEEP is used, are much reduced. The factors leading to these problems are:

1. A large tidal volume.
2. A long inspiratory time.
3. An inspiratory plateau.
4. PEEP.

A *low* mean intrathoracic pressure is produced by:
1. A small tidal volume.

2. A short inspiratory time.
3. No inspiratory plateau.
4. No PEEP.

A tidal volume of 30–300 ml is used with a respiratory rate of 120–240 per minute, though 200 per minute is probably the optimum.

There is a variety of means of introducing the jet — from an intravenous cannula inserted into an endotracheal connector or through the cricothyroid membrane, to a narrow-gauge catheter inserted into the trachea.

Fluidic, rather than electrical, mechanical or pneumatic devices, would seem to be the most suitable for cycling high-frequency ventilators, and one such device is shown in Fig. 11.42, and a diagram of a fluidic switching system with a pneumatic actuator is shown in Fig. 11.43.

It is interesting to note that recent attempts at insufflation anaesthesia with a continuous flow of gases via a tracheal catheter have had results less favourable than those reported several decades ago. A possible explanation for this discrepancy is that while modern pressure regulators give a steady flow, older models were prone to oscillate. Perhaps high-frequency ventilation was being used unwittingly.

In a single chapter it is impossible to describe

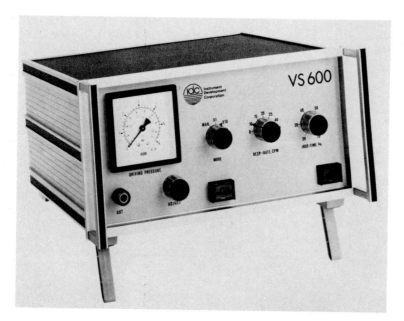

Figure 11.42   A high-frequency jet ventilator.

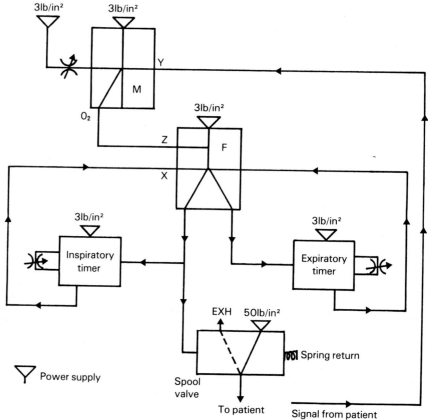

Figure 11.43   A fluidically controlled ventilator. Compressed air or oxygen at a pressure of 3 lb/in² supplies two fluidic logic elements and two fluidic timers. The element F is a flip-flop logic, and outputs of which control the inspiratory and expiratory timers. During inspiration the output of F is applied to the spool valve and the 50 lb/in² supply is directed to the patient. The change to the expiratory phase will occur either as a result of the output from the inspiratory timer at X, or as a result of the pressure in the patient's airway rising to such an extent that it passes through Y, causing the fluidic element M to switch to the output O₂ and thus produce a signal Z which causes the bistable element to switch to the expiratory mode. EXH = exhaust.

more than a few of the very many ventilators now available.

Most of those that have been described are mainly, but not exclusively, designed for use in anaesthesia rather than intensive care. Each is taken as an example of a particular mode of operation or application. For a more comprehensive review of ventilators the reader should consult a text such as *Automatic Ventilation of the Lungs* by Mushin, Rendell-Baker, Thompson and Mapleson (Blackwell Scientific, 1980).

Humidification of Gases

When a patient is treated on a ventilator over a prolonged period of time it is necessary to humidify the dry gases in order to prevent damage to his respiratory tract, which could arise because his respiratory mucosa, which normally humidifies the inspired air, is bypassed by the endotracheal or tracheostomy tube. The gases from cylinders are dry, as opposed to atmospheric air which, except when very cold, contains a considerable amount of water vapour.

Most ventilators, with the exception of some of the minute volume dividers, are suitable for use in conjunction with humidifiers, details of which are given in Chapter 13.

The position of the humidifier in the breathing system is of importance when considering the sterilization of the ventilator. Humidifiers can become reservoirs of infection, especially on closed-circuit ventilators, and provision should be made either for the installation of a bacterial filter or for the detaching, emptying and sterilization of the humidifier; alternatively, the humidifier may be used in situ to vaporize sterilizing agents to treat the whole ventilator.

Sterilization of the Interior of Ventilators

Sterilization is particularly important when a ventilator has been used on a patient with a respiratory infection. In the case of many ventilators, such as the Blease Pulmoflator, P5 or P11T, full sterilization is difficult, or impossible, without a complete mechanical dismantle and overhaul of the apparatus, and reliance may be better placed on bacterial filters.

The breathing attachments carrying air or gases to and from the patient may be sterilized by one of the methods described below, but contaminated moisture may remain in the exhaust limb and give rise to contamination of the gases being vented to the atmosphere. A bacterial filter may be used to prevent such contamination. Bacterial filters must be re-sterilized or replaced at regular intervals to prevent them becoming reservoirs of infection, helping to spread rather than to prevent it. A bacterial filter may also become blocked with particulate matter or condensed water and act as a resistance to the flow of gases. The Williams anaesthetic filter (Fig. 11.44) may be sterilized by autoclaving or by using ethylene oxide. This should be done between cases or after every 72 hours of use.

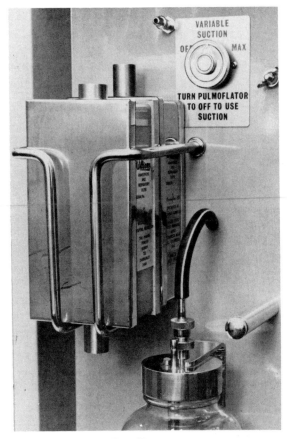

Figure 11.44 The Williams filter.

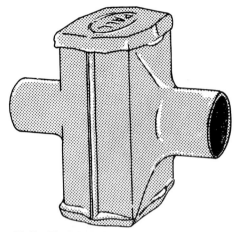

Figure 11.45   The Pall Ultipor disposable bacterial filter.

More recently, disposable bacterial filters, such as the Pall Ultipor (Fig. 11.45), have been developed. These are constructed of hydrophobic material and are not only efficient as filters but present very low resistance and are inexpensive. Some ventilators, such as the Blease 5050 (Fig. 11.24), have been designed in such a way that the whole breathing system can be removed and autoclaved. A bacterial filter at the point where the exhaust gases pass to the 'box' may be used to prevent the contamination of those parts of the ventilator that cannot be sterilized. It should be remembered that not only the breathing attachment but also the whole ventilator, including the interior of the casing, may need to be decontaminated.

Ventilators may be classified by considering the suitability of the breathing system for sterilization. In Class 1 ventilators, engine-driven ventilators with a closed circuit (Fig. 11.46), the whole ventilator may become contaminated if used on closed circuit. If it has been used without rebreathing, only the expiratory portion needs treatment. A filter fitted at F would prevent contamination. Although Class 2 ventilators, which are gas driven (Fig. 11.46) do not permit rebreathing, the patient's expired air is returned to the ventilator for control and sometimes measurement of tidal volume. The expiratory limb acts as a reservoir of infection, which will later be discharged into the ambient atmosphere though not directly to the patient. Again a filter fitted at F would prevent contamination.

In Class 3, 4 and 5 ventilators (Fig 11.46), only a small portion of the ventilator requires sterilization, and often this is very easy to perform. Some types are suitable for autoclaving.

The decision as to when to sterilize a ventilator is a clinical one, but most anaesthetists agree that this should be done after all prolonged cases where respiratory infection is present.

Many anaesthetic ventilators in the operating theatre are never sterilized, and although this negligence should not be condoned it must be accepted that sterilization after every case is not practical where the construction of the ventilator renders the process time consuming and complicated. The more common use of filters would seem prudent.

The breathing tubes and reservoir bags should be decontaminated in the same way as those on the anaesthetic machine at the end of every day's work, if not more often.

Before any ventilator or component part is sterilized, the manufacturer's instructions should be consulted. Agents such as formaldehyde and hydrogen peroxide which may be suitable for one ventilator may cause irreparable damage to another.

Accessories that may be Used in Conjunction with Ventilators

Alarm giving warning of failure

An apnoea alarm may be connected to a ventilator to give a warning of failure, e.g. due to interruption of the power supply. If such an alarm is activated by airway pressure, it also indicates the accidental disconnection of the ventilator from the patient.

It is necessary to make provision for the alarm to operate even when the mains electric supply fails. Figure 11.47 shows the East Ventilarm pressure monitor, which claims to give warning of the failure of the ventilator, leaks from the circuit, and excess pressure owing, for example, to obstruction of the breathing system. This type of monitor is more useful in the intensive care ward, where patients are treated by ventilation over prolonged periods and where continuous observation of ventilator and patient may be difficult to ensure.

Ventilation rate meter

The ventilation rate meter indicates the frequency in

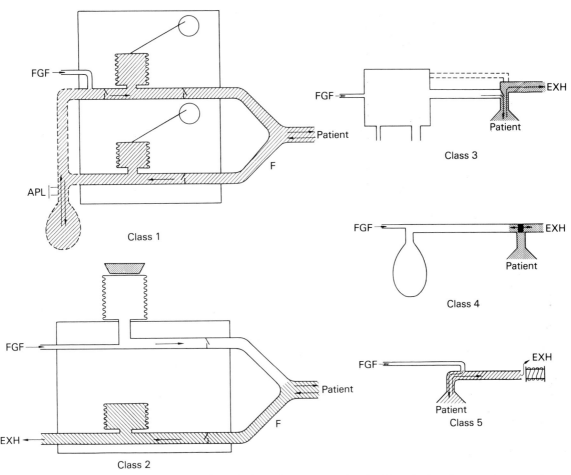

Figure 11.46 Classification of ventilators according to the breathing system employed, with particular reference to the extent of contamination by the patient and the need for sterilization. FGF = fresh gas flow. EXH = exhaust (to scavenging system, if required).

Class 1—Engine-driven closed-circuit anaesthetic ventilators, such as the Cape Waine. Since the expired gases are stored in a reservoir and then returned to the inspiratory side, the whole of the breathing system becomes contaminated and requires sterilization. The filter shown in Fig. 11.45 may be fitted at F to prevent such contamination. If the reservoir bag is removed and there is no rebreathing, then only the expiratory side becomes contaminated.

Class 2—Gas-driven ventilators, such as the Manley MN2 or MP2. Only the expiratory side becomes contaminated. In the case of the MP3, this may be detached for sterilization.

Class 3—Gas-driven ventilators, such as the Bird Mark 7. Only the expiratory valve becomes contaminated and may easily be sterilized.

Class 4—Minute volume dividers, such as the East–Freeman automatic vent. Only the valve itself and the expiratory limb become contaminated.

Class 5—The mechanical thumb. The whole attachment except for the fresh gas delivery tube becomes contaminated.

cycles per minute of the ventilator and, in conjunction with measurement of the tidal volume, gives an indication of the minute volume.

Spirometer

It may be necessary to measure the patient's tidal volume during ventilation. This should be done by connecting a spirometer to the expiratory limb of the

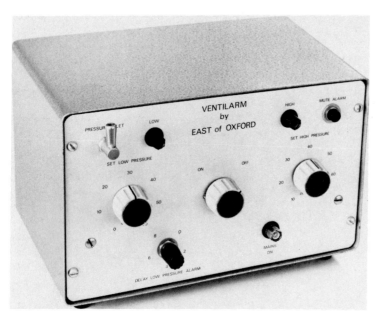

Figure 11.47   The East Ventilarm.

breathing system. Measurements on the inspiratory side may be rendered inaccurate by reason of losses or leaks from the system. These losses may be due to a leak from around the endotracheal tube or from any other part of the breathing attachment. Elongation, under pressure, of the breathing tubes and also a small element of compression of the gases also cause 'losses' of stroke volume. The loss due to compression may well amount to 100 ml in ventilators where the apparatus volume is high. These losses are far less evident in the expiratory side, since the pressure is nearer to atmospheric.

The Wright respiration monitor is shown on p. 270.

Accessories for positive end-expiratory pressure (PEEP)

Some slowing of the gas flow during expiration or even a PEEP may be required to prevent trapping or terminal airway closure in the patient. This may be achieved either by installing a flow restrictor or a spring-loaded valve in the expiratory side of the breathing system or by creating a positive pressure as in the Blease cycling mechanism.

Selection of a Ventilator for a Particular Situation

There are two main considerations to be borne in mind. First, the selection of a ventilator will depend on whether it is to be used as part of an anaesthetic technique or for long-term ventilation of a patient in the intensive care ward, Secondly, the pneumatic characteristics of the ventilator should be considered.

A classification of ventilators by Grogono describes the ability of the ventilator to perform according to the settings made. The three functions, minute volume, tidal volume and inspiratory flow rate are considered separately. Each is described as being either *stable* or *flexible*. For example, in a minute volume divider, the minute volume delivered to the patient equals the minute volume input of the driving gases, i.e. it is stable. In a motor-driven ventilator, such as the Cape Waine, the stroke volume is set and, as it is a constant volume generator, this volume is always achieved; therefore it too is stable. With a Manley ventilator, if the bellows pressure is low, the tidal volume will be flexible, since the bellows may not be emptied at each stroke. But if the pressure is high, the bellows will completely close at each stroke and the tidal volume will be stable.

When classifying ventilators in this way it is important to consider not only stability or flexibility with respect to the compliance of the patient, but also the effect of leaks on the efficiency of ventilation. For instance, in the case of a constant volume generator such as the Cape Waine, a leak will result in a reduced tidal volume. On the other hand, the airway pressure gives a good indication of changes in the patient's compliance, and this is useful particularly in the intensive care ward. Other ventilators may, however, compensate for leaks.

Features in respect of which ventilators may be classified

1. *Application.* Intensive care — anaesthesia.
2. *Breathing system.* Closed — open — T-piece.
3. *Driving force.* Compressed air or gas — electric motor — minute volume dividers.
4. *Function.* Constant pressure — constant volume — constant flow.
5. *Method of cycling.* Time — volume — pressure — patient triggering.
6. *Respiratory pattern.* Fixed — variable — negative phase — plateau — positive end-expiratory pressure.
7. *Performance.* Flexible/stable.
8. *Sterilization.* Impossible — difficult — simple.
9. *Portability.*
10. *Paediatric system.* Primary design — by adaptation.

12

Equipment for Paediatric Anaesthesia*

Various items of equipment required for paediatric anaesthesia have already been described in the appropriate chapters. It is important to understand the reasons why these differ from those employed for anaesthetizing adults. When selecting apparatus for paediatric anaesthesia, account must be taken of the physiological, anatomical and mechanical factors involved, which differ from those that present when adults are being anaesthetized.

Physiological differences between adults and children

In neonates and small infants, the respiratory pattern tends to be sinusoidal, there being no expiratory pause. This would render inefficient a system such as the Mapleson A, in which the voiding of expired gases during the expiratory pause is important.

The alveolar ventilation in small infants needs to be about double that of an adult, on a weight-for-weight basis.

The respiratory rate is high, with a small tidal volume, so that dead space, whether it be physiological or that of the apparatus, becomes a high proportion of the tidal volume. Even a small dead space may render ventilation inefficient, thereby adding to the work required in breathing. The fast

respiratory rate, with a relatively high peak inspiratory flow rate, requires rapid changes in gas flow. If the volume of the breathing system is high, this requires considerable kinetic energy in repeatedly reversing the direction of flow of the gases within it. Resistance to flow is also an important factor.

From a consideration of the foregoing, it will be appreciated that a scaled-down version of a breathing system designed for, and satisfactory in, adult anaesthetic techniques is not necessarily suitable for infants.

Heat loss may be an important factor in the management of infants, and steps may have to be taken to warm the inspired gases, ambient atmosphere and infusion solutions, and radiant heaters and insulating or heated blankets may have to be used. A further cause of heat loss is that involved when dry, rather than humidified, gases are delivered to the patient, and work is done in the normal physiological process of humidification within the respiratory tract.

Anatomical differences between adults and children

The air passages of an infant being narrow, the external diameter of paediatric endotracheal tubes is small. The wall of the tube, which must be sufficiently robust to prevent obstruction by kinking or compression, occupies a considerable proportion of its cross-sectional area, so that the lumen is small even compared with that of the trachea. Thus the effective diameter of the air passages may be reduced by intubation to a proportionately greater degree in infants than in adults.

The anatomy of the larynx of an infant or small child is different from that of an adult. In the former the narrowest part is at the cricoid ring and is circular in cross section. For this reason a plain, rather than a cuffed, tube is appropriate and one may be chosen which is a snug fit, thus permitting minimal leakage.

Mechanical factors for consideration in paediatric anaesthesia

Even when scaled down, the type of breathing attachments and components employed for adults are too cumbersome and have too high a dead space for use in infants. It should be remembered too, that

---

* For the purposes of this chapter the patient is defined as a neonate up to the age of one month, as an infant from one month to two years, as a young child from two to seven years, as a child from seven to 14 years, and as a young adult from 14 to 18 years.

242

if the diameter of a tubular component is reduced by half the resistance to laminar gas flow is increased sixteen-fold (resistance $\propto 1/r^4$, where r is the radius of the tube). In addition, the flow velocity is quadrupled for the same flow rate (litres per minute), and hence there is the likelihood of causing turbulence which increases even further the resistance.

For small children, therefore, specially designed breathing systems and components are used. For children over the age of three years (15 kg) or so the Magill attachment (Mapleson A) may be used for techniques employing spontaneous ventilation, although some paediatric systems are suitable for larger children.

The Anaesthetic Machine

The choice of an anesthetic machine is not difficult. A continuous flow machine is needed: intermittent flow or draw-over machines require too much inspiratory effort by the patient and are therefore unsuitable for small children, with the single exception that in dental-chair anaesthesia of short duration, varying flow machines, such as the McKesson intermittent flow machine, the AE or the Walton Five, may be used provided that the 'pressure' control is advanced sufficiently to give an adequate fresh gas flow (FGF) rate.

The vaporizer should be of a type that gives an accurate percentage of vapour, even when low flow rates are used. Nevertheless, in most instances a relatively high FGF rate is employed.

There should be a pressure relief valve at the end of the back bar, particularly where the regulated pressure is high (i.e. 60 lb/in², ~ 4 bar). Perhaps this should open at 60 cmH2O pressure, though arrangements for it to be more heavily loaded or provided with a manual over-ride should be made in order to facilitate the treatment of small patients with very poor pulmonary compliance or to drive minute volume dividers. It has been suggested that such a pressure relief valve be fitted with a whistle to give warning of its operation.

Breathing Systems

The T-piece system

As mentioned above the breathing system requires special consideration, especially in the case of neonates and small infants. The majority of anaesthetists consider that very small patients, especially those in poor physical condition, should not be required to breathe spontaneously for more than short periods of time, and that IPPV should be used for most procedures. The *Ayre's T-piece* (Fig. 7.12), especially as modified by Jackson Rees (Fig. 7.14), is the most appropriate breathing attachment. It is equally efficient for both spontaneous and controlled ventilation. The absence of valves, which inevitably present resistance, and its simplicity make it most attractive.

Many modifications of this system have been developed and the *Stellenbosch Universal T-piece system* (Fig. 12.1) has certain interesting refinements. It is a complete anaesthesia kit for children up to the age of about five years and uses both facepiece and endotracheal methods. It includes a modification of the Ayre's T-piece and also of the Jackson Rees modification of that system. The T-piece itself has been redesigned in such a way that

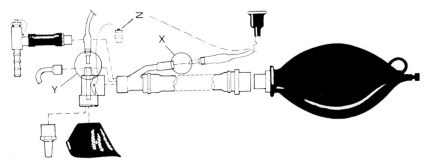

Figure 12.1 The Stellenbosch Universal T-piece system (see text). X and Y are the alternative sites for the fresh gas inflow; Z is a bung to occlude the unused port.

the fresh gas entry is directed towards the patient, so that the fresh gas stream remains separated from the expired stream. It may be connected directly to a modified Magill endotracheal connector, or may be attached to a right-angled facepiece mount. A port on the facepiece mount is normally occluded by a bung but could be used for suction, or it may be used for the introduction of the fresh gas inflow so as to reduce the dead space. If this is done, the port on the T-piece should be occluded by the same bung. The facepiece mount has an external diameter to fit a facepiece and an internal diameter to fit an endotracheal adaptor. The expiratory limb consists of a 12 mm internal diameter plastic tube of 500 mm length and 50 ml capacity. It terminates in a 15 mm male plastic connection which accepts a double-ended bag of somewhere between 500 and 1000 ml capacity. Alternatively, it may be connected to a ventilator. The tail end of this bag is connected to a special outlet which, if left unattended, will allow excess gases to escape. If a thumb is placed over an aperture in the plastic attachment to this bag, it will occlude the outlet and facilitate artificial ventilation by squeezing the bag.

This attachment may therefore be used in several methods of administering anaesthesia to children of up to about five years of age. It also includes a scavenging system which can be attached to the expiratory end of the T-piece system, complete with double-ended bag.

The Bethune T-piece (Fig. 12.2) is somewhat similar in performance to the Ayre's T-piece but presents less dead space.

In the T-piece system with spontaneous ventilation, rebreathing can be prevented by the provision of an adequate FGF rate; if the latter is too low, it may occur. The necessary FGF rate varies not only with the size of the patient but also with the design of the T-piece. Provided that the expiratory limb has a capacity at least as great as the patient's tidal volume, 250 ml/min per kg body weight should be adequate. This approximates to 2.5 times the patient's minute volume. If the capacity of the expiratory limb is less than the tidal volume, a higher FGF rate is required, and in the extreme, where the expiratory limb is merely an orifice and has no capacity, the FGF rate would need to equal the peak inspiratory flow rate to avoid the ingress of air through the expiratory limb, which dilutes the anaesthetic gases.

During spontaneous ventilation the bag on the Rees T-piece is a useful indicator of the breathing. In order to prevent total collapse or over-filling of the bag, the tail may be partially occluded by a fine pair of forceps, a paper clip or a small piece of adhesive plaster. Various factors influence the excursion of the bag and it is not possible to make an accurate assessment of tidal volume simply by watching it.

The Digby Leigh system (Fig. 12.3)

The Digby Leigh system positively prevents rebreathing and may be used for spontaneous ventilation in patients of up to two or three years of age. There are two unidirectional valves which, being constructed of mica, are fragile but nevertheless very light and present very little resistance. The fresh gases enter the distal end of the reservoir bag, and the delivery tube continues through almost the

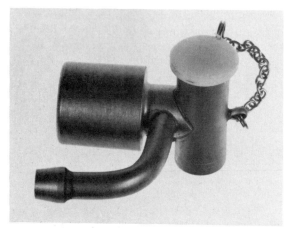

Figure 12.2 The Bethune T-piece.

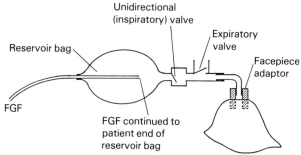

Figure 12.3 The Digby Leigh non-rebreathing system. FGF = fresh gas flow.

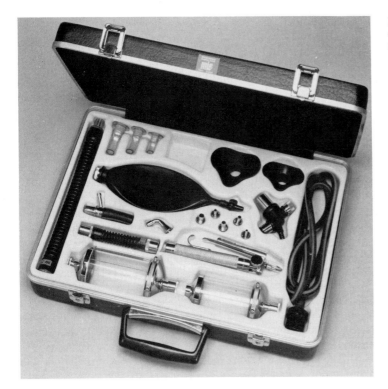

Figure 12.4   The MIE compendium of components for various paediatric breathing systems.

whole length of the bag, so that the freshest gases pass through the patient, thus accelerating any change in their composition which the anaesthetist might make. From the reservoir the gases pass to the patient via the inspiratory valve, which cannot be observed since it is situated within a metal enclosure. There is no spring or adjustment to either the inspiratory or the expiratory valve disc and the only means of closing the expiratory valve is by pressure from a finger — taking great care not to damage it. This attachment is, therefore, inappropriate for IPPV. The expiratory valve is very sensitive and if not correctly orientated, will not operate properly. The valve body ends in a female taper into which either a facepiece mount or an endotracheal connector may be inserted.

In spite of the mechanical difficulty mentioned above, the Digby Leigh system is popular with many anaesthetists for techniques employing spontaneous ventilation in infants and small children.

Some manufacturers produce compendia of fittings, such as that shown in Fig. 12.4, which may be connected up by the anaesthetist to form a variety of breathing systems. If these are used, it must be ensured that they are suitably assembled and that the basic principles, such as the reduction of dead space and the prevention of rebreathing without CO_2 absorption, are observed. They are capable of being assembled incorrectly, with dangerous consequences.

The Magill attachment (Mapleson A)

The ordinary adult Magill attachment may be used in children over two years of age. It will be less efficient when used for children of this age as opposed to adults, since there may be a difference in respiratory pattern, as mentioned above, and also the APL (expiratory) valve is less efficient. The FGF should be at least as high as the patient's minute volume or even somewhat higher. If the standard two-litre reservoir bag is replaced by one of smaller capacity (though at least as great as the patient's tidal volume), the respiratory movements may be more easily observed.

The normal APL valve could be removed and replaced by a Ruben or Ambu-E valve in order to make this into a non-rebreathing attachment. However, the above valves are not so efficient with small patients due to their resistance and 'slip'. (The 'slip' refers to the leakage of gas past the valve, particularly during a change in the respiratory cycle.)

As is the case with adults, the Magill attachment is not recommended for prolonged periods of IPPV.

Closed systems

In the days when cyclopropane, which is explosive and costly, was commonly used there was a preference for closed systems. 'To-and-fro' absorption systems with a Waters' canister or similar device did not prove altogether satisfactory. This is because there was a large dead space, which increased as the soda lime at the patient end of the canister became exhausted, because of the possibility of the inhalation of soda lime dust and because of the cumbersome arrangement when the absorber had to be placed close to the patient's head.

Adult circle absorbers can be used for children, but it is preferable to use breathing systems with scaled-down components and tubing, in order to overcome the inertia of large volumes of gases. Special face-piece mounts overcame the problems of weight and, by incorporating a chimney, reduced the dead space (see Fig. 7.73). More modern, lightweight plastic tubing and components, in which the need for antistatic precautions has been obviated by the use of non-explosive anaesthetic agents, lend themselves to more suitable breathing attachments for paediatric work. With the increasing awareness of atmospheric pollution and the use of scavenging systems, there may be a return of the popularity of closed systems. The work done in breathing would be reduced and the efficiency of the system would be considerably increased by the employment of a Revell's circulator (Fig. 7.73), or Jorgensen's venturi circulator (Fig. 7.77).

The Components of the Breathing Attachment

1. *Reservoir bags.* These may be smaller than the usual two-litre bag used for adults, 0.5 or 1.0 litre bags being the most popular. The capacity of the bag must be not less than the patient's tidal volume. The material of which it is constructed

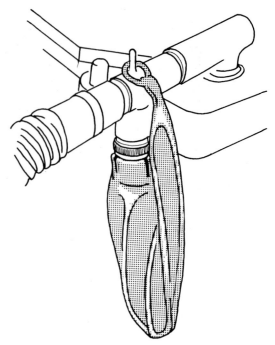

Figure 12.5   A reservoir bag may be folded upon itself to reduce its capacity.

must not be too stiff. Larger bags often have a loop at the lower end which may be hung on a hook, thereby folding the bag in two and thus reducing its capacity (Fig. 12.5). A reduction of capacity does not in any way improve the efficiency of the system from the point of view of rebreathing, etc. — it merely serves to make the movement easier to observe.

2. *Corrugated hose.* The new plastic hoses available are considerably lighter than the old rubber or neoprene ones. They therefore drag far less on the face-piece or tracheal tube. They may also be of smaller diameter. Some plastic hoses have the disadvantage that although they may be easily coiled up, they offer resistance to twisting along their long axis (Fig. 12.6). This leads to movement of the hose being transmitted to the face-piece or tracheal tube, which is undesirable.

3. *APL (expiratory) valves.* The Heidbrink valve may offer too much resistance for an infant. There may also be a leak. Resistance can be reduced by inserting a safety pin, as shown in Fig. 12.7, or by removing the spring. The latter manoeuvre may lead to unacceptable leakage if

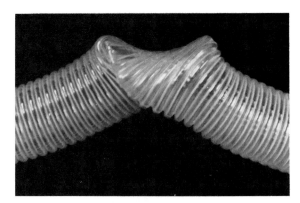

Figure 12.6 A lightweight corrugated hose may become twisted along its long axis and as a result become obstructed. This is because it is not flexible around its long axis.

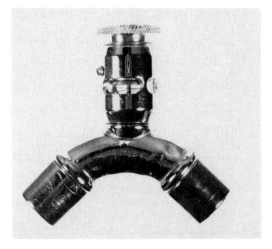

Figure 12.8 The Inglis paediatric expiratory valve.

the valve is orientated in such a position that gravity tends to cause it to open. There are several smaller, lighter valves, such as the Inglis (Fig. 12.8) and the Rendell-Baker (Fig. 12.9) the latter being made of plastic and having a chimney to reduce dead space.

4. *Facepieces* for neonates and infants, an example of which is shown in Fig. 7.37, are usually anatomically moulded to fit the face as closely as possible. Considerable experience in the selection of a facepiece of exactly the right size is required to achieve a good fit but without

obstructing the nares. Flaps and inflated pads are not used, as the smooth, round and soft tissues of the patient's face usually facilitate a good fit.

For larger infants and children a facepiece with a flap, such as the Everseal, may be used. The dead space is often reduced by employing a relatively large facepiece, into which the face fits, rather than a small one which perches on top of it (Fig. 7.38). It will be noted that the entry from the breathing attachment is positioned immediately over the airway.

5. *Facepiece mounts*. The 'chimney' used with the Revell's and other circulators is described on p. 166.

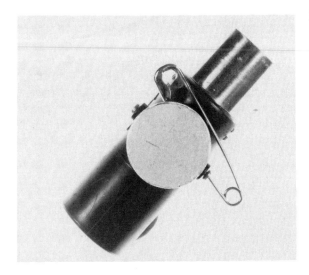

Figure 12.7 A safety pin inserted between the disc and the seating of an APL valve in order to reduce its resistance.

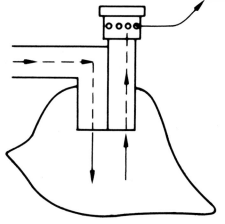

Figure 12.9 The Rendell-Baker paediatric system, which includes a chimney and a low-resistance expiratory valve.

6. *Endotracheal connectors.* The 'International 15' plastic connectors (adaptors) are deservedly popular. They come in a wide range of sizes (Fig. 7.64) to fit any tube, and at the other end have a 15 mm male taper to fit the standard components of the breathing attachment. A catheter mount is not required and abrupt angulation is prevented. They are light and so cheap that they may be regarded as disposable. If autoclaved, they are often distorted and will not fit properly. Whatever connector is used, it should present as little resistance as possible. Any curve should be smooth and the internal diameter should be not less than that of the tube. This may sometimes be achieved by pushing the end of the tube into a larger connector and fixing it securely with tape.

7. *Endotracheal tubes.* These are described in Chapter 7. They are now available in such a wide variety that general guidance is all that is appropriate here. Figs 7.39–7.55 show examples of various tubes. Points to consider when selecting a particular type of tube are as follows:

(a) *Red rubber or plastic.* Many of the old red rubber tubes were irritant to the larynx and trachea and predisposed to the encrustation of the tube and damage to the trachea. Plastic tubes do not have such a harmful effect. Many anasthetists fail to realize that, as is the case with plastic tubes, red rubber ones may soften as they warm up in the patient's air passages, so predisposing to kinking.

(b) *Tubes of silicone rubber (Silastic),* which with care will survive many re-sterilizations and long storage, have now replaced those of latex, which perish rapidly.

(c) There are several anatomically shaped tubes — the earlier red rubber ones, such as the Oxford (Fig. 7.45) which was originally designed for neurosurgical anaesthesia, and the later plastic ones, such as the RAE oral and nasal plastic tubes (Fig. 12.10), which were designed for a variety of surgical procedures. When using such tubes care must be taken to ensure that they are not too long and therefore enter the right main bronchus.

(d) The Enderby tube (Fig. 7.48) is not only armoured but also tapered. The distal portion is a snug fit in the larynx, whereas the wider proximal part offers less resistance. The consequent extra capacity does not pose measurable problems of increased dead space.

(e) Armoured tubes are useful when there is a possibility of compression by the surgeon, or where movement of the head and neck may lead to such an acute angulation of the tube that it might kink.

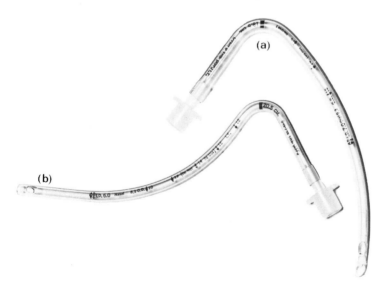

Figure 12.10   The RAE preformed endotracheal tubes. (a) Oral. (b) Nasal.

Formerly, armoured tubes were constructed of latex or red rubber, which perishes rapidly — but recently Silastic armoured tubes have been developed.

(f) Where intubation is to be prolonged, as in the intensive care unit, nasal tubes may be preferable. Not only are they less restrictive to access to the mouth, e.g. for tube feeding, they are also less prone to movement within the trachea and thus to traumatizing the delicate mucosa in that area, as they are splinted by the nose and nasopharynx.

(g) There is no place for cuffed tubes in the treatment of neonates and infants. As stated above, a plain tube may be selected that fits the air passages with minimum leakage.

(h) The fixing of a tube in position is all important. 'Four-point' fixation with adhesive tape is usually satisfactory for oral tubes, but the self-adhesive device shown in Fig.

12.11 is particularly useful for smaller sized tubes.

A prediction of the size of endotracheal tube required may be taken from Table 12.1, though of

Table 12.1 Diameters of endotracheal tubes for various ages

Age of patient	Internal diameter of tube (mm)
Preterm	2.5
At birth	3.0 or 3.5
Six months	4.0
One year	4.5
Over one year	According to formula: $\dfrac{\text{Age in years}}{4} + 4.5$

From Jackson Rees G. and Cecil Gray T. *Paediatric Anaesthesia – Trends in Current Practice*. London: Butterworths (1981).

Table 12.2 Endotracheal tubes: correct lengths for given diameters

Nasal tubes	
Diameter (mm)	Length (cm)
2.5	13.0
3.0	13.0
3.5	14.0
4.0	14.5
4.5	15.0
5.0	16.5
5.5	17.0
6.0	17.5
6.5	18.5
7.0	19.0
8.0	19.5

Oral tubes	
Diameter (mm)	Length (cm)
2.5	10.5
3.0	10.5
3.5	11.0
4.0	12.0
4.5	13.5
5.0	14.0
5.5	14.5
6.0	15.0
6.5	16.0
7.0	17.5
8.0	18.5

From Jackson Rees G. and Cecil Gray T. *Paediatric Anaesthesia – Trends in Current Practice*. London: Butterworths (1981).

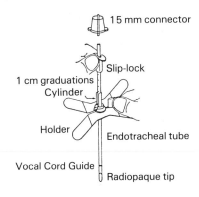

15 mm connector
Slip-lock
1 cm graduations
Cylinder
Holder
Endotracheal tube
Vocal Cord Guide
Radiopaque tip

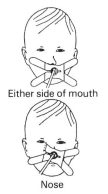

Either side of mouth

Nose

Figure 12.11 The RSP endotracheal tube holder.

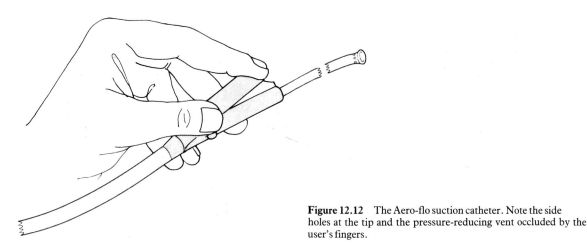

Figure 12.12   The Aero-flo suction catheter. Note the side holes at the tip and the pressure-reducing vent occluded by the user's fingers.

course there may be considerable variation in the size of patients at any age. The length of tube required may also vary, but the figures given in Table 12.2 may be taken as a general guide.

Laryngoscopes

Over the age of about 1½ years the standard adult MacIntosh curved laryngoscope is satisfactory. The curved infant blade does not, in fact, offer any advantages.

For the smaller patients, a straight bladed instrument is usually preferred. Two patterns are shown in Fig. 22.4. The fact that so many types exist is evidence that no single one suits all anaesthetists or situations. Two of the problems encountered in neonates and infants are the large tongue and the floppy epiglottis. Anatomical abnormalities encountered in neonates may render intubation very difficult.

Suction Equipment

When treating neonates and infants a relatively low-power vaccum should be used, in spite of the fact that a very narrow catheter may be needed to aspirate viscous secretions. Too high a vacuum could result in pulmonary atelectasis and damage to the delicate mucosa could result from the employ-

ment of a catheter with an inappropriate termination, performing a 'suction biopsy'! The Aero-flo catheter (Fig. 12.12) is so designed that, by virtue of its side holes, its tip remains in the mid cavity and does not attach itself to the tracheal wall.

Ventilators

Chapter 11 describes ventilators in general and includes automatic anaesthetic ventilators which may be used for children, infants and neonates. However, there are some practical points which might well be considered here.

The simplest way to achieve IPPV in infants and neonates is to employ a T-piece system and intermittently occlude the expiratory limb with the thumb. The disadvantage of this system is that the inspiratory flow rate is limited to that of the FGF. Whereas this may be satisfactory for short anaesthetics, it may be considered to fall short of the ideal for long-term ventilation.

'T-piece occluder' ventilators such as the Sheffield (Fig. 11.12) and the Amsterdam (Fig. 11.13) are therefore of limited value. The addition of a bag to the expiratory limb, as in the Rees T-piece, allows a much higher inspiratory flow rate with manually controlled ventilation or when used in conjunction with a mechnical ventilator, such as the Blease, employing the 'bag in a bottle' principle (Fig. 12.13). This is because during the inspiratory phase the FGF is augmented by the gases that have been

Table 12.3 Choice of breathing system, according to age and anaesthetic techniques

Age of patient	Spontaneous ventilation	IPPV
Neonates (up to 1 month)	Rees T-piece	Rees T-piece manually or as 'bag in a bottle'
Infants (1 month to 2 years)	Rees T-piece Stellenbosch Rendell-Baker Digby-Leigh	Paediatric minute volume divider
Young children (2–7 years)	Digby-Leigh Stellenbosch Mapleson A (? reduced dead space) (= Magill)	Adult ventilator capable of precise control with high rate and small stroke volume
Children (7–14 years)	Mapleson A (= Magill or Lack)	

displaced from the expiratory limb as a result of the bag being squeezed.

Table 12.3 summarizes the type of breathing system generally recommended according to the age of the patient and the anaesthetic technique required.

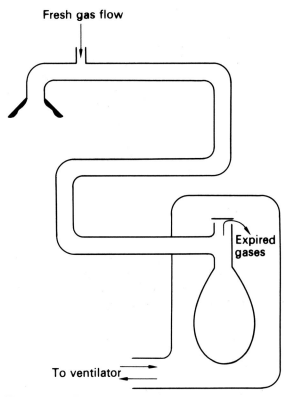

Fresh gas flow

Expired gases

To ventilator

Figure 12.13   The 'bag in a bottle' principle. This may be used to connect an adult ventilator to a paediatric T-piece system.

13
Humidifiers

Humidity is the term used to describe the amount of water vapour present in the air or in the gases concerned. The amount of water that a gas can carrry depends on its temperature. For example, a cubic metre (m^3) of air can carry about 10 g of water as vapour at 10 °C (50 °F), but when warmed to 22 °C (72 °F) it can carry twice as much, and three times as much at 30 °C (86 °F).

For the rest of this chapter, unless otherwise stated, the humidity of *air* will be considered, but the same considerations apply to anaesthetic gases.

Definitions

The *absolute humidity* is the mass of water vapour present in a unit volume of air. It is usually measured in grams per cubic metre (g/m^3).

The maximum mass of water vapour that can be carried in a cubic metre of air at a particular temperature will be referred to in this book as the humidity at saturation (Fig. 13.1). The *relative humidity* is the ratio between the absolute humidity and the humidity at saturation at the same temperature. It is usually expressed as a percentage.

The implications of the above facts and definitions are sufficiently important to justify the consideration of some examples, since the former are not always fully understood.

1. Suppose that the temperature of the air in a room is 15 °C (59 °F) and that it has a relative humidity of 50%. The humidity at saturation at this temperature is about 13 g/m^3; the actual amount of water vapour in the air is, therefore, 6.5 g/m^3.

   At body temperature (37 °C) the humidity at saturation is about 43 g/m^3. Therefore, when the temperature of the air in the same room is raised to body temperature its relative humidity is (6.5 ÷ 43) × 100 %, i.e. approximately 15%. If the air is to be saturated with water vapour within the body, the respiratory epithelium must vaporize 43 − 6.5 = 36.5 g of water per cubic metre of room air inhaled. And as 1 m^3 is 1000 litres, so 36.5 mg of water are required per litre of inspired air.

2. If a humidifier saturates air at room temperature, and then that air is warmed to body temperature, the absolute humidity is unchanged but the relative humidity will fall to only about 30%.

3. If air is saturated with water vapour at body temperature, i.e. in a 'warm' humidifier, and is then allowed to cool to room temperature before it reaches the patient, some of the water vapour will condense. When the air is eventually rewarmed in the patient's respiratory tract, the relative humidity will again be only 30%. From this it will be seen that if it is desired to humidify the inspired air so that it will have a relative humidity of 100% at body temperature, it will either have to be supersaturated at the lower temperature or will have to be maintained after humidification at body temperature. Supersaturation may be achieved by adding to the air a mist or fog of minute droplets of water, which vaporize when the relative humidity falls.

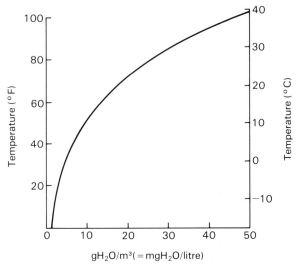

Figure 13.1 Graph showing the mass of water that is carried at saturated vapour pressure in terms of grams of water per cubic metre of air.

It should be understood that humidification refers to the addition to the air of water in the form of either vapour or nebulized droplets. The addition of excessive water in the form of droplets to the inspired air could harm the patient by waterlogging.

The Importance of Humidification

Air or gases need to be humidified for the following reasons:

1. If the natural humidifying process in a patient is by-passed by an endotracheal or tracheostomy tube and the patient is given dry gases to breathe, damage will result from the drying of the respiratory tract. Whereas this is not very important in short administration, it can be most serious in patients who are subjected to prolonged treatment on ventilators. As mentioned in the previous chapter, neonates and infants, especially those in poor condition, can be saved work if their inspired air is already humidified and warmed.

2. The atmosphere of the operating theatre, for which there is usually air conditioning, should be kept at a suitable level of relative humidity. This should be between 50 and 70%. Too high a humidity results in a most uncomfortable and tiring atmosphere for the staff, and too low a relative humidity can increase the risk of explosion due to static electricity. The ventilation and humidifying equipment used in operating theatres does not come within the scope of this book.

   For the surface administration of drugs, as in spraying the larynx with local analgesic solution, a nebulizer may be used.

Classification of Humidifiers

The various devices used may be classfied in four ways. First, they may be either active or passive. The active devices are those that require power to drive them. This may either be electric power, as in the ultrasonic nebulizer, or the power of a jet of air or gas, as in the venturi type, which can be used to humidify oxygen from the cylinder or pipeline. The 'bubble bottle', in which the gases simply bubble through water, is an example of a passive humidifier, as is the 'artificial nose', which will be described below.

Second, they may be classified according to whether they produce pure vapour on the one hand, or droplets of water, however small, on the other. The latter are generally referred to as *nebulizers*, the term *humidifier* referring strictly to the former. There is a great deal of variation in the size of the droplets produced by nebulizers and this will be discussed later.

Third, humidifiers may be classified as either hot or cold. Those that are heated can produce air at body temperature, or even higher, which is saturated with water vapour. Needless to say, caution must be taken to prevent scalding of the patient by air that has been heated to a temperature above that of the body.

Some cold nebulizers produce such a profusion of droplets that even when the air has been warmed in the body to body temperature, the droplets are sufficient in mass to produce 100% humidity.

Finally, nebulizers and humidifiers can be classified into groups, depending on whether they are intended to deliver their gases or vapours to a breathing system, or whether they are intended to humidify the atmosphere at large.

Nebulization of liquids may also be employed to disperse sterilizing agents for the decontamination of the breathing system of ventilators and anaesthetic machines. Similar nebulizers known as 'fogging machines' (Fig. 17.2) are used to disperse disinfectant around the entire operating theatre and anaesthetic room.

Some medicaments are best administered by being nebulized in the inspired air. However, unless the droplet size is very small, not exceeding 1 μm, they do not reach the alveoli but are deposited in the bronchial tree and may be ineffectual. The scope for this type of medication is, therefore, limited, unless there is close control of droplet size.

Examples of Humidifiers

1. A simple bottle humidifier (Fig. 13.2), such as the Boyle's bottle, may be used in an anaesthetic machine. If the air passes over the surface of the

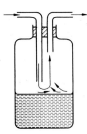

Figure 13.2   A simple bottle humidifier.

water, a modest degree of vaporization takes place. Unless there is a very large surface area of water, and the flow rate is very low, however, the air is by no means saturated with water vapour. Improvements to this type of humidifier may be made by either bubbling the air through the water or immersing wicks in the water in much the same way as in vaporizers for volatile anaesthetic agents (Fig. 13.3). To further increase humidification the bottle may be housed in a heated jacket or even contain an electric heating element (Fig. 13.4).

In the case of heated humidifiers, the temperature of the water is thermostatically controlled and it is a general practice to install two thermostats in series with each other (Fig. 13.5) so that if one thermostat were to fail, the other would still cut off the electric supply before a temperature that might cause the patient to be scalded were reached. After use, this type of humidifier may be intentionally sterilized by boiling water inside it, using a bypass switch to cut out the thermostats. The outlet and delivery tube from a heated humidifier should be lagged if possible, to reduce cooling which would result in the condensation of some of the water vapour. Ideally, a temperature sensor should be installed at the patient end of the delivery tube.

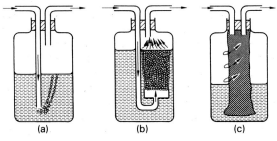

(a)	(b)	(c)

Figure 13.3   Methods of increasing humidification. (a) and (b) By bubbling gases through water, using, in (b), a sintered filter, which breaks the air up into a very large number of small bubbles, to maximize the rate of vaporization. (c) By immersing a wick.

Where the gases are bubbled through water, provision should be made to prevent the accidental reverse connection of the bottle, which would cause the water to be forced along the delivery tube to the patient. Two precautions are generally taken to prevent such an accident: a 'trap' or empty bottle B of the same capacity as the 'bubble bottle' A is interposed between the latter and the patient (Fig. 13.6), and the humidifier is always kept at a lower level than the patient, so that, in the event of an accident, there is no risk of water running down the tubes and scalding or even drowning the patient.

2. Water vapour or steam may be produced simply by boiling water. This is not a satisfactory method for use in conjunction with anaesthetic apparatus, but may, as a mere makeshift method, be quite useful in the treatment of a patient, especially in his own home, by humidifying the whole atmosphere of the room. Simple steam therapy achieved by boiling water is not usually appropriate in hospitals, and the danger of scalding the patient should be remembered.

3. A jet of air or gases may be used to entrain water drawn up from a reservoir (Fig. 13.7). As the water enters the jet it is broken up into a large number of droplets, i.e. it is nebulized. This principle is used in simple sprays for administering topical analgesics and it is also used to humidify the inspired air in ventilators. Such nebulizers create large droplets, but if these are made to impinge on a solid 'anvil', they are broken up into smaller ones.

4. The water may also be broken up into a large number of small droplets by causing a fine jet to impinge upon one or more objects, such as pins, while subjected to a moving air stream. This system is used in the humidification system in the air conditioning plant for an operating theatre, and also in some medical nebulizers.

5. In ultrasonic nebulizers (Fig. 13.8), water is broken up into droplets or fine particles by a continual sonic bombardment generated by a high-frequency resonator.

When considering nebulizers, thought must be given to the size of the particles of water. Too large a droplet will fall out and be deposited on the breathing tube rather than passing down to the patient's lungs, while too fine a particle will be carried right down almost to the alveoli but will not sufficiently

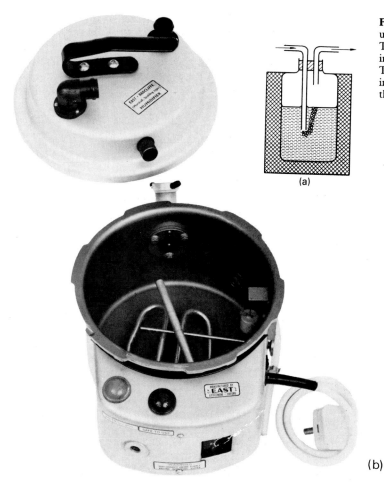

Figure 13.4 (a) A hot-water jacket may be used to increase the rate of vaporization. (b) The Marshall Spalding humidifier, which incorporates an electric heating element. This humidifier may be sterilized by intentionally boiling the water inside it. Note the appropriate warning lights.

humidify the patient's tracheal and bronchial mucosa. Ultrasonic nebulizers are useful for the dispersal of antiseptics when sterilizing anaesthetic machines and ventilators and some may be connected directly to the breathing system. However, problems have been experienced when using them for the humidification of gases because the amount

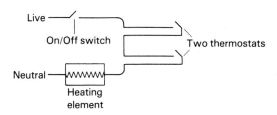

Figure 13.5 An electric heater should have two thermostats in series to reduce the risk of accidental overheating.

of water nebulized was excessive and virtually drowned the patient.

Two types of ultrasonic nebulizer require further comment. In one, a drop of water is allowed to fall on the vibrating 'transducer' and is broken up into small droplets (which one manufacturer claims are of uniform size, around 1 μm). In the other, the transducer is submerged and droplets of a variety of sizes, usually in excess of 1 μm, are produced. Since the volume of a sphere is proportional to the third power of the radius, it will be appreciated that a 2 μm droplet is eight times as heavy as a 1 μm one, and will therefore 'fall out' far more quickly. If the 'submerged' type is allowed to run dry, irreparable damage to the transducer may result. Various measures to prevent such damage are incorporated in some models.

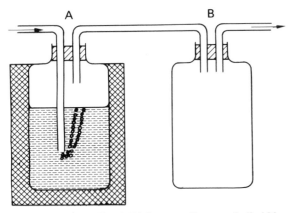

Figure 13.6 A 'trap' bottle B is interposed between the 'bubble bottle' A and the patient to prevent water reaching the patient in the event of the accidental reverse connection of the humidifier.

6. In the 'hot-rod' humidifier, water is fed on to a heated surface. The heater is electrically energized, and may be surmounted by a block of material such as porcelain, which ensures immediate vaporization. The volume of water may be metered so as to ensure the production of, say, 75% relative humidity at 37 °C. Thus if the incoming gases are fresh and unhumidified, or if they are merely room air with some pre-existing humidity, the output will be adequately, but not excessively, humidified. The reservoir of water may be in the form of a plastic infusion bag, as shown in Fig. 13.9. The breathing attachment may be coaxially arranged so that the expired gases in the outer portion help to prevent cooling of the inspired gases within the inner tube. The tubing may be detached for sterilization by autoclaving.

7. The heat and moisture exchanger (HME), also known as the 'vapour condenser/humidifier' and the 'artificial nose', is a passive device, and therefore cannot achieve full humidification. It is adequate where the latter is not required.

It consists of a chamber containing a screen, through which the respiratory gases pass in each direction (Fig. 13.10). The screen may consist of layers of wire mesh, a block of hygroscopic foam or a spiral of corrugated aluminium foil or specially formulated paper. Its operation is as follows. During exhalation the warm moist expired gases impinge on the cooler, dryer screen and the water vapour condenses; the specific heat of the expired gases, and, more important, the latent heat of the water, warm the screen. Thus at the start of inhalation the relatively cooler and dryer inspired gases are warmed and humidified as they pass through the screen. This in turn cools and dries the screen, ready for the next expiratory phase.

HMEs are available in several forms. Some are disposable, some may be autoclaved complete, and others consist of a reusable chamber with a disposable screen. One problem with the last type is that it tends to leak, which is a problem with IPPV. They also come with a range of fittings, mainly with 15 mm and 22 mm tapers, and as a rule fit directly onto the tracheostomy or endotracheal tube. Flexible and swivelling connectors are available, but they tend to add to one of the problems found in the use of HMEs, namely the increase of dead space. Where IPPV is used, this can be accommodated by increasing the tidal volume, but with spontaneous breathing it may be a problem. The dead space of some types is as high as 90 ml, but in others it is as low as 10 ml.

Some manufacturers claim a relative humidity in the trachea of as high as 80% at 37 °C (i.e. 36 mg of water per litre), but an independent investigation has found, at best, 70% at 33 °C (24 mg of water per litre). One explanation of this discrepancy may be

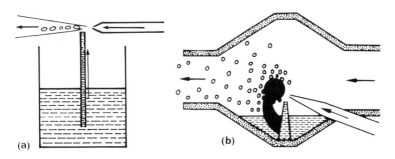

Figure 13.7 The principle of a nebulizer. (a) By employing the Bernoulli effect, a jet of air may be used to draw a liquid up a small tube from a reservoir and to entrain it as droplets. (b) The droplets may be made to impinge on an 'anvil', so causing them to be broken up into still smaller droplets.

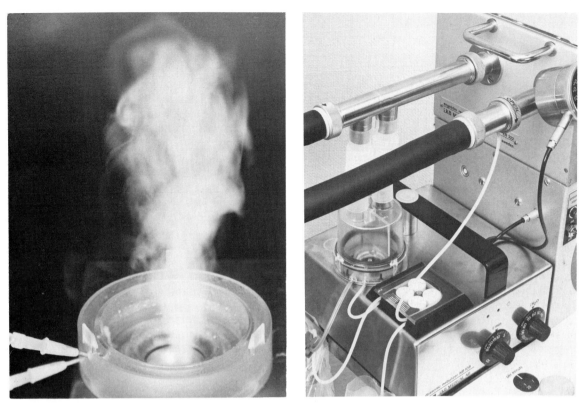

Figure 13.8 (a) A cloud of droplets emerging from an ultrasonic nebulizer. (b) The delivery of the correct volume of water by a peristaltic pump in the NB 108 nebulizer.

Figure 13.9 The principle of a 'Hot-rod' humidifier. Water from the reservoir (which may be in infusion bottle or bag) is metered through a solenoid valve in the drip gate, at a rate determined by a pulse generator in the drip speed controller. Drops of water therefore fall at a predetermined rate onto the porous sleeve that surrounds the hot rod. This is situated in an enclosure which is continuous with the breathing system and the ventilator. The breathing system is of the coaxial type, the expired gases passing through the outer tube, thereby reducing heat loss from the humidified gases. The rod temperature controller is influenced by a temperature sensor at the patient end of the breathing system.

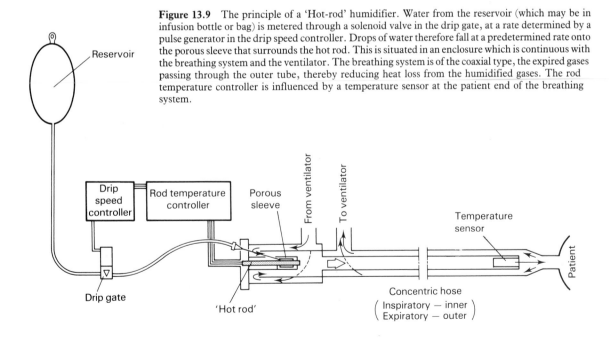

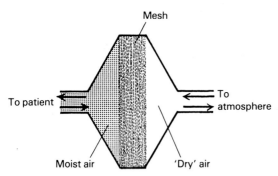

Figure 13.10   The heat and moisture exchanger ('artificial nose' vapour condenser/humidifier).

that the HME is most efficient at low tidal volumes — of an order considerably smaller than that used in clinical practice. Some improvement may be made, provided that the dead space volume is low, by installing two HMEs in series. Resistance to the gas flow is doubled, but when IPPV is being used, this is not a serious problem. The pressure drop across a single unit with a flow rate of 50 *l*/min, which is by no means less than the usual peak inspiratory flow rate, may be as low as 0.4 cmH₂O in some of the larger models (dead space = 90 ml), whereas it may be as high as 4.0 cm in some of the low dead space types.

The vapour output of the HME may be improved by using some other form of humidification, or by using room air, which already carries some water vapour (perhaps 10 ml/litre). However, nebulizers should not be employed in conjunction with the HME, especially when they are used to carry medicaments.

Finally, the HME may become infected, so it should be re-sterilized or changed at appropriate intervals — say, every 24 hours.

The HME does not replace the active humidifier where complete humidification is required. However, where a low relative humidity is clinically acceptable it may be used, with the advantages that it is inexpensive, simple and immune to such accidents as over-heating, drowning the patient, electrical failure, etc. Also, it avoids having to use a large volume of possibly infected water and the mechanical difficulties that may arise when a patient has to be transported.

On the other hand, during long operations, of several hours duration, where the present practice is to use dry gases from the cylinder or pipeline, with a high fresh gas flow, an HME would do much to reduce the damage done to the mucosa of the patient's air passages.

The HME still smacks of the attempts over the ages to produce perpetual motion; where partial humidification only is required, it succeeds!

General Principles

During the course of an anaesthetic the anaesthetist may make repeated readings of the appropriate functions, but an instrument can give a continuous reading, a permanent record and even, if desired, a warning signal if the function strays outside certain preset limits. This procedure is known as monitoring (from the Latin word *monere* meaning 'to warn'). Monitors may be used to analyse the gases and vapours in an anaesthetic system, to confirm the correct functioning of a ventilator and to check the performance of vaporizers and the mixed gas concentrations of anaesthetic machines.

One should avoid surrounding the patient with so many gadgets that it is impossible to get near enough to make ordinary clinical observations. It should be remembered, too, that the value of a monitor depends on its reliability and accuracy as well as on

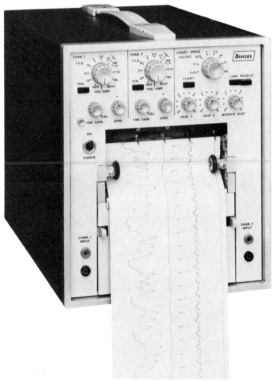

Figure 14.1 A printout recorder that may be used for several functions simultaneously.

the ability of the anaesthetist to interpret correctly the information obtained from it. Monitors can fail or give false readings, and the patient's safety may depend on the anaesthetist's ability to detect this and make appropriate deductions. There is no substitute for the anaesthetist keeping constant vigilance himself.

The term 'parameter' has recently become commonly misused in medicine to describe measurements of functions such as arterial or venous pressure, pulse rate, temperature, partial pressures of gases, etc. The real meaning of 'parameter' is difficult to define and means rather different things to physicists and mathematicians. It may be taken to be a factor common to a number of equations or situations, and may be used as an arbitrary constant that defines or assists in defining the relationship between other variables and quantifies them.

The descriptions that follow relate to instruments used to measure various functions. Often more than one of these functions can be measured at any one time. Printout records can be made, and with the more elaborate recorders (Fig. 14.1) several channels are available to give simultaneous recordings of all the measurements required. The part of the instrument that senses a physical or physiological function and converts it into an electric or other signal is known as a 'transducer'.

For the purposes of this chapter the monitoring of functions is considered in the order in which gases

---

* As stated in the Preface, the description of monitoring equipment in this edition is restricted to that of anaesthetic equipment. The monitoring of bodily functions, such as pulse rate, blood pressure, blood gases, temperature, etc., has become such a vast subject that it now justifies a complete volume on its own, and is not, therefore, included here.

flow. The circumstances are discussed first, the items of test equipment being described later in the chapter.

The only ways in which we can check the contents of a cylinder are by weighing it or by noting the pressure within it. These are described in Chapter 3.

At the pipeline outlet the responsibility for checking the identity and purity of gases is the province of the hospital engineer and pharmacist. (This refers particularly to Great Britain and details may be found in HTM 22.) There may, however, be occasions when in an emergency situation the anaesthetist is called upon to verify the identity of gases delivered by a particular pipeline outlet. The possession of a gas differentiator, such as that shown in (Fig. 14.4), will prove most useful in this event. The maintenance of adequate pressure in pipelines is discussed in Chapter 4, but where intermittent flow machines are used in conjunction with mini-pipelines, particular care should be taken by the anaesthetist to check, and if necessary adjust, the regulated pressure. The McKesson, in particular, requires an accurate line pressure in order to assure the correct oxygen percentage in the mixed gases.

When we come to the monitoring of the output of the anaesthetic machine, we have to consider not only the correct identity of gases in the fixed pipeline, but also the correct connections of the flexible hoses and the internal pathways of the machine itself — both of which have been the location of crossed connections.

The composition of the gases at the outlet of the machine may be checked by an oxygen analyser (such as that shown in Fig. 14.5 or 14.6), a discriminator (such as that mentioned above and shown in Fig. 14.4) or a whistle discriminator (see Fig. 14.9).

When the vapour concentration of volatile anaesthetic agents is measured at the outlet of the anaesthetic machine inaccuracies may occur if steps have not been taken to mix the gases thoroughly. A mixing chamber in the form of a long tube in which there are baffles or some form of mesh may be used. Without adequate mixing, 'streaming' may occur, in which case the concentration of vapour may be greater on one side of the gaseous pathway than on the other.

Earlier halothane analysers, such as the Hook and Tucker (see Fig. 14.10), took about twenty minutes to warm up and stabilize, and needed frequent recalibration.

The most sophisticated instrument for measuring vapour concentration is the mass spectrometer, but this is too costly and bulky for use in day-to-day anaesthesia. More practical instruments are the Dräger Narcotest (see Fig. 14.11) for halothane only and the Engström Emma (see Fig. 14.12) for several vapours, either of which may be used to continuously monitor the concentration during anaesthesia. They may be permanently included in the breathing attachment. The Riken interferometer (see Fig. 14.13), which may be used only to take intermittent samples of gas, has a wide range of applications. It is portable and simple to use. For checking, rather than continual monitoring, it is probably the most convenient and cost-effective instrument available.

In the past few years there has been a return of popularity for closed and semi-closed systems with rebreathing. This is partly due to the arousal of interest in the problems of atmospheric pollution. Oxygen monitors of the galvanic (fuel cell) type may conveniently be included in the circle system, as may halothane analysers such as the Engström

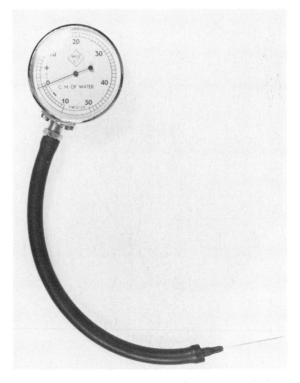

Figure 14.2   A 'water gauge' manometer, which is connected to the breathing attachment via an intravenous needle.

Emma. If an infrared analyser, such as the Hook and Tucker, is used, the gases that have been sampled should be discarded and not returned to the breathing system, since the halothane will have been degraded. In addition, it may be required to monitor the level of carbon dioxide in either the expired air or somewhere within the circle system. This may be done with a capnograph (such as that shown in Fig. 14.14).

It may be required to monitor the tidal or minute volume of a patient who is breathing spontaneously, or the stroke volume and pressure produced by a ventilator. Tidal volume may be read from a Wright respirometer (see Fig. 14.18), which should preferably not be kept permanently connected to the breathing system, since there might otherwise be problems from condensed water vapour. Some ventilators have an arrangement whereby the expired air may be temporarily switched to a Wright respirometer and voided to the atmosphere; as soon as the pressure on the switch is released, it will return to the closed mode. For continuous monitoring, the Wright respiration monitor (see Fig. 14.19) is more

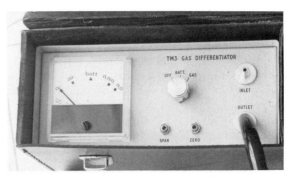

Figure 14.4   The Bedfont TM3 gas differentiator.

appropriate. During IPPV it is the expired volume that should be measured, since this will take account of any losses due to leaks.

An airway manometer may be an integral part of the anaesthetic ventilator, but if it is not, a simple manometer may be connected via a needle which is inserted into the catheter mount (Fig. 14.2). This is an extremely simple and efficient method of measuring airway pressures.

There are many ventilator alarms available that will detect either a pressure rising above a preset limit, which would suggest some form of obstruction, or a lack of pressure for a preset length of time, which would indicate a disconnection. Such an alarm is shown in Fig. 11.47.

For testing a ventilator, a lung simulator, such as that shown in Fig. 14.3 may be used. These simulators can indicate tidal volume and airway pressure, and can also be adjusted so as to include a leak or airway obstruction. The compliance of the simulator may also be varied.

Examples of Monitoring and Measuring Equipment

The Bedfont TM3 gas differentiator (Fig. 14.4)

The Bedfont TM3 gas differentiator can distinguish between oxygen, compressed air, nitrous oxide and Entonox (50% nitrous oxide + 50% oxygen). It may be used, for example, to verify the gases emerging from a pipeline outlet. It works on the principle that the gases have different thermal conductivities. The sample of gas to be tested may either be led in through a tube at a rate of 0.5–1 *l*/min or may be

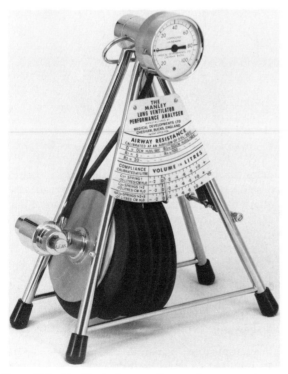

Figure 14.3   The Manley lung ventilator performance analyser.

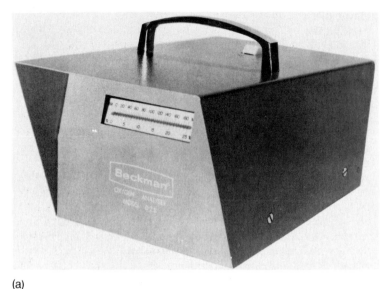

(a)

Figure 14.5   (a) The Beckman paramagnetic oxygen analyser. (b) Working principles. Two hollow glass spheres S, filled with nitrogen, are each suspended between two magnets M. If oxygen is present, it is attracted by the magnetic field and displaces the spheres, the amount of displacement being indicated by the movement of a light beam, which is reflected from a small mirror, mounted on the suspension between the spheres, to a suitably calibrated scale.

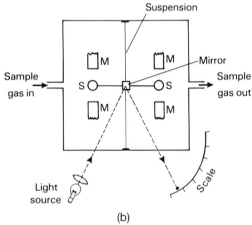

(b)

introduced by a bulb aspirator. The response time is about 20 s. No percentages are indicated, and the presence of carbon dioxide, other gases or anaesthetic vapours could invalidate the result.

The gas differentiator is therefore useful for checking the identity of gases on an anaesthetic machine or following any work done on the pipeline system. It is not used for monitoring during the course of an anaesthetic.

The paramagnetic oxygen analyser (Fig. 14.5)

The paramagnetic oxygen analyser which depends for its operation on the fact that oxygen has magnetic properties, resembles a string galvanometer: the

mirror reflects a beam of light from a small battery-operated lamp to a glass scale which is calibrated both in mmHg partial pressure and as a percentage. The lamp is illuminated when a small microswitch is kept depressed.

It is more useful for making spot checks of the percentage of oxygen rather than for continual monitoring during the course of anaesthesia or oxygen therapy.

The galvanic (fuel cell) oxygen analyser (Fig. 14.6)

The galvanic oxygen analyser depends for its operation on the principle of measuring the potential produced by an oxygen-sensitive fuel cell. Some cells, such as the Teledyne C1 cell, are suitable for measuring the concentration of oxygen in enriched air, whilst others, such as the Teledyne C2 cell, are suitable for measuring oxygen percentages in mixtures of anaesthetic gases containing nitrous oxide and the volatile agents. The analyser is calibrated from 0 to 100% oxygen, but in common with the paramagnetic analyser it is, in fact, the partial pressure that is measured. There is usually a control for calibrating the output, and a red line usually marks 21%, the point against which atmospheric air may be calibrated. The fuel cell may be housed in a T-piece with 22 mm tapers so that it can be incorporated in a breathing attachment to give a continuous indication of the percentage of oxygen.

The device shown in Fig. 14.7 also incorporates alarms which may be set to give warning if the percentage of oxygen falls below, or rises above, preset limits. It is advisable to turn the monitor off when it is not in use and to exclude the fuel cell from air or other sources of oxygen — as a rule it is connected to the monitor by a plug which may be removed from the appropriate socket. Fuel cells have to be replaced at intervals of about six months in general use, and they are costly — currently about £50 in Great Britain. The C2 cell, which would be needed for use during anaesthesia, may have a working life of less than half that of the C1. A battery is required only if there is a warning device.

The polarographic oxygen analyser (Fig. 14.8)

The polarographic oxygen analyser resembles the galvanic oxygen analyser, but the sensor is an oxygen electrode, which requires the application of a potential for it to operate. A battery is therefore required even if there is no warning device. Its response is more rapid than that of the galvanic type and although its purchase price may be a little

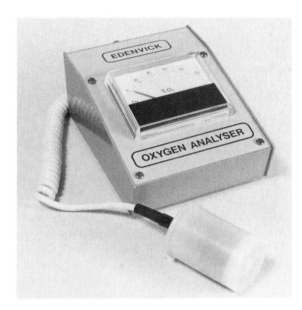

Figure 14.6   A galvanic (fuel cell) oxygen analyser.

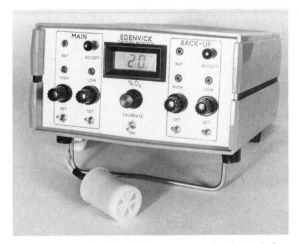

Figure 14.7   A galvanic (fuel cell) oxygen monitor in which the electronic warning devices are duplicated for extra safety.

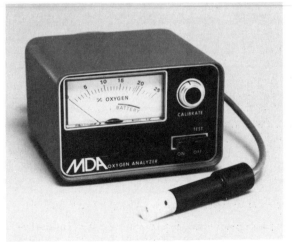

Figure 14.8   A polarographic oxygen analyser.

higher, its annual running cost in terms of the replacement of the electrodes is considerably less. For oxygen therapy it is, therefore, the more appropriate of the two. Unfortunately, the electrode is sensitive to nitrous oxide and in some cases may give a false, dangerously high reading for oxygen. It is, therefore, less appropriate for use in anaesthesia.

Where only an occasional check of oxygen concentration is required, the paramagnetic oxygen analyser is more suitable, since there is only an easily obtainable battery to be replaced and maintenance is inexpensive. If a galvanic or polarographic oxygen analyser is used only occasionally, it is all too frequently found that the cell is exhausted and that a replacement is not immediately available.

The whistle discriminator (Fig. 14.9)

This very simple device was designed to check that the nitrous oxide and oxygen supplied from an anaesthetic machine had not been accidentally crossed over. It consists of a plastic body with a 22 mm taper that may be fitted directly onto the outlet of the anaesthetic machine, and a small whistle which sounds when gases pass through it. After it is attached to the anaesthetic machine, the oxygen flow control valve is opened until the flow rate is 8

l/min. The pitch of the whistle is then noted. The oxygen is then turned off and the nitrous oxide flow control valve opened to the same flow rate. Once the oxygen in the back bar and internal tubing of the machine has been voided, nitrous oxide will reach the whistle and the pitch of the note will change to a lower tone. Thus, by noting this lowering of pitch it may be confirmed that the nitrous oxide and oxygen are correctly connected.

If unequal flow rates of nitrous oxide and oxygen are employed, there may be a discrepancy in the tone; in any case, the difference in pitch is not very great and will not be easily confirmed by those who are tone deaf. This device does, however, go one further than the simple single hose test in that it confirms the identity of the two gases, provided, of course, that the gases concerned are pure oxygen and pure nitrous oxide.

An alternative method of testing the oxygen supply is as follows:
1. The oxygen pipeline is disconnected.
2. The reserve cylinder is turned on and a flow rate of 8 l/min is set.
3. Without altering the flow rate, the cylinder is turned off and the pipeline reconnected.
4. There should be no change in pitch.

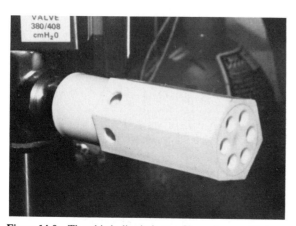

Figure 14.9 The whistle discriminator. Since nitrous oxide is denser than oxygen, the pitch of the sound produced by the whistle is lower for the former than for the latter. In either case the flowmeter is set at 8 l/min. If oxygen is drawn first from a cylinder and then from the pipeline, the pitch should not change. If oxygen is drawn from either the pipeline or the cylinder and then replaced by nitrous oxide, the tone of the whistle will change to a lower pitch.

The Hook and Tucker halothane meter (Fig. 14.10)

The earliest method of measuring halothane concentration, either in the breathing attachment or when testing a vaporizer in the laboratory, was by using the Hook and Tucker halothane meter. This works on the principle of the absorption of ultraviolet light by halothane vapour. A small internal suction pump draws the sample of vapour into the test chamber, it having first passed through a liquid trap and a desiccant. The sample should be voided after analysis rather than returned to the breathing attachment, because there may be small amounts of toxic degeneration products present.

Although the Hook and Tucker has the advantage that it can be used continuously during anaesthesia, it has the disadvantage that it takes about twenty minutes to warm up and stabilize and even then, in the author's experience, frequent recalibration is necessary. When used to check the output of vaporizers in the laboratory, the best system is to line up a

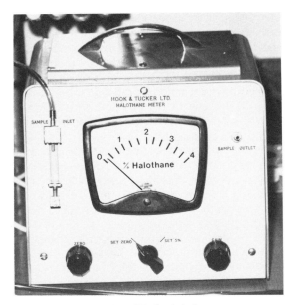

Figure 14.10 The Hook and Tucker halothane meter.

number of anaesthetic machines and test the halothane output of their vaporizers in succession, so that any that are inaccurate will be seen to be the 'odd man out'.

The Hook and Tucker halothane meter has now been superseded by more suitable instruments, and is no longer manufactured, but it is still supported by the manufacturers.

The Dräger Narcotest halothane indicator
(Fig. 14.11)

The Dräger Narcotest halothane indicator is a relatively simple device which depends on the absorption of the vapours of various anaesthetic agents by silicone rubber. The gases containing the vapour circulate around strands of the rubber, and being absorbed by it alter its length and modulus of elasticity. A bimetallic strip acts so as to compensate for changes in temperature. There is a clamp which may be used to secure the needle during transportation.

The Dräger has the advantage that it requires no power and may be kept continually in line during an anaesthetic. It has the disadvantage that the highest concentration of halothane indicated is 3%. Although it is calibrated for the latter agent, there are conversion factors that enable it to be used for other agents, such as enflurane, methoxyflurane and

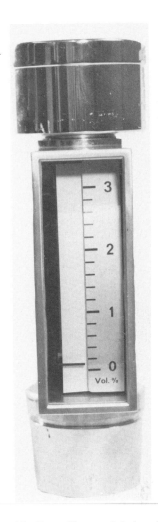

Figure 14.11 The Dräger Narcotest halothane indicator.

diethyl ether. Nitrous oxide also has an effect, and if the carrier gas consists of nitrous oxide and oxygen in a ratio of 3 : 1, the reading on the halothane scale will be increased by 0.25%. Alternatively, the needle may be readjusted to zero with the gas mixture.

The Engström Emma anaesthetic vapour analyser (Fig. 14.12)

The Engström Emma anaesthetic vapour analyser incorporates a transducer head in which there are two quartz crystals, both of which are exposed to the sample of vapour to be measured. One of them is

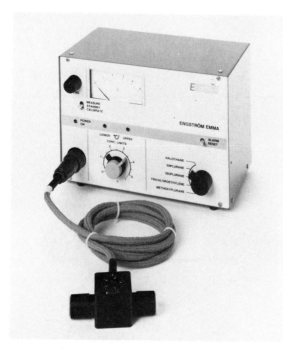

Figure 14.12   The Engström Emma anaesthetic vapour analyser.

coated with a special oil and therefore absorbs volatile anaesthetic agents. This increases the mass of the crystal and as a result the frequency at which it oscillates is changed: measurement of the concentration of anaesthetic vapours is made by a comparison of the frequencies of the two crystals. The oil is permanent and should not need servicing or replenishing.

Nitrous oxide produces a very small false reading, at worst less than + 0.2% on the meter scale. If one is using nitrous oxide mixtures, the machine can be set to zero for the appropriate nitrous oxide percentage and the readings will then be true. Carbon dioxide has no appreciable effect.

The transducers need to be matched to the analyser. On each transducer there is a disc showing a scale, which, having been set to one particular number, is fixed by a screw. In order to make a new transducer compatible, the analyser is switched to 'calibrate', and if the scale reading does not coincide with the setting on the disc, the electronics of the analyser should be brought into line by adjusting a small screw which is located in a hole in the right-hand panel of the apparatus.

It is advisable not to use ether with this analyser, since there is a heater in the transducer head and this could ignite the vapour. The response time of the instrument is one-tenth of a second. The switch may be set to 'standby'.

There are two audible alarms, one for an upper limit and the other for a lower limit, and these can be adjusted to such extremes that they will not sound under any circumstances. There are also two visible alarms, in the form of red lights. A function switch may be set to 'standby', thus maintaining the heat in the transducer head, but with the alarms switched off.

The frequency of the oscillator is about 9 kHz, and may be interfered with by surgical diathermy.

One of the advantages of this analyser over, for example, the Hook and Tucker, is that it does not merely take a small sample from the gas flow — the entire gas flow passes through the transducer head — and there are therefore less problems with inaccuracies due to streaming, etc.

If the transducer is installed in the expiratory limb of a breathing attachment, water vapour may be absorbed by the non-oily crystal and produce a low reading.

The Engström Emma measures the concentration of any substance that is absorbed by the oil in one of the two transducers, and since all volatile anaesthetic agents are oil-soluble, they can be detected. However, the device is incapable of distinguishing one agent from another. It will therefore be most useful in checking the performance of individual vaporizers, and calibration for agents that may be introduced in the future should not prove a problem. When used in the breathing attachment during clinical anaesthesia, problems may be encountered when more than one agent is present in distinguishing between one and the other.

The Riken gas indicator (Fig. 14.13)

The Riken gas indicator is an interferometer (interference-refractometer). It depends for its operation on the fact that there is a difference between the refractive index of clean air and that of air containing another gas. Light from a small lamp bulb is condensed into a beam, which is split into two parallel beams by prisms. Each parallel beam then passes through a chamber, one of which contains clean air and the other the sample of gas to be

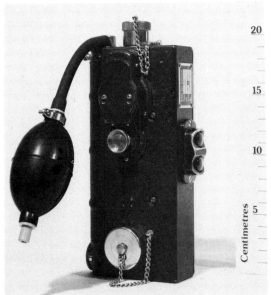

(a)

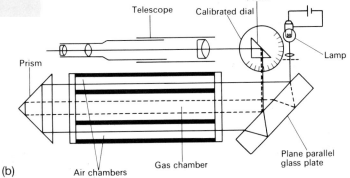

(b)

Figure 14.13   (a) The Riken gas indicator. (b) Working principles.

analysed. There is a difference in the effective length of the paths taken by the two beams, which, when they are brought together again, causes the appearance of an interference fringe that includes two characteristic black lines, one of which is taken as the reference. The position of the reference line may be moved by a control knob until it falls on a reference point on the scale, when the sampling chamber is filled with air. By means of a small manual aspirator the sample of gas is then drawn into the sampling chamber and this causes a change in the position of the reference line on the scale. The displacement is proportional to the concentration of the gas. There is a vernier scale with which to obtain a more precise reading.

The interferometer may be calibrated for any required gas or vapour: one calibrated for halothane in oxygen may be used for other vapours by refer-

ence to a conversion table. Although it is not convenient for repeated or continuous measurements during anaesthesia, the Riken gas indicator is a most satisfactory instrument for checking the calibration of vaporizers for any known anaesthetic agent. The battery and bulb are easy to replace.

Checking of anaesthetic vaporizers

Very often there are complaints from anaesthetists that a vaporizer does not appear to be giving the correct concentration. In nearly every case it is eventually found that the vaporizer is, in fact, performing satisfactorily. One of the problems is that the human nose is extremely inefficient at estimating vapour concentration. This is due in part to the fact that it very quickly acclimatizes to the odour, and also to the fact that the strong smell of thymol,

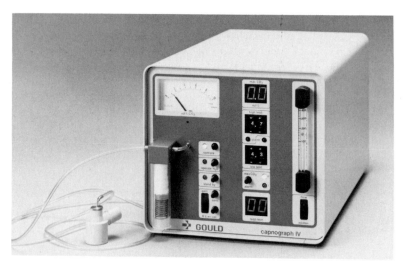

Figure 14.14   A capnograph.

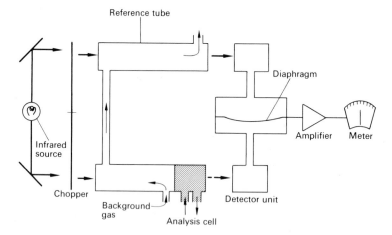

Figure 14.15   Working principles of the infra-red gas analyser.

which has become concentrated in the vaporizer, can be misleading. Again it is common that there has been some form of human error in the anaesthetic technique, such as the oxygen bypass being turned on.

The capnograph (Fig. 14.14)

Infrared gas analysers, which work on the Luft principle (Fig. 14.15), may be used to measure the concentration of gases and vapours. Infrared rays are passed through two parallel identical channels — one of which contains the pure gas or vapour and the other the sample of unknown concentration. The heating effect of the infrared rays from the two channels, which have been filtered to a different

extent, is compared and the electronic circuitry gives a read-out or recording of the vapour concentration.

Such an analyser is used for many different

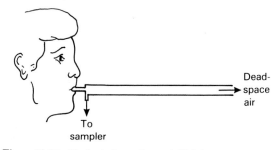

Figure 14.16   Method of sampling end tidal air.

vapours in research, but is particularly useful for estimating the carbon dioxide concentration in expired gases.

The capnograph is a large and expensive piece of equipment. However, it does give a direct and immediate indication of carbon dioxide in expired gases. It may therefore be connected into the breathing system during anaesthesia.

Simpler carbon dioxide analysers depend on the removal from the system of a sample of gases for analysis. For this purpose it is important that the correct sampling technique is followed. During the early part of expiration the gases sampled are those that occupied the dead space and have not been in the alveoli nor undergone respiratory exchange. It is therefore necessary to take an end expiratory sample.

One way of achieving this is to have the patient

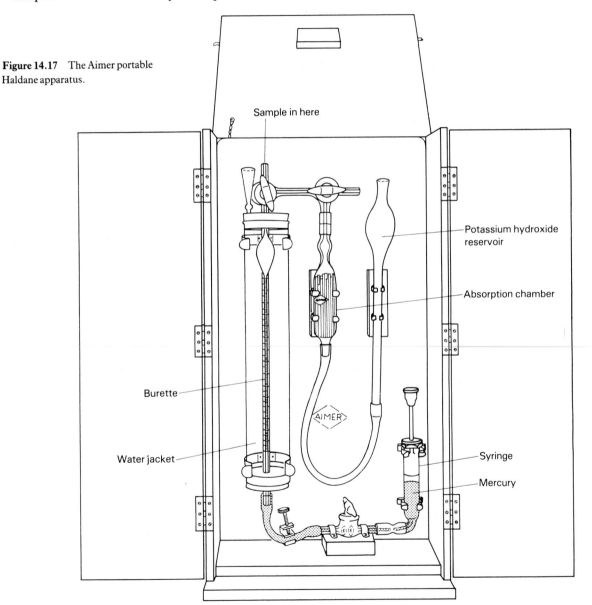

Figure 14.17 The Aimer portable Haldane apparatus.

Sample in here

Potassium hydroxide reservoir

Absorption chamber

Burette

Water jacket

Syringe

Mercury

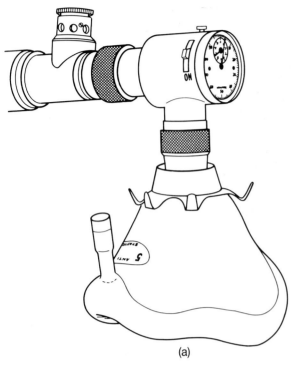

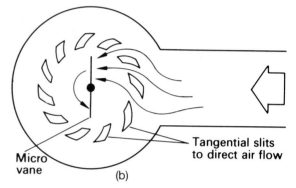

Figure 14.18 (a) The Wright respirometer. (b) Working principles.

Micro vane　(b)　Tangential slits to direct air flow

(a)

exhale through a long tube in which there is a side arm at the proximal end (Fig. 14.16). The sample is taken at the end of expiration.

Methods of estimating the carbon dioxide concentration in such a sample include the chemical absorption of the carbon dioxide by bringing the sample into contact with a solution of sodium hydroxide. The reduction in volume of the sample indicates the volume of carbon dioxide absorbed and a simple calculation then gives the percentage of the gas in the original mixture.

In the Aimer modified portable Haldane apparatus (Fig. 14.17) the sample is taken from a breathing bag into a calibrated burette. It is then exposed to potassium hydroxide solution until all the carbon dioxide has been absorbed, when the calibration, which gives the percentage of carbon dioxide in the original sample, is noted.

The Wright respirometer (Fig. 14.18)

The Wright respirometer is a small but efficient anemometer which measures the volume of gas that passes through it. The gas passes through oblique slits in the casing of a chamber and then impinges on a double vane. Through a series of gear wheels, the number of rotations of the vane is recorded on a dial which is calibrated to show the volume of gas. There is a brake which may be applied until the recording is to be commenced, and also a push button which returns the pointers to zero. One of the problems of measuring expired gases is that they contain water vapour, which condenses on the internal parts of the respirometer. In order to prevent the gear wheels and their bearings from becoming corroded by this moisture, the Wright respirometer has a mercurial seal interposed between them and the vane. It is also so constructed that only gases entering by the radial port cause movement of the vane, so that if it were mounted in a to-and-fro part of the breathing system, as when attached to the catheter mount, only gases passing in one direction would be measured.

The Wright respiration monitor (Fig. 14.19)

The Wright respiration monitor has a transducer with a vane similar to that of the Wright respirometer, but by means of an electric current gives a meter reading to indicate either the tidal or the

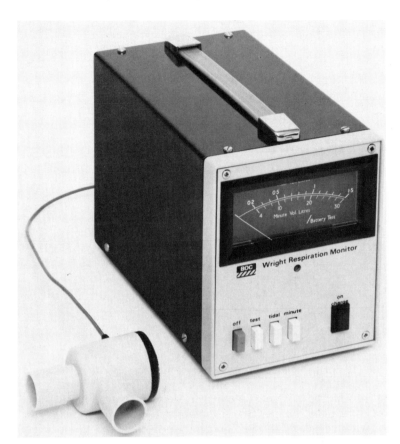

Figure 14.19 The Wright respiration monitor.

minute volume, as may be required. It can operate either from the mains, or from its own battery, which is rechargeable from the mains.

Calibrated positive pressure bellows

These may be part of a ventilator and measure stroke volume, but they may be inaccurate because:
1. There may be a leak in the breathing attachment, or due to underinflation of the cuff of the endo-tracheal tube.
2. There may be distension of the wide-bore hose, resulting in the loss of some of the volume delivered from the bellows.
3. The gases are compressed in the breathing

attachment, which in the case of some ventilators has a capacity of several litres.

For any of these reasons the volume of the gas entering the patient may be less than that delivered by the bellows. As mentioned above, measurements of the *expired* volume are not subject to these inaccuracies and are therefore more reliable.

Anemometers as described above are not as accurate as displacement meters (the same as 'town gas' meters) and other spirometers, but the latter are used in research rather than in routine anaesthetic practice and are not, therefore, within the scope of this book. Their large size renders them cumbersome to use.

15

Atmospheric Pollution

Although at the time that this goes to press there is a paucity of definite evidence, it does seem that women who work in the operating department and the wives of men who work in the operating department may suffer from an increased rate of involuntary infertility and of spontaneous abortion. The suggestion that they suffer a higher incidence of certain malignant growths and of fetal abnormalities is not so well supported.

The conclusion that these misfortunes are due to the inhalation of anaesthetic agents was merely presumptive until experiments by teams such as Moyes et al. showed that female rats exposed, and the partners of male rats exposed, to trace quantities of nitrous oxide, produced litters of smaller number and of smaller sized offspring than the control animals. Various questions, including that of species difference, remain to be answered: but the evidence is suggestive. The significance of the more recent discovery that chronic exposure to nitrous oxide may interfere with methionine synthase has yet to be evaluated, but it does add to the argument in favour of removing waste gases from the atmosphere of the operating theatre.

Earlier theories impugned halothane as the causative agent. This led to the development of the Aldasorber (Fig. 15.18), in which halothane is absorbed by activated charcoal. However, if nitrous oxide is 'to blame', it would seem that this exercise was fruitless, at least so far as the increased rate of involuntary infertility and the prevention of spontaneous abortion are concerned. However, there has been evidence, and frequent complaints by anaesthetists, that poorly ventilated rooms, contaminated with anaesthetic vapours of whatever nature, lead to drowsiness, poor performance and malaise.

At the time of writing we still await the British Standard and ISO regulations, though the preparation of these is understood to be at an advanced stage. In the meantime it is possible only to examine the evidence already published and to hazard a guess as to the provisions that will be advocated in the appropriate publications.

The Extent of Pollution

This depends on five factors:
1. The amount of anaesthetic vapours employed.
2. The size and layout of the operating theatre and any other place where anaesthetic vapours are used.
3. The efficiency of the scavenging system.
4. The efficiency of the air conditioning and ventilating systems.
5. The amount of leakage from the anaesthetic equipment.

The extent of pollution is difficult to estimate. Detectors that measure trace quantities of vapours and gases are available, but these are expensive and it is unlikely that they will be purchased by the majority of hospital authorities. Even when available, they must be employed with care, since levels of pollution may vary greatly between different locations in one room. Samples may be taken for analysis in laboratories elsewhere either quickly from each of several locations in the room, or more slowly, over the course of several hours, using a special container carried by the anaesthetist. The problems of sampling by these techniques are exemplified by Austin et al (*British Journal of Anaesthesia*, vol. 50, pp.1109–1112, 1978). The retention of nitrous oxide in samples of nitrous oxide in air held in disposable plastic syringes, glass syringes and custom-made nylon film bags were studied by means of gas chromatography at intervals of 90 minutes, 24 hours, 48 hours and 120 hours, after filling the containers. After 24 hours the nylon bags retained a mean concentration of 94.5% of the original concentration of nitrous oxide. The disposable plastic syringes and glass syringes were unsatisfactory and retained only 80% after 90 minutes. These values decreased to 51% and 31% of the original concentration of nitrous oxide at 24 and 48 hours respectively. It is therefore obvious that it is very important to choose the correct type of container when sampling and sending away for analysis air contaminated with nitrous oxide. The efficiency of this system has been improved by employing absorbent materials within the containers, such as the Adsorba personal monitor.

It is expected that the 'safe' level of nitrous oxide will be found to be less than 200 ppm (parts per million) in the vicinity of the anaesthetist and 100 ppm at the extract grille of the ventilating system. In the USA the levels recommended by the National Institute for Occupational Safety and Health (NIOSH) are 25 ppm in the operating room and 50 ppm in the dental operatory.

The amount of anaesthetic vapours employed

This may vary considerably. At one extreme is the non-rebreathing system used commonly in Great Britain, where there is a fresh gas flow of about 8 l/min, of which 70% may be nitrous oxide, and to which the vapour of halothane or other agents may be added. Many anaesthetists in Great Britain feel that the employment of high flow rates contributes to simplicity and safety, and are not deterred from using them on economic grounds, since they do not, personally, have to defray the cost of drugs used in the National Health Service.

At the other end of the scale are those who employ local and regional analgesia and total intravenous anaesthesia, or low flow and closed systems. Discussion of the relative merits of these techniques as they affect the patient is not within the scope of this book.

The size of the premises

'Dental chair' anaesthetics for extractions are frequently administered in small rooms. This, in itself, is probably of little importance, since they are of only short duration and most dentists employ general anaesthetics only occasionally, so exposure of the personnel (except the travelling anaesthetist!) is limited. However, the advent of inhalational methods for relative analgesia and sedation has resulted in much more prolonged exposure. In these techniques high flow rates of nitrous oxide may be used. This is discussed in greater detail in Chapter 9.

The efficiency of the air conditioning system

The frequency of air changes is often quoted. A figure of twenty per hour is usually considered satisfactory. However, the circulation of air throughout the theatre is often uneven, and frequently the recovery area, where the patient exhales anaesthetic agents, is poorly ventilated and there may be no arrangements for scavenging. The nurse attending the patient is often in direct line with his exhaled gases. There are two further considerations. The first is that some air conditioning systems are wholly or partly recirculating, and may result in the vapours from one location polluting another. The second is that thought must be given to the siting of the external outlet of the extract system, which again may pollute other areas in which people work.

Leakage

However efficient a scavenging system may be, its purposes will be defeated if gases and vapours are permitted to escape from the apparatus. Overt leaks from the high-pressure and regulated-pressure parts of the anaesthetic machine may be easily detected. Leaks from the breathing attachment may be less obvious, however, and may even be due to diffusion through the rubber or neoprene parts. The latter often absorb significant quantities of some of the volatile agents during the administration of one anaesthetic — only to release them during the next. For this reason new and unused breathing attachments should be used for the administration of an anaesthetic to a patient who exhibits sensitivity to a particular anaesthetic agent, for instance in the case of malignant hyperpyrexia.

Leakage may also result from carelessness when vaporizers are refilled.

Before a rush is made to devise and install scavenging systems, it might be better to give priority to the improvement of existing ventilating systems and to determining which, if any, of the anaesthetic agents are responsible for the misfortunes that befall those who work in operating departments.

Scavenging Systems

There are many systems designed to transport the

waste gases and vapours from the breathing system and to discharge them at some safe, remote location. To simply pass a hose through the wall to the outside of the building, or to insert a tube from the piped vacuum system within the distal limb of a T-piece in the breathing attachment, would, as shown below, be satisfactory only in a very few instances. It is quite evident that a universally efficient system is required.

In the absence of the early publication of authoritative advice on methods of scavenging, a number of manufacturers and individuals have developed and advocated scavenging systems which, even if they prove efficient in the operatories for which they were designed (and this is by no means always so!), are not applicable to all other situations. Perhaps the difficulty of designing a system that can be universally installed with a prospect of satisfactory operation has been responsible for the long delay in the publication of the appropriate standards and codes of practice. It would perhaps be wise to await these sources of advice before embarking on the installation of complicated and expensive systems for the disposal of anaesthetic gases and vapours.

Perhaps at this juncture we should consider the requirements of the system and the various items of equipment that have been developed to meet these needs. There must be a *collecting system* which conveys the waste gases via a *transfer tubing* to a *receiving system*. From this they have to pass via a *disposal tubing* to the *disposal system*, which may be active, semi-active (assisted) or passive. Two or more of these components may be embodied in one single item of equipment.

The principles involved, and details of equipment currently available can, perhaps, be better understood if they are discussed in an order in reverse to that in which the gases flow.

The disposal system

ACTIVE SYSTEMS

Active systems employ apparatus that, using some form of power, purposefully moves the waste gases and expels them to the outside atmosphere. Those systems that are used solely for scavenging are termed 'dedicated' systems, to distinguish them from those that are intended primarily for other purposes. The most popular active systems employ one of the following:

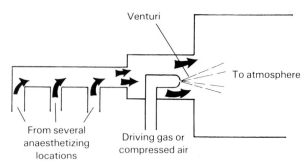

Figure 15.1　A venturi system for the disposal of waste anaesthetic gases.

1. A fan within the fixed pipework 'behind the wall', which may serve either a single operating theatre or a whole suite, such as an operating theatre, anaesthetic (induction) room and recovery room.
2. A venturi system (Fig. 15.1) powered by compressed air, installed as above, 'behind the wall'.
3. An ejector for each disposal point, which is mounted on the wall and acts as an interface between the flexible hose and the rigid pipework.
4. A system such as the ejector flowmeter, which is attached to each anaesthetic machine (Fig. 15.7).

The use of the existing hospital piped vacuum system has often been advocated, but may often be unsatisfactory because:
1. Scavenging requires a high flow with low pressure, whereas the piped vacuum in a hospital is usually a low-flow, high-pressure system.
2. The extra demand upon the medical vacuum for this purpose may result in other users being deprived of an adequate medical vacuum in an emergency.
3. The displacement (flow rate) of the vacuum line may be inadequate to cope with the high flow rate and pulsating nature of the output of some ventilators.
4. The outlet from the vacuum system may be so located that the expired gases would pollute areas where other personnel are working.
5. There is danger that an excessive vacuum may be applied to the patient, as shown in Fig. 15.20 (b).

Use of dedicated vacuum lines for scavenging
The above remarks notwithstanding, high-pressure, low-displacement suction lines can be installed as a separate and dedicated service for scavenging, espe-

cially when a new hospital is being built. This should not only be separate from the general piped vacuum service, but there must be no possibility of interchangeability of the probes and other fittings between them. Consideration must also be given to the type of pump used and the position of the outlet.

Whatever type of high-vacuum system is used, an adequate air-break is essential in order to prevent the accidental application of a dangerous degree of vacuum to the patient. Problems have also occurred when excessive vacuum emptied the reservoir bag on the breathing attachment.

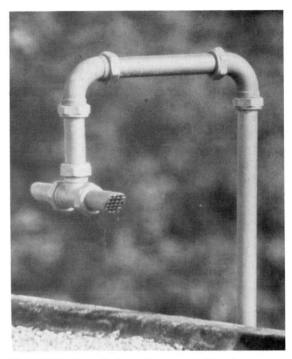
Figure 15.2   A ventile for passive waste gas disposal.

SEMI-ACTIVE (ASSISTED) SYSTEMS

In semi-active systems the expired gases are delivered into the ducts of the extract side of the air conditioning plant. Owing to differences in layout and design, the pressures and flow rates in these systems vary greatly and they may be by no means always efficient. Before the ventilation system is employed it should be ensured that it is not of a recirculating type and that exhaust air is not voided where it may be inhaled by others!

PASSIVE SYSTEMS

In passive systems a tube — albeit wide-bore — passes through one of the walls or the roof of the building and terminates in a ventile (Fig. 15.2). A ventile is a device which depends on the wind to entrain the exhaust gases or air and therefore expedite their voidance. Unfortunately the passive system can be relied upon to operate satisfactorily only when the outlet is installed in a suitable position and when the wind is blowing from the desired quarter. It may be affected by the juxtaposition of other buildings. Under adverse conditions the flow may be in the opposite direction, and, because it would be possible for the scavenged gases from one operating theatre to be expelled into another, each point must have its individual ventile. Branching of the pipework is unsatisfactory. Usually the system terminates on the roof. As the waste gases pass to the cooler areas above the ceiling of the operating theatre they become denser, thus tending to slow their flow, and water vapour may condense and run back down to the theatre, possibly carrying infection. A water trap is therefore essential.

The receiving system

The exhaled gases emerge from the breathing system intermittently, their volume and flow pattern varying according to the type of apparatus in use. For example, with spontaneous respiration there may be a fresh gas flow of, say, 8 l/min, and therefore that is the volume of gases to be scavenged per minute; however, the peak flow rate, during the period that the APL valve is open, may be much higher. On the other hand, the Blease Pulmoflator not only has a minute volume of expired gases, but also, mixed with them, driving air which may be in excess of 70 l/min. The combined peak flow rate of these, during the expiratory phase, is therefore very high.

It would be difficult to design a disposal system that could cope with these great fluctuations. Therefore the receiving system contains a reservoir for the expired and driving gases, from which they are passed more evenly to the disposal system. The container may be either a reservoir bag or an open-ended vessel of rigid material. There may be problems with the latter — for instance, if it is con-

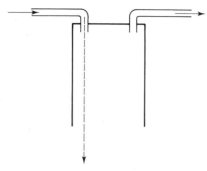

Figure 15.3   A receiving system constructed in such a way that a bolus of gas may pass straight out through the open end.

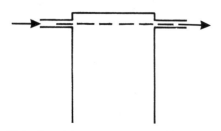

Figure 15.4   A receiving system constructed in such a way that a bolus of gas tends to pass straight into the transfer tubing.

structed as shown in Fig. 15.3, the gases emerging from some of the breathing systems and ventilators may flow with such a velocity that they pass as a 'bolus' straight out of the open end. If, however, the arrangement is as shown in Fig. 15.4, the bolus enters the disposal tubing directly.

If the reservoir is in the form of a closed bag, it is necessary to install two safety valves: one that opens to allow the escape of gases if the pressure within the system rises above a predetermined level, say, 10 cmH2O (~1 kPa), to guard against accidents in which a part of the tubing could be obstructed; and the other that opens at a subatmospheric pressure of 0.5 cmH2O (50Pa), to admit atmospheric air if the demand of the disposal system becomes excessive. This is also known as the 'patient safety protection system' or 'interface system'. In one instance the absence of this provision led to a situation where the closure of the APL valve was prevented and the reservoir bag of the breathing attachment promptly emptied!

As an alternative, an 'air-break' (Fig. 15.5) may be installed, as a fixture on the wall or pendant. This performs the function of the receiver, over- and underpressure relief valves and the disposal tubing.

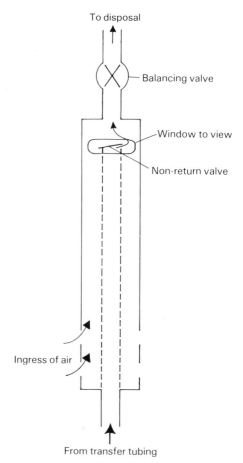

Figure 15.5   An air-break, which allows for the ingress of air to satisfy any excess demand by the disposal system. It performs the functions of both the receiving system and the disposal tubing.

The transfer tube is all that is required. If one disposal system serves more than one air-break, a balancing valve in each air-break is necessary.

The receiving system may be mounted on the anaesthetic apparatus, fixed to the wall of the operating theatre or placed in some intermediate position. Whichever is the case, the transfer tubing between the collecting system and the receiving system should be fitted with either 30 mm or 19 mm tapered connections. The disposal tubing, if detachable, should have fittings *other than* 30 mm, 19 mm, or 22 mm tapers in order to prevent interchangeability with any other part of the anaesthetic apparatus.

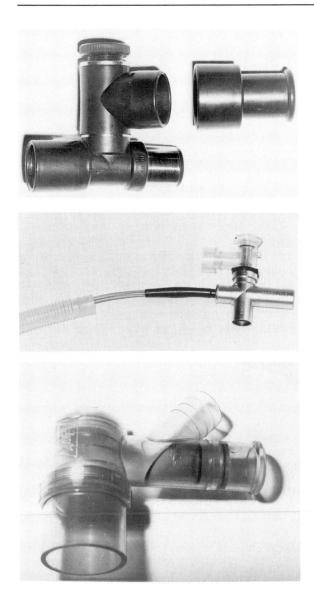
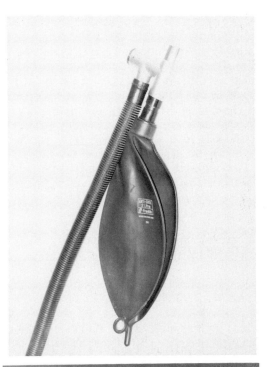
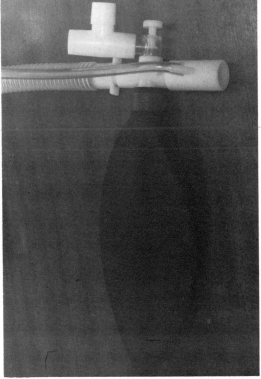

Figure 15.6 Various collecting systems.

The collecting system

The collecting system collects the gases leaving the
anaesthetic equipment. It may consist of a shroud
which surrounds a Heidbrink APL (expiratory)
valve, as shown in Fig 15.6, or it may be a purpose-
made device such as the Enderby valve (Fig. 7.7).
When the latter was installed at the patient end of
the breathing attachment it proved to be very heavy
in use, dragging on the facepiece or endotracheal

tube. To prevent this, breathing attachments such as the Bain and Lack in which the APL valve is situated at the machine end, were developed.

There remain some systems from which it is difficult to collect expired gases, such as the Rees T-piece, in which there is simply an open end to the bag. Here, as in the recovery area, a patient proximity system is employed. One such method is to rest the bag in a large funnel, from which the vacuum system drains a high flow rate of ambient air. Such arrangements may be objectionable due to the noise they make, and their efficiency is questionable.

Breathing Attachments

The advent of scavenging has led to the introduction of many new or modified breathing systems. This is for two reasons.

First, systems such as the Mapleson A (Magill attachment) have the APL valve at the patient end of the corrugated hose. The addition to these of collecting systems with their associated tubing resulted in the placing of weighty components in such a position that they would cause a heavy drag (see above). Systems in which they were mounted at the machine end became preferable.

Secondly, some new systems dispose of the traditional APL valve in favour of a device such as the ejector flowmeter (see Fig. 15.7), or the 'valveless' Samson breathing system (see Fig. 7.3).

Coaxial breathing attachments

The best known of the modified breathing attachments are the Bain and Lack attachments, both of which are examples of coaxial systems, sometimes referred to as TWT (tube within a tube) systems. It is noteworthy that the original Mapleson-D system, with a narrow external tube delivering the fresh gases very close to the patient end, had been popular as early as 1950, because it was said to 'deliver the fresh gases to a point as close to the patient as possible'.

In the newer and more modern forms, the breathing attachment is constructed of coaxial tubes and it is important to distinguish between the Lack and Bain attachments.

The Lack attachment (see Fig. 7.9) is essentially a Mapleson-A system (Magill attachment) and its characteristics are similar to those of the Mapleson A (see p. 122). The Bain attachment (see Fig. 7.8) is essentially a Mapleson-D system and its characteristics are similar to those of the Mapleson D (see p. 125).

The Lack attachment will therefore be most efficient for spontaneous ventilation, whilst the Bain is more suitable for controlled ventilation (See pp. 122–129).

These attachments are convenient to use and compact in design, but the internal tube is not readily visible and may be subjected to kinking, which could lead to obstruction, or to disconnection. An accident resulting from the kinking of the internal tube has already been reported. Some Lack and Bain attachments have been constructed with components that are not all of antistatic material, and in 1982 an explosion occurred in a Bain-type attachment of which the outer tubing was nonconductive. In this case the anaesthetic agent used was cyclopropane, but fortunately the accident occurred after the end of the administration, and the anaesthetic machine had been transferred to a corridor outside the operating theatre.

MOUNTING OF COAXIAL BREATHING ATTACHMENTS

Whereas the Lack attachment may be mounted directly onto the 22 mm male tapered outlet of an anaesthetic machine, the Bain attachment cannot. The coaxial tubing of the latter, which is intended to be disposable, can, however be mounted on a special adaptor which, in turn, fits the 22 mm outlet of the anaesthetic machine (see Fig. 7.8c). On the side branch of this adaptor may be mounted an ordinary APL (expiratory) valve or an antipollution APL valve in the form of a collecting system, and a reservoir bag. It should be noted that although the adaptor, APL valve and reservoir bag are not intended to be disposable, they can become infected from a patient during the course of an anaesthetic and should therefore be resterilized as required.

'Valveless' breathing systems

Because an APL valve must inevitably present some resistance to expiration and also because the attachment of the collecting system to it may present mechanical difficulties, various 'valveless' breathing systems have been devised. Two such systems are described below.

THE SAMSON BREATHING SYSTEM

The Samson breathing system resembles most of the traditional systems used with spontaneous ventilation including those modified for paediatric anaesthesia. The APL spring-loaded disc valve has been replaced by an orifice, the effective diameter of which may be varied (see Fig. 7.3). The various forms of this system are all intended for use with scavenging, suitable arrangements having been made for both active and passive systems.

THE HAFNIA BREATHING SYSTEMS

In the Hafnia breathing systems, which are modifications of the Mapleson-A, -B, -C and -D and closed-circuit systems, the APL valve is replaced by a relatively narrow tube through which excess gases are evacuated by an ejector flowmeter. The advantages claimed for the Hafnia are that scavenging is efficient and that owing to the constant active evacuation of excess gases, the pressure within the breathing attachment is kept at ambient and there is minimal resistance to expiration. If one considers the modification of the Mapleson-A system, (see Fig. 7.75), one finds that whereas during spontaneous breathing with the traditional form the fresh gas flow (FGF) may be reduced to less than the patient's minute volume without rebreathing, in the Hafnia modification the FGF rate to prevent an increase of PCO_2 has to be 135% of the patient's minute volume. This is because in the former the APL valve opens only at intervals to permit the escape of expired gases, while in the latter evacuation is continuous and at times during the cycle fresh gases are withdrawn. Further use of the Hafnia system is required before a full evaluation may be made, but the requirement for a high FGF rate cannot be avoided.

Collecting valves

The earliest commercially produced collecting valve was that designed by Enderby (see Fig. 7.7). Others have since been designed and commercially pro-

duced (see Fig. 15.6). There have also been a number of 'home-made' collecting valves, which were made of various forms of plastic and were often constructed from waste products such as used syringes, syringe containers, etc. Some of these were heavy and unsuitable for installation at the patient end of the breathing attachment, but were satisfactory if mounted on the anaesthetic machine; others were flimsy.

However necessary these may be, it is a pity that they do not produce a whistling noise as does the Heidbrink valve, which hitherto has been a boon to the anaesthetist concerned with observing the patient during spontaneous ventilation. Manufacturers promised the fitting of 'acoustic windows' in the breathing attachment, but these have so far not been forthcoming.

The ejector flowmeter (Fig. 15.7)

The ejector flowmeter assists the removal of waste anaesthetic gases from the breathing attachment. It

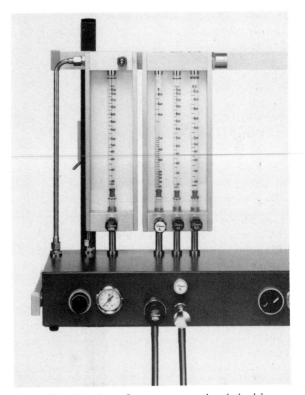

Figure 15.7   The ejector flowmeter mounted on the back bar.

consists of an ejector (venturi) powered by compressed air or oxygen at a pressure of at least 1 bar (100 kPa). The entrained gases pass through a flowmeter, their rate being controlled by a flow control valve. By careful adjustment of this valve the rate of withdrawal of gases from the breathing attachment can be equated to that of the FGF, thus maintaining a status quo within the breathing attachment, with neither under- nor overpressure. The resistance to expiration is reduced virtually to zero. Since this is an active system, a passive disposal system may be used. There may be condensation of water vapour, and therefore a water trap, which may be filled with silica gel, is fitted.

To give some idea of the performance of the ejector flowmeter, 2.4 l/min of driving gas at a pressure of 1 kg/cm^2 (~1 bar) would be required to remove 7.5 l/min of waste gases.

An ejector flowmeter is of use not only to equate the evacuation of waste gases with the FGF, but also to verify that the ejector is functioning correctly. In one investigation concerning over 100 ejectors without flowmeters it was found about half were failing to achieve the expected performance, and one was actually blowing 4.5 l of air plus the waste gases into the atmosphere of the theatre!

The significance of atmospheric pollution and the general principles of methods by which it may be reduced having been discussed, some examples of the equipment available will now be described.

Examples of Scavenging Systems

The Penlon system

In the Penlon system there are a number of components from which those that are necessary to meet the local requirements may be chosen. They may be used in conjunction with an active, assisted or passive disposal system.

The collecting system consists of either a special APL valve or a direct connection to an expiratory port, for example of a ventilator.

Transfer tubing
The inlet connector of the transfer tubing has a 30 mm female taper and may incorporate a positive pressure relief valve which opens at a pressure of

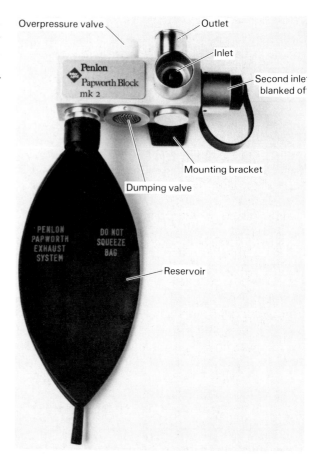

Figure 15.8 The Papworth block. This is a receiving system, which is usually mounted on the anaesthetic machine, but may also be mounted on the wall. There are two inlets, the second of which may be blanked off when not in use. The outlet is connected via the disposal tubing to the disposal system. Note that there is an overpressure valve and a dumping valve.

10 cmH$_2$O. The tubing itself is 22 mm plastic hose, and the outlet has a 30 mm male taper.

There are three different devices for the reception of waste gases and their disposal:

1. THE PAPWORTH BLOCK (Fig. 15.8)

This is a receiving system with a 2 l reservoir bag, two inlets with a 30 mm female taper, and an outlet for a push-on 32 mm hose. There is an overpressure relief valve which opens at 10 cmH$_2$O pressure and a dumping valve which opens at 0.5 cmH$_2$O subatmospheric. A V-plate bracket enables the Pap-

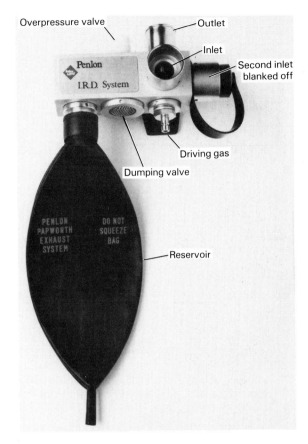

Overpressure valve

Outlet

Inlet

Second inlet blanked off

Penlon
I.R.D. System

Driving gas

Dumping valve

PENLON PAPWORTH EXHAUST SYSTEM   DO NOT SQUEEZE BAG

Reservoir

Figure 15.9 The Penlon integrated receiving and disposal system. This may be mounted on the anaesthetic machine itself. The model illustrated here contains a venturi driven by compressed gas and which expels the waste anaesthetic gases via an otherwise passive disposal system. There is another version in which the waste gases are removed by the piped medical vacuum plant. Note that there are two inlets, and that if only one is in use, the other is blanked off by a specially provided plug.

worth block to be mounted either on an anaesthetic machine or on the wall. There is also a bung to occlude the second inlet if only one transfer tube is in use. It is noteworthy that the reservoir bag is labelled 'Do not squeeze bag'.

2. THE PENLON INTEGRATED RECEIVING AND DISPOSAL UNIT (Fig. 15.9)

This unit is intended to be attached to an anaesthetic machine and to replace the Papworth safety block. It is similar to the above, except that it has the addition

of a venturi flow inducer and therefore fulfils the role of an active disposal system. The venturi requires 3–4 *l*/min of driving gas, at a pressure of 400 kPa. It can handle up to 60 *l*/min of waste gases without imposing any positive pressure upon the transfer system.

3. THE PENLON PURGE (Fig. 15.10)

This consists of a wall-mounted venturi, again using 3–4 *l*/min of driving gas, at 400 kPa. It is connected to the Papworth receiving block by a 32 mm corrugated hose, and the outlet is a 35 mm parallel tube for fitting to the copper pipe of the passive system.

THE PENLON GRILLE ATTACHMENT (Fig. 15.11)

This is an attachment that can be screwed to the extract grille of the ventilating system. It may have a protruding or a flush 35 mm parallel connection. It is common practice to lead the gases through a short length of 35 mm pipe from the grille attachment to a position further within the ventilating duct, thus assuring that there is efficient scavenging.

The Eastox antipollution system

The components of the Eastox anti-pollution system are intended to be assembled in such a way as to suit any particular circumstance and to be connected to whichever type of disposal system is available. They include a scavenging APL valve (Fig. 15.12), a collecting block system (Fig. 15.13), a reservoir-type receiving system and the appropriate tubing. The collecting block has two inlets for waste gases, such as the attachment for spontaneous breathing on the anaesthetic machine and the outlet from a ventilator. There are also a dumping valve and an over-pressure valve. The reservoir (Fig. 15.14) consists of a large container that is open at the lower end.

If a passive disposal system is used, the waste gases may be collected into the collecting block and then transferred directly to the disposal system. Where there is an active or semi-active system the reservoir is interposed between the collecting block and the disposal system. It may be mounted either on the anaesthetic machine or on the wall.

Certain design features of the reservoir-type receiving system are worthy of mention. First, the

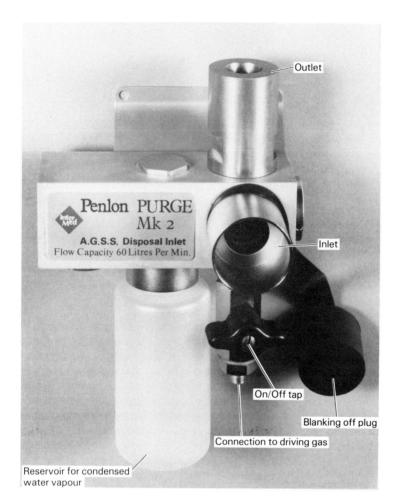

Figure 15.10   The Penlon purge. This is a wall-mounted system, which contains a venturi which entrains waste anaesthetic gases and expels them via an otherwise passive disposal system. The requirements for the driving gas are 4 *l*/min, at a pressure of 400 kPa ($\sim$ 60 lb/in^2), to dispose of up to 60 *l*/min of waste gases. There is a reservoir to accommodate condensed water vapour which might run back from a passive disposal system.

holes drilled in the side wall towards the lower end would allow the ingress of air or efflux of gases under excess pressure if the open end were occluded, for instance if it were stood on a flat surface. Secondly, the inlet port is directed horizontally, pointing directly towards the exit port. This is important when one considers the fast-moving bolus of gas that may be passed through it rapidly, for example from the exhaust of a ventilator. If it were to pass vertically into the reservoir, it might be shot straight out of the open end, however large the capacity of the reservoir might be.

By selecting the appropriate components from the above, most types of breathing system or ventilator may be connected to any type of disposal system.

The Gardner antipollution system (Fig. 15.15)

The Gardner anti-pollution system is intended to be used in conjunction with either the hospital vacuum system or a dedicated high-pressure vacuum system installed for this purpose. It includes a large, transparent sealed container, which has the following features:

An inlet port through which the collecting system delivers gases directly to the interior of the container.

An outlet port connected to the vacuum system.

An 'adjuster' to control the rate of evacuation.

An overpressure relief valve.

A dumping valve.

Within the container there is a 0.75 *l* reservoir bag, the interior of which is isolated from the con-

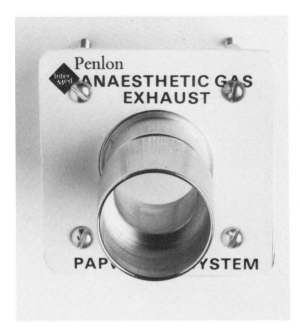

Figure 15.11   The Penlon grille attachment. This is attached to an existing extract grille of the ventilating system by screws or toggle bolts. There is a 30 mm female taper connection to accept the disposal tubing.

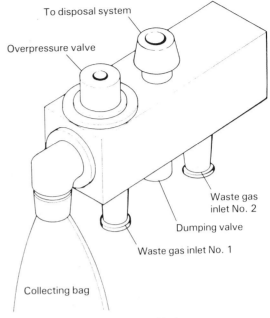

Figure 15.13   The Eastox collecting block.

tainer but open to the ambient atmosphere. Ambient air leaves and enters the bag in phase with the pulses of waste anaesthetic gases entering and leaving the container.

The Medec Gasovac scavenging system

This system is intended primarily for use with an active disposal system employing either a dedicated high vacuum line or the general hospital medical vacuum. The receiving system consists of a 'bag in a bottle' but with a number of interesting refinements (Fig. 15.16).

The exhaust gases pass through a flow restrictor to the vacuum line. Before they encounter the flow restrictor they pass two tees, one of which is to a reservoir bag and the other to a side limb. Ambient air is drawn through the 'exchanger' in order to comply with the filling and emptying of the bag

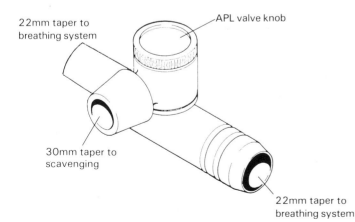

Figure 15.12   The Eastox scavenging APL valve.

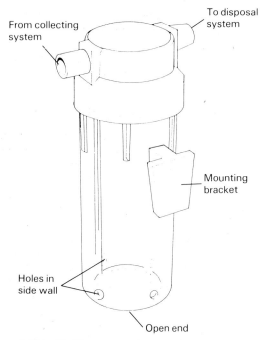

Figure 15.14   The Eastox reservoir.

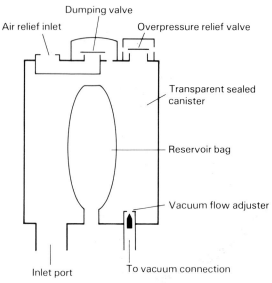

Figure 15.15   The Gardner anti-pollution system.

during the phases of respiration, and also passes, as required, up the side limb to satisfy excess vacuum. The system also includes an overpressure valve and a dumping valve.

The vacuum displacement is said to range between 10 and 18 *l*/min, which would be satisfactory for breathing systems with spontaneous ventilation, controlled ventilation with minute volume dividers, and also with closed, rebreathing systems. It would

not, however, be satisfactory for use with ventilators that have a high efflux of driving compressed air or oxygen.

The general caveat with regard to the use of a piped vacuum system for scavenging must be regarded. In other words, it must be ascertained that the vacuum pumps would not be damaged by the evacuation of large volumes of gases containing the vapours of anaesthetic agents, and that the discharge point is appropriately located.

With non-recycling air conditioning systems or with separate dedicated fan extract systems, wide-bore tubing is used in place of the narrow-bore

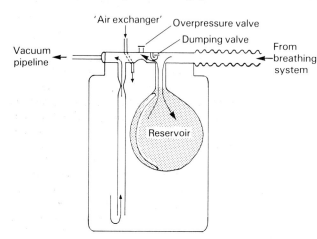

Figure 15.16   The working principles of the Medec Gasovac system (see text).

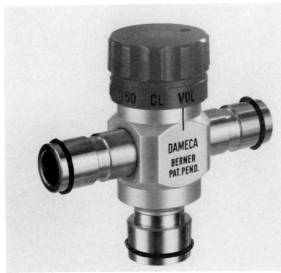

(a)

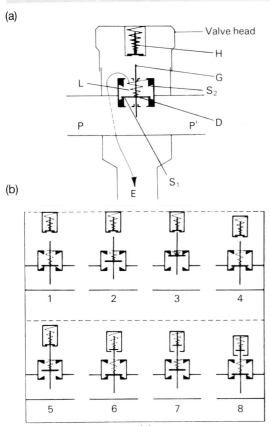

(b)

(c)

Figure 15.17   (a) The Berner valve. (b) & (c) Working principles (see text).

tubing to the vacuum plant, and the flow restrictor is removed. Caution should also be exercised in using this equipment with inflammable anaesthetic agents such as cyclopropane and ether, and the maker's instructions should be observed if these are employed.

The Berner valve (Dameca) (Fig. 15.17)

The Berner valve can be used with spontaneous, assisted or controlled ventilation. Its mode of operation can perhaps be best understood if its components are considered one at a time. The two ports P and P' (Fig. 15.17b) are connected within the breathing system. In this instance P is connected to the patient and P' to a reservoir bag and the fresh gas flow. The head of the valve is mounted on a screw thread and thus may be screwed up and down. Let us start with it screwed fully up. At rest, the valve disc D, which is mounted on a guide G, is kept in contact with the lower seating S_1 by the light spring L (Fig. 15.17c (**1**)). When the pressure in the breathing system reaches 1.5 cmH₂O, D is lifted to a midway position (Fig. 15.17c (**2**)), allowing excess gases to escape. During spontaneous inspiration the valve remains closed by the action of L, so preventing the admission of atmospheric air.

If the breathing bag is compressed sharply, so as to cause an increase of pressure within the system in excess of 3 cmH₂O, D rises so far that it engages upon the upper seating S_2, again closing the valve and thus permitting controlled or assisted ventilation (Fig. 15.17c (**3**)).

A problem arises, however, in that if the pressure within the system were to be *maintained* at over 3 cmH₂O (as could happen during controlled ventilation, or during spontaneous ventilation as a result of the patient coughing), the escape of excess gas from the system would be prevented, because D would be kept permanently seated on S_2. To prevent this there is a second spring H, of higher tension, attached to the valve head. When the valve head is screwed down from its uppermost position (marked 'VOL'), H and its plate impinge upon G and oppose the upward movement of D towards S_2 (Fig. 15.17c (**5**)). The pressure is progressively increased as the head is screwed further and when it is completely down to the 'CL' position (Fig. 15.17c (**8**)) pressure on the guide is such that D is kept permanently seated on S_1 and the valve is completely closed. By screwing the head down only as far as 'SP' (Fig.

15.17c (**4**)), the permanent closure of D on S₂ is prevented.

Since the pressure in the patient's air passages, and in the breathing system, varies with the degree of inflation of the lungs, the tidal volume may be selected by adjusting the valve head (and thereby the tension in H) so that the valve opens at the appropriate pressure, allowing excess gases to escape (Fig. 15.17c (**6**) & (**7**)). Under these circumstances the tidal volume at any particular setting will be constant, provided that the patient's compliance does not alter. The valve head is calibrated for pressures of 5, 20, 35 and 50 cmH₂O.

The expired gases are taken away through a port E, to which a length of corrugated hose may be attached to act as a reservoir. The vacuum hose used to achieve scavenging may be introduced either into the downstream end of the corrugated hose or to a small side-branch, which is fitted to the back of the valve body in some models.

Absorption systems

Alternative methods may be employed for the removal of the vapours of volatile anaesthetic agents from waste gases. Activated charcoal, in canisters of 1 kg, absorbs halothane vapour efficiently. It has a low resistance and may be incorporated in the expiratory limb of a breathing system (Fig. 15.18). The canister increases in weight as the halothane is absorbed, and this may be monitored by a spring balance on which it is mounted. When the weight reaches the level stated, it should be discarded. Care must be taken to ensure that it is disposed of in a safe location, where it will not permit the halothane to be released and pollute the atmosphere breathed by other people. Used canisters should not be allowed to fall into the hands of drug addicts, who have been known to heat them in order to gain the release of halothane. Indeed, the use of heat to release the halothane has been employed in one type of canister, which being made of suitable metal, may be placed in the autoclave in order to discharge it. If this system is employed, one must, again, ensure that the discharge of halothane-laden steam from the autoclave is to a safe location.

Unfortunately recent research incriminating nitrous oxide rather than the volatile anaesthetic agents has rendered the employment of the relatively simple Aldasorber less appropriate.

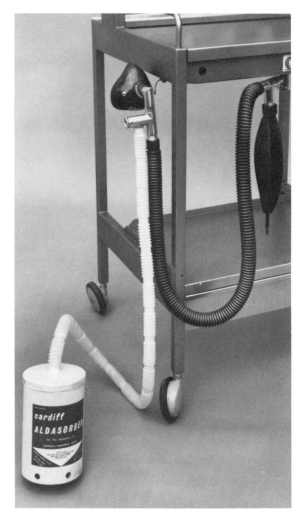

Figure 15.18   The Aldasorber.

Improvised systems

In the absence of a disposal system, it is still possible to make arrangements to lessen the exposure of the anaesthetist to waste anaesthetic gases. When the Mapleson-A system (Magill attachment) is used, and also during dental chair anaesthesia, there is a tendency for the expiratory valve to discharge waste gases in a position very close to the nose and mouth of the anaesthetist.

To prevent this it may be replaced by systems such as those shown in Figs 15.19 and 15.20. The

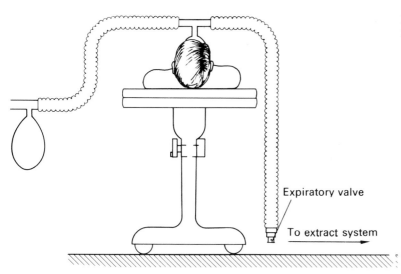

Figure 15.19   A simple method for removing exhaled gases.

Expiratory valve

To extract system

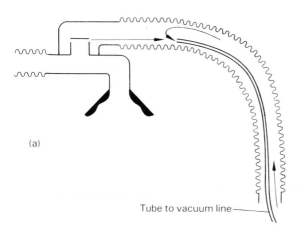

(a)

Tube to vacuum line

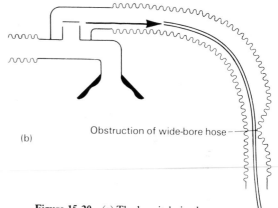

(b)

Obstruction of wide-bore hose

Figure 15.20   (a) The hospital piped vacuum line used for scavenging. The standard length of corrugated hose acts as a reservoir. (b) An obstruction of the corrugated hose could result in an excessive vacuum being applied to the patient.

former may be assembled from the original reservoir bag, the twin tubing and Y-piece of a circle absorber and an expiratory valve at the end of the distal limb. The waste gases are discharged at floor level and therefore do not pollute the air breathed by the personnel to the same extent as before.

The use of the vacuum line was described and its disadvantages enumerated on p. 274. Figure 15.20 shows how it may be used and also how an excessive vacuum may be accidentally applied to the patient.

16

Medical Suction Apparatus

The three essential parts of a suction apparatus are:
1. The source of the vacuum.
2. The reservoir.
3. The delivery tubing (which may include a nozzle or a catheter). Other refinements that modify performance are discussed later.

The efficiency of a suction apparatus depends on:
1. The displacement, i.e. the volume of air (measured at atmospheric pressure and usually expressed in l/min), that the pump is able to move.
2. The degree of negative (subatmospheric) pressure that can be produced by the pump, with particular regard to the time taken to achieve it.
3. The length and diameter of the delivery tube.

The Source of the Vacuum

An electric or other motor may be used to drive a mechanical pump, various forms of which are shown in Fig. 16.1.

Figure 16.1a shows a piston pump, which is capable of creating a high vacuum, but in portable models has a rather low displacement. Figure 16.1b shows a diaphragm pump, which is a variation of the piston pump and is rather simpler. Figure 16.1c shows a rotary pump, which may be designed to produce a very high displacement, as in the high-volume aspirator (Fig. 16.2), which works on the principle of a vacuum cleaner. And Fig. 16.1d shows a high-pressure rotary pump.

Note that the pumps shown in Fig. 16.1a and d usually require hydraulic oil, the level of which should be periodically inspected, and topped up, as required.

A bellows (Fig. 16.3) may be used to draw in air from one direction and expel it in another, as in the foot-operated suction apparatus (Fig. 16.4). A rubber bulb resembling an enema syringe may be used in the same way.

Pneumatically driven pumps usually work on the injector (venturi) principle. They may be driven by compressed air, oxygen, steam, water or 'gas' from an aerosol can. A high displacement or a high-vacuum pressure may be achieved, depending on the design of the injector. When driven from an oxygen cylinder, these pumps are usually wasteful of oxygen, but they have the virtue of being portable (Fig. 16.5).

A piped vacuum service may be installed using a high-capacity pump connected to a large reservoir in a central position. The patient end of the pipeline is fitted with a self-closing, non-interchangeable valve similar to that on the oxygen and nitrous oxide pipelines, to which the reservoir bottle and delivery tube may be attached. There should be a trap or other device to prevent liquid or solid matter being drawn into the pipeline system, where it could cause a blockage that would be difficult to relieve. A pressure regulator may also be fitted at this point to reduce the degree of vacuum applied to the patient. The central pump, which operates intermittently to maintain the vacuum in the central reservoir, is controlled by a pressure switch. It is common practice to install two pumps so that one may be in use while the other is undergoing maintenance. (See Chapter 4.)

Traps should be installed in the various branches of a large piped system to intercept any liquid or solid accidentally aspirated into it. The output of the vacuum pump should be either discharged to the exterior at a suitable site or fitted with a filter to prevent the spread of infection.

The Reservoir

Whatever the source of the vacuum, the size of the reservoir is important. Sufficient capacity should be allowed for all the matter to be aspirated. Too big a reservoir, however, will not only be cumbersome, but will also increase the time taken for vacuum

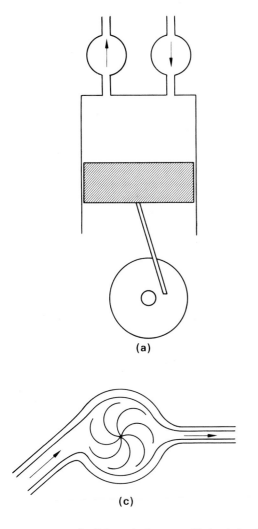

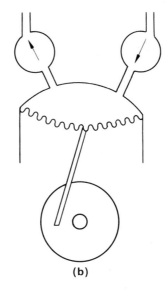

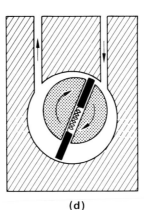

Figure 16.1 Vacuum pumps. (a) A piston pump. (b) A diaphragm pump. (c) A rotary vane 'vacuum cleaner' pump. (d) A high-pressure rotary vane pump.

(a)

(b)

(c)

(d)

pressure to build up in it, even if the inlet for the delivery tube is completely occluded.

The rim of the jar should be free from chips, and the sealing washer should be in good order. A common cause of failure in suction apparatus is a leak at this point. Jars should be graduated so that the volume of an aspirate such as blood can be measured. In the case of large jars it is wise to select a model that has a neck wide enough to admit the hand in order to facilitate cleaning. Recently jars made of polycarbonate have been developed and these are more satisfactory.

The Delivery Tubing

The diameter and length of the delivery tubing should allow the greatest possible amount of suction at the 'patient end'. Reference to the behaviour of fluids, which is set out on p. 11 et seq. will show that the resistance of the delivery tube is reduced by keeping it as wide and as short as possible. Whereas a tube of about 6 mm (¼ in.) diameter may present little resistance to air, it will considerably impede the passage of blood, mucus or vomit.

The flow of air alone through the delivery tube may be laminar, but when it is mixed with liquids or bits of solid matter it is likely to become turbulent,

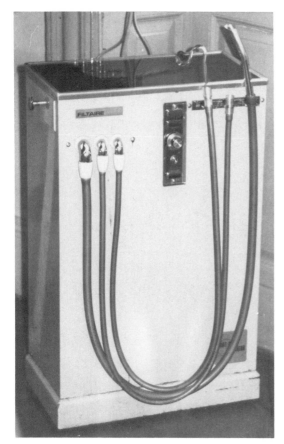

Figure 16.2 A high-volume aspirator, which is used particularly in the dental operatory.

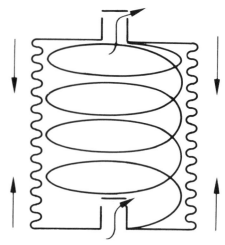

Figure 16.3 The bellows and spring pump. The bellows is closed by the pressure of the foot and reopened by the recoil of the spring.

which case provision may be made to admit air into the delivery tube or bottle by means of a bleed valve or hole. If there is a hole in the proximal end of the suction end or catheter, it may be occluded when required by a finger (Fig. 16.6). This is particularly useful when performing endobronchial suction. The advantage of placing the bleed valve or hole at this point is that it does not reduce the suction through the delivery tube.

Many of the 'disposable' plastic suction ends can be cleaned and resterilized by autoclaving, provided that care is taken to avoid distortion.

further increasing the resistance. The wall of the tube should be sufficiently firm to prevent collapse or kinking.

The suction nozzle or catheter

It may be necessary to use a long, narrow catheter, as, for example, in bronchial suction, but otherwise excessive length should be avoided. Suction 'ends' should taper to the nozzle so that as much of the length as possible may be of wide diameter. The shape of the tip should be smooth so as to prevent damage to delicate surfaces, and it is sometimes desirable to have two or more holes so that suction will continue if one is blocked, possibly by sucking the mucous membrane into it. This type of blockage is more common when the pressure is too high, in

Refinements to Medical Suction Apparatus

The following refinements may be added to a suction apparatus, in the positions indicated in Fig. 16.7.

A cut-off valve
This is fitted inside the reservoir jar, and usually consists of a float which, being lifted by the rising level of liquid, operates a valve to shut off the connection with the suction source. Its purpose is to prevent liquid from a full reservoir entering the pump and causing failure. Sometimes it operates by admitting outside air rather than liquid from the jar

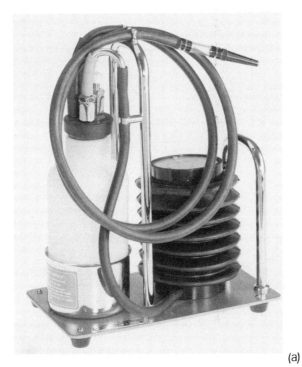
(a)

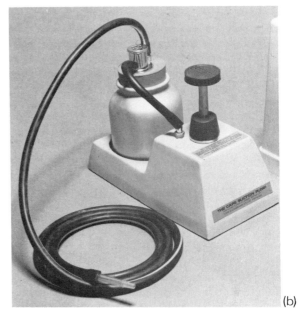
(b)

Figure 16.4   Foot operated suction pumps. (a) The Ambu. (b) The Cape.

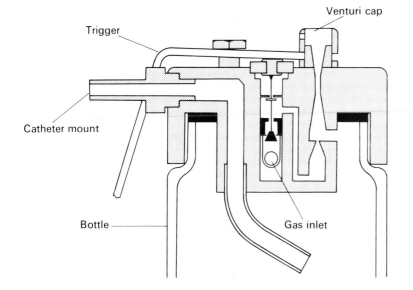

Figure 16.5   An injector suction unit.

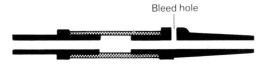

Figure 16.6   The bleed hole in a suction nozzle, which can be occluded by the operator's finger. Note that there may be a transparent window to allow the operator to observe the material that is being aspirated.

freely to the vacuum source.

Occasionally a cut-off valve, having been closed, is held closed by the vacuum acting on it. It is necessary after emptying the reservoir either to stop the vacuum source or to pull the float down again and so reopen the valve.

A bacterial filter

This may (in fact, should) be fitted to prevent air that has been contaminated during its passage through the apparatus from infecting the atmosphere when it is blown out of the pump. It is best placed between the reservoir and the pump so as to protect the latter. A container packed with cotton wool makes a fairly efficient filter — provided that it is dry. If it becomes wet, it will be ineffective, and may also obstruct the air flow. Filters should be changed at regular intervals, depending on their size, or they simply become a reservoir of infection. If there is no filter, a little disinfectant solution may be used in the reservoir, but this is not very effective.

A vacuum control valve

A vacuum control valve may be fitted between the pump and the reservoir. This is a bleed valve which, when opened, admits air, thereby reducing the degree of vacuum.

A vacuum gauge

These gauges, which are normally calibrated from 0 to 760 mmHg, are fitted to the tubing between the vacuum control valve and the reservoir, or on the top of the reservoir itself. Note that modern vacuum gauges are calibrated so that the needle moves in a counter-clockwise direction as the vacuum increases. However, there are still many in use that are calibrated clockwise.

Foam prevention

Foam may sometimes be a problem since it causes closure of the cut-off valve when the reservoir is far from full, or it may pass to the filter and even the pump, causing failure. Foam may be suppressed by the addition of methylated spirit to the reservoir (remember explosion risk) or, more effectively, by silicone-based emulsions such as Foamtrol.

A stop valve

This valve may be used to occlude the delivery tubing close to the nozzle. It allows the build-up of a vacuum during a standby period and is particularly useful when the pump gives a low displacement.

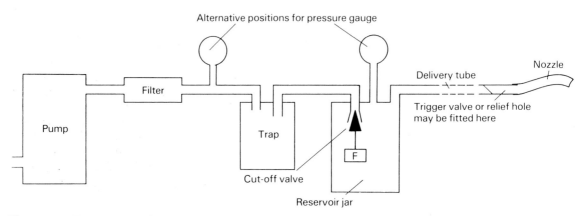

Figure 16.7   The components of a portable suction apparatus. The pump may be protected from infected material, which could be drawn from the reservoir jar, by a trap or filter. There is a cut-off valve within the reservoir jar, which operates when the level of fluid in the jar is sufficiently high to raise the float F, so as to prevent any foreign material being aspirated into the pump. There are alternative positions for the pressure gauge. A trigger valve may be fitted close to the nozzle in order to maintain a constant standby vacuum in the reservoir jar.

Two reservoir jars

There are two ways in which two jars rather than one might be used. In one arrangement there is a switching arrangement that enables the second jar to be used and the first one to be isolated when it is full, or if there is a leak owing to a faulty washer or chipped jar. This is of particular use when large volumes of fluid, such as ascites, are being aspirated. In the second arrangement the jars are in series so that if the first jar is overfilled, the overflow goes harmlessly to the second jar rather than into the vacuum pump or the pipeline.

Unfortunately the mechanical principles, though simple, are not always appreciated by the theatre staff, and misconnection is common.

When selecting a suction apparatus for a particular purpose the following points should be considered:

1. Must it be portable? If so, foot suction or cylinder with an injector? If not, electric motor or pipeline?
2. Is a high displacement needed?
3. Is a high vacuum needed?
4. What size should the reservoir be?

It is also important to ascertain in the case of an electrically driven suction machine whether it is rated for continuous or intermittent use, since many are intended for intermittent operation only, and prolonged periods of operation could cause electrical or mechanical failure. Such units are often labelled appropriately.

'High volume aspirators', which use a pump similar to a vacuum cleaner, usually have three delivery tubes of different diameters or with different nozzles (Fig. 16.2). Under no circumstances should the nozzles not in use be obstructed, since the free air passing through them is needed to cool the motor, which may otherwise overheat. These aspirators are most commonly used in the dental operatory, especially where a jet of water or airborne spray is used for cooling during the operation of the high-speed turbine drill.

Pipeline Vacuum Units

Piped vacuum systems are now installed in most major hospitals. The 'behind the wall' equipment

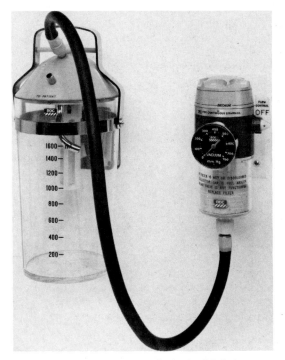

Figure 16.8 A pipeline vacuum unit. On the right is the controller, which is plugged directly into a flush fitting outlet, which is obscured in this picture. On the left is the reservoir jar.

and terminal outlets are described in Chapter 4. There are two types of local vacuum unit:

1. Free-standing floor units, often with two large reservoir bottles, used for surgical purposes in the operating theatre.
2. Those that are wall mounted and often plug directly into the pipeline outlet, as shown In Fig. 16.8, and have a single reservoir jar. These may be either (a) high vacuum, for short-term use for the aspiration of vomitus, secretions, etc. (for which a high pressure and high displacement are required) or (b) low pressure for prolonged suction of body cavities. The latter has in recent years to a large extent been replaced by Portovac and Readyvac concertina drainage systems, where no external power source is needed.

Standards and Tests

Individual surgical suction apparatus

Electrically operated high-vacuum, high air displacement types are covered by BS 4199, Part 1 of 1967, and electrically operated apparatus for continuous drainage by BS 4199, Part 2 of 1968.

1. HIGH-VACUUM APPARATUS

The above standard requires that this apparatus should develop, within ten seconds of switching on, a vacuum of 500 mmHg ($\sim$ 660 mbar) below atmospheric pressure, and that at that pressure, and without suction tubing attached, it should displace 25 l/min of free air. This may be sufficient for surgical purposes, but for use in the anaesthetic and recovery location, where vomitus may have to be speedily aspirated, a flow rate of at least 35 l/min is desirable and a negative pressure of at least 600 mmHg ($\sim$ 800 mbar), and if possible higher, is desirable.

2. LOW-VACUUM APPARATUS

This is used for the continuous drainage of body cavities, and the maximum permissible negative pressure is 180 mmHg ($\sim$ 240 mbar), but should not fall below 150 mmHg ($\sim$ 200 mbar). The pressure gauge is calibrated for 0–200 mmHg.

BS 4199, Part 2 specifies two types, one with a low air flow of not less than 0.3 l/min and the other with a high air flow of not less than 20 l/min.

Testing

A simple test to prove the efficiency of a high-vacuum suction apparatus is performed as follows. A litre or so of water, so hot that the hand can only just be immersed in it, is placed in the reservoir jar, which is then replaced in position. The vacuum source is then turned on and the delivery tube completely occluded. By the time the vacuum has built up to its maximum the water should be boiling.

Although it is generally agreed that all items, such as endotracheal tubes and airways, that come into direct contact with the patient should be sterilized, there remains a considerable divergence of opinion as to the degree of sterility required for anaesthetic machines and ventilators. Whereas in some hospitals anaesthetic ventilators and the breathing attachments of anaesthetic machines are regularly sterilized, in others this is seldom done. The fact that there is little evidence of cross-infection of patients when sterilization is neglected in general anaesthetic practice should not be allowed to condone such negligence. There are certain circumstances in which thorough cleansing and sterilization are universally accepted as necessary. Such occasions are when a patient with a virulent infection or tuberculosis has been anaesthetized, or when a patient with a respiratory infection has been maintained on a ventilator in an intensive care ward. In such cases special precautions may be taken, and these are discussed later. It can be argued that any patient who is ventilated over a prolonged period becomes infected, and so does the ventilator. In practice a compromise is drawn between complete sterilization after each case, on the one hand, and what may be regarded as the minimum required, on the other. Most instances of cross-infection from ventilators that have been reported are from intensive care wards where patients are on prolonged treatment, rather than from the operating theatre. Undoubtedly the risk of cross-infection is increased where little time elapses between cases.

At this juncture we should distinguish between decontamination, disinfection and sterilization. *Decontamination* consists of the physical removal of infected matter and can be referred to as a thorough washing or scrubbing. It renders an object both bacteriologically and ethically more acceptable and does not necessarily require high temperatures or chemical agents. Modern decontamination devices include the automatic washing machine and the ultrasonic washer. Some detergents are particularly useful; for example, it is claimed that 'Neodex gets under and lifts off contaminating material'. Certainly, if dirty airways and endotracheal tubes are dropped into a solution of Neodex (20 ml/5 *l* of water) immediately after use, they appear very clean when they are removed at the end of the day's work. *Disinfection* implies the removal or killing of most or all infective organisms, with the exception of the

17

Sterilization of Anaesthetic Apparatus

most resistant ones such as spores. This is regarded as suitable for many purposes and may be done by cold chemical methods or pasteurization, which is particularly suitable for materials that do not well withstand the higher temperatures of autoclaving. *Sterilization* infers the killing of all organisms, including spores, but the methods employed either require expensive and sophisticated equipment (irradiation) or the employment of temperatures that damage the article being sterilized.

Note that not all methods of sterilization or disinfection remove such things as chemical contamination. The term 'decontamination' has often been used erroneously where 'disinfection' was more appropriate since no attempt at the removal of the contaminant was included in the attempts at destruction of the contaminating organisms.

The stages in the process are therefore:
1. General cleaning and decontamination, and then, if required,
2. Disinfection, or
3. Sterilization.

Decontamination

A system for the decontamination of the corrugated hose, reservoir bags, facepieces, airways and endotracheal tubes, as well as other small items of anaesthetic equipment, is available in the form of the Scotts' SL40 anaesthetic apparatus decontaminator (Fig. 17.1). This machine resembles a dishwasher

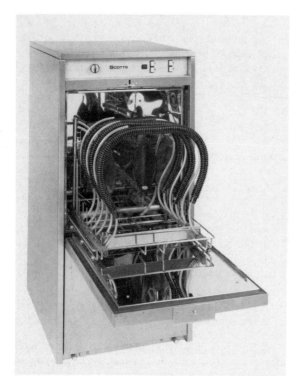

Figure 17.1   The Scotts' SL40 anaesthetic apparatus decontaminator. Note that different trays may be used in the same machine to wash and disinfect other equipment, including surgical instruments.

and cleans the equipment and then pasteurizes it by raising the temperature to 80 °C and holding it at that level for 10 minutes. The pasteurization combines the process of decontamination with disinfection. An earlier model employed Cidex, but this proved to be uneconomical.

Of particular use for small pieces of equipment, and for equipment of intricate shape, is the ultrasonic washer. This consists of a bath of water in which the objects are immersed and in which they are subjected to ultrasonic vibration. The water contains detergent, and for specialized purposes, as in the dental operatory, other chemicals, such as ammonia, which may be used to break up the resins and alginates which are common contaminators.

If no further treatment in the way of disinfection or sterilization is required, articles such as facepieces may then be thoroughly washed and rinsed in hot water and then hung up to dry.

Disinfection

One of the most suitable methods for the disinfection of anaesthetic equipment is *pasteurization*. This consists of heating the article to a temperature of 70 °C for 20 min or 80 °C for 10 min. It is most conveniently done in a water bath but may also be done in the low-pressure autoclave (see below). It is not so efficient as boiling, but does kill most infective agents and is usually considered adequate for perishable articles and where absolute sterility is not necessarily required. Whereas plastic and rubber articles may soon lose their shape and antistatic properties as a result of repeated boiling, they are less damaged by pasteurization. The antistatic properties may be restored by the weekly application of a spray such as Croxtine (BOC).

One of the problems arising in the use of the water tank or sterilizer is that rigid discipline is required to ensure that it continues for the necessary length of time. Not only must the temperature be maintained but one must also prevent the addition of extra items while the process is continuing, thus recontaminating those already being treated.

Boiling

Relatively small articles, including facepieces, may be boiled in water for five minutes. This is a fairly efficient method of disinfection, provided that one maintains the discipline mentioned above for pasteurization. Boiling is satisfactory for any article made entirely of metal and also for those made of rubber or neoprene. The process should be timed from the point where the water returns to the boiling point after the introduction of the last item to be treated. Large, cold metal articles may lower the temperature significantly!

Chemical methods of disinfection

Formaldehyde (H·CHO) vapour is only moderately efficient as a disinfectant and requires the presence of water vapour. It is essential that there is sufficient generation and circulation of the formaldehyde vapour. Paraformaldehyde tablets contain 95% formaldehyde in polymerized form and no more than 5% residue. Their action depends on sublimation, which takes many hours to complete and may be inefficient. The nebulization of formalin solution (which contains at least 38% w/w of formaldehyde) is a more efficient means of generating sufficient vapour. A high vapour concentration of formaldehyde is required to ensure satisfactory sterilization.

A method of autoclaving with low-pressure, low-temperature steam together with formaldehyde has recently been introduced and is described below.

Alcohol has in the past been considered to be a fairly efficient sterilizing agent. It may be used in the form of 70% ethyl alcohol or 70% isopropyl alcohol, in water. Watery mixtures of alcohol are more efficient than pure alcohol. A 'quick lick' of alcohol is probably useless except as a cleanser.

Chlorhexidine (Hibitane) may be used in varying concentrations. It is a non-detergent chemical disinfectant. Facepieces may be soaked for half an hour in a 0.05% solution in water. Quicker sterilizing (2 min) may be attained by using a 0.5% solution in 70% alcohol. This solution is also useful for swabbing down equipment such as anaesthetic machines. Detergent chemicals should be avoided since they may cause damage to the rubber parts of anaesthetic apparatus.

Chloroxylenol (Dettol) has frequently been used, particularly for facepieces. A dilute solution should be used and the facepieces must be rinsed in clear water for 2 hr after immersion. However, there is a danger that the patient may develop skin rashes of the face as a result of sensitivity to chloroxylenol, which is absorbed into the rubber of the facepiece; so this agent is best avoided.

Cidex, a glutaraldehyde solution which requires to be mixed with an activator before use, claims a very high bacteriological range and is active against various spores. The solution may be kept in use for up to 14 days. It is very expensive, but is popular for the disinfection of items such as endoscopic instruments.

Mists or fogs of sterilizing agents may be used for equipment such as ventilators, which draw the air through them, or even for an entire room full of equipment. In the case of ventilators, the agents are best nebulized in an ultrasonic nebulizer (Fig. 13.8). Care must be taken to make sure that the nebulizer does not run dry, since some types may be damaged if this happens. Larger fogging machines (Fig. 17.2) are available, which are capable of treating a whole operating theatre. Recently, doubt has been ex-

pressed as to the efficiency of fogging a whole theatre. Also, evidence has been reported of damage to electrical apparatus by corrosion. However, it is described here since the principle is satisfactory and it is the nature of the disinfectants themselves that presents problems. The advent of new agents may bring fogging back into vogue.

For ventilators, solutions such as 70% alcohol or Stericol, a mixture of dimethyl phenols in an alcoholic/anionic detergent base, which contains 18% phenols v/v, or hydrogen peroxide, may be used. Resiguard, which contains 1% picloxydine digluconate, 11% octylphenoxy polyethoxyethanol and 12% benzalkonium chloride, is used for sterilizing operating theatres as a whole, but is probably better not used in the ultrasonic nebulizer for the purpose of sterilizing ventilators. Alcohol may be nebulized and passed through a ventilator, but the risk of explosion must be considered. During the process, ventilators should be left running and drawing the sterilizing agent through all the parts that are to be sterilized.

The ventilators should then be run for several hours in fresh air, to clear all the sterilizing agent from the tubing and internal parts of the breathing systems.

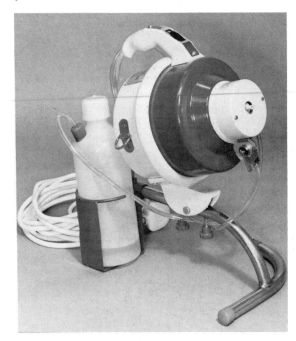

Figure 17.2 A fogging machine.

Another system uses a fumigation cabinet. Figure 17.3) shows the Dräger Purfactor cabinet, built into the structure of an operating theatre suite. Small articles may first be hung up on nozzles through which the fumigating vapour passes, and then larger items such as anaesthetic machines are wheeled in. A special disinfecting agent is first introduced into the cabinet and then expelled through a vent pipe. Residual traces of vapour are then removed and the contents of the cabinet rinsed and then dried in hot air. The disadvantage of this method is that the whole process takes 2½ hr and some preparation is required beforehand.

This principle may be enlarged to form a complete 'formalin room' into which several ventilators may be wheeled. They are set in motion so that the disinfectant vapours are drawn into all the parts of the ventilator that may be contaminated. The location of the exhaust from this room needs careful consideration.

Sterilization

Autoclaving

In autoclaving, the most effective method of sterilization, the articles to be treated are placed in a chamber with a close fitting door. Steam is admitted not only to the chamber, but also to the jacket surrounding it, in order to raise the temperature within. The various stages of the process are usually controlled automatically and finish with a vacuum stage in which the remaining moisture is removed. Small portable autoclaves generate their own steam by electricity and are independent of the boiler house.

The steam is at a temperature considerably above the boiling point of water and therefore at a high pressure. The time required depends on both the pressure and temperature developed, as shown below:

Time	Pressure		Temperature
30 min	15 lb/in²	1.05 kg/cm²	122 °C
10 min	20 lb/in²	1.46 kg/cm²	126 °C
3 min	30 lb/in²	2.11 kg/cm²	134 °C

Articles such as facepieces, which consist of canvas covered by rubber, are liable to be damaged, but red rubber endotracheal tubes may be autoclaved perhaps ten or twenty times. Many plastic items are likely to be damaged. Articles may be prepacked in envelopes or boxes of suitable material before autoclaving, and chemical 'tellers', in the form of Browne's tubes (which contain a liquid that changes colour after the appropriate temperature treatment) or Thermalog strips (which act in the same manner), may be included in the pack to demonstrate that the heat process has been adequate and sterilization is complete. Alternatively, the pack may be sealed with adhesive tape that shows, by colour changes, that the heat process has been adequate.

Autoclaving is the most efficient, quickest, simplest and probably the most cost-efficient means of sterilization for use in the hospital. Other methods of sterilization, mentioned below, are appropraite only when autoclaving is contraindicated.

Dry heating

Some articles are suitable for sterilization by dry heat. They may be wrapped in special kraft paper and then placed in a thermostatically controlled hot air oven at 150–170 °C for 20–30 min. This method is not suitable for plastics or rubber. All-glass syringes may be sterilized by dry heat provided that the temperature is raised and lowered slowly to prevent breakage by uneven expansion. Most lubricants deteriorate and should not be used on syringes. Metal plungers should be removed from the barrel of the syringe before heating, or the latter will be fractured. It is the method of choice for some ophthalmic instruments.

Ethylene oxide or propylene oxide gas may be used for sterilizing equipment and in particular those articles that are damaged by other methods. The difficulty is that a special sterilizer is required. This consists of a chamber resembling an autoclave, in which both humidity and temperature are controlled. The process is expensive and takes several hours. Ethylene oxide is very inflammable and is used in a 5–10% mixture with a gas such as carbon dioxide or 'Arcton 12' (dichlorodifluromethane) to prevent explosion risk. Heat and water vapour are also required. The expense and mechanical difficulties of this method usually limit it to use in specialist

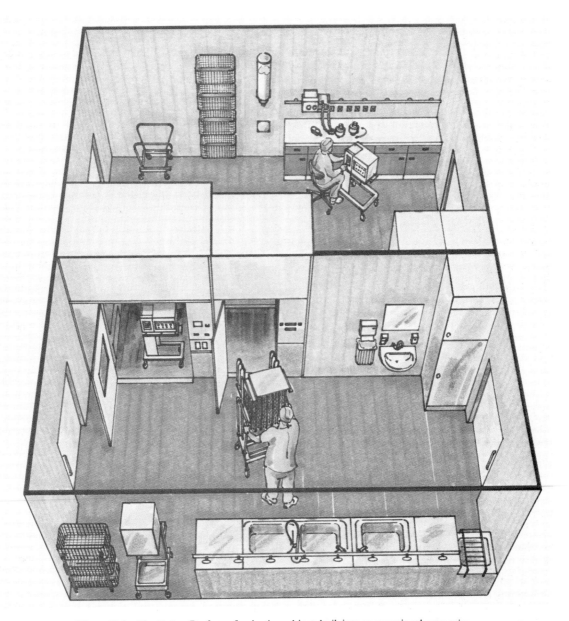

Figure 17.3   The Dräger Purfactor fumigation cabinet, built into an operating theatre suite.

departments and for perishable items.

Provided that it is properly used, ethylene oxide is an efficient sterilizing agent, but makeshift arrangements such as enclosing large items of equipment in plastic bags, may prove unsatisfactory.

After sterilization in ethylene oxide, a period of 5–7 days must elapse before the gas is entirely eliminated from rubber and plastic. This period of 'elution' may be speeded by the use of an aeration chamber.

Ethylene oxide cannot be used to sterilize polystyrene, since it has an adverse effect on this material.

Gamma irradiation

The use of γ-rays requires a large, expensive and sophisticated plant, which is appropriate to the sterilzation of large quantities of disposable goods, rather than the resterilization of individual pieces of equipment in repeated use. This method is quite inappropriate for any but the largest of hospital groups and will not therefore be described here.

Resterilization of Disposable Articles

Many articles such as syringes, needles, suction catheters and Ryle's tubes are made of plastic and are supplied sterile in envelopes or other protective packing. They are intended to be used once and then thrown away. Although it is not always desirable or economical, it is often possible to clean and resterilize such articles. Some of the plastic items are not suitable for autoclaving, but many types may be boiled or pasteurized. Plastic items that have been sterilized by gamma irradiation must on no account be resterilized with ethylene oxide, since toxic substances may be produced.

In the case of syringes and needles, boiling or sterilizing with formalin vapour is considered inadequate, since there is a risk of the transmission of homologous serum jaundice. For this reason most authorities consider that the resterilization by boiling of plastic disposable syringes is dangerous and all such intravenous equipment should be discarded after use. However, provided that the labour costs are not too high, there would seem to be no contraindication to the resterilization of nasogastric tubes, suction catheters, etc. Many types of plastic suction catheters and nozzles may be autoclaved provided that they are carefully packed to prevent distortion.

There is no doubt that many of the plastic disposable articles now used in hospitals are better than the original non-disposable types and also make for an economy in labour costs. However, the 'disposable' habit has become so firmly engrained in hospital personnel that many things are thrown away when they could, more economically, be resterilized and used again.

Routine Sterilization of Anaesthetic Equipment

Anaesthetic machines

At the end of every day's work the external surfaces of the anaesthetic machine should be thoroughly cleaned with a solution containing soap or 70% alcohol or with a suitable disinfectant solution, such as 0.5% chlorhexidine (Hibitane) in 70% alcohol. The breathing attachments should be removed and the corrugated hose, rebreathing bags, expiratory valves, elbows and catheter mounts thoroughly washed in hot soapy water, rinsed and hung up to dry. The immersion of these parts in any form of detergent solution is not advised, since the surface of the rubber parts may be damaged. They may safely be soaked in a solution of 0.1% chlorhexidine in water for 1 hr. If the anaesthetic machine is not to be used immediately, it is better to cover it after cleansing.

At intervals the breathing attachments, tubing, fittings, etc. should be autoclaved. This is by far the most satisfactory method of sterilization, but its too frequent use may result in softening of the rubber parts and a reduction of their antistatic properties. Rubber breathing bags may be damaged by autoclaving. Increasing use is being made of neoprene, a synthetic substance which stands up better to heat treatment.

Circle absorbers

Some circle absorbers are constructed of materials that would be damaged by heat sterilization, in which case the following is advised. The rebreathing bag and corrugated hose should be treated as above. The glass domes on the unidirectional valves may be unscrewed and the valve discs carefully removed and cleaned and the dome wiped out with a spiritous solution, such as 70% alcohol, or a 0.5% chlorhexidine solution. When refitting the dome one should make sure that the sealing washer is in place. From time to time the soda lime canister should be emptied and thoroughly cleaned. This is partly in the interest of sterility, and partly to remove small particles of soda lime from the thread of the canister, which otherwise would cause corrosion and wear and might prevent an air-tight fit.

The contamination of circle absorbers may be reduced if, during use, the hoses are allowed to fall in a deep U-loop. This tends to cause droplets of moisture containing infection to 'fall out' before they reach the absorber. Bacterial filters, as described in Chapter 11, may be used to protect the absorber from infection.

Many modern circle absorbers may be autoclaved, and this is obviously more satisfactory.

Elbows, expiratory valves, catheter mounts and small fittings that are made partly of rubber

These may be soaked in chlorhexidine solution or boiled. Autoclaving may cause the rubber to deteriorate rapidly in some makes, whilst in others the manufacturers recommend it. They may be pasteurized in the decontaminator shown in Fig. 17.1.

Ventilators

The tubing and reservoir bag should be removed and treated in the same manner as the anaesthetic machines. The exterior of the ventilator should be swabbed down in an antiseptic solution, such as alcohol or chlorhexidine, and carefully dried. (For further details of sterilization see Chapter 11, where different types of ventilators are classified from the point of view of sterilization. It should be remembered that there are three parts of a ventilator requiring separate consideration, namely (a) the air or gas passages, a distinction between the inspiratory and expiratory sides being sometimes possible, (b) the exterior of the cabinet, and (c) the space within the cabinet but outside the respirator pathways, which may become contaminated by expiratory gases.) In respect of the above it should be remembered that the infection that contaminates a ventilator during one operation may be distributed around the theatre during the next — therefore contamination of the ventilator is to be avoided.

Facepieces

Immediately after use facepieces should be dropped into a bucket containing soap solution. A suitable concentration is 5–10 ml of spirit soap per litre of water. At the end of every day's work the facepieces should be taken out, thoroughly washed in a hot soapy solution, rinsed in hot water and hung up to dry. They should not be cleaned with detergents or with substances such as trilene, since these tend to damage the surface and make them sticky. (This damage is particularly likely in the case of facepieces made of rubber with a silicone finish.) Facepieces should not be autoclaved, since with many types not only may the rubber perish, but also structural damage may occur.

Endotracheal tubes (red rubber) and airways

Endotracheal tubes and airways should also be dropped into the bucket of soap solution immediately after use. They should later be cleaned out with a long narrow brush specially made for the purpose (Fig. 17.4), thoroughly rinsed and then either autoclaved or boiled for 3 min. Autoclaving is undoubtedly the most efficient method of sterilization, but endotracheal tubes tend to become soft with repeated treatment in this manner and do no usually stand up to many more than ten or twenty

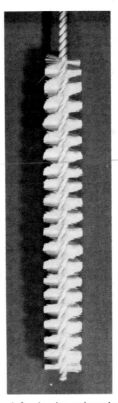

Figure 17.4 A brush for cleaning endotracheal tubes, etc.

treatments. Connectors are best removed from the tubes before heat treatment to prevent permanent stretching. The cuff should be tested to ensure that there are no leaks at some time during the process.

Airways and endotracheal tubes made of latex rubber and thermoplastic materials require careful handling during autoclaving or boiling. Plastic articles, in particular, are liable to lose their shape when heated, and until perfectly cold again should not be distorted in any way. Armoured endotracheal tubes should be handled with especial care, since if they are crushed with forceps, the armour will be distorted and the lumen of the tube diminished.

Silicone rubber armoured tubes often have a self-sealing attachment on the cuff inflation tube. In this case it should be confirmed that no water or air remains in the cuff, or that the self-sealing end be maintained open by a dummy syringe, otherwise during autoclaving the cuff may become over-distended and rupture.

Perspex articles

Perspex articles, such as transparent soda lime canisters, should not be heat treated, but after washing may be wiped out with a 70% alcohol (not chloroform, which dissolves Perspex) or 0.9% chlorhexidine solution.

Special Precautions for Infected Cases

Where a patient who is known to have a virulent respiratory infection is to be anaesthetized, special precautions may be taken. If a semi-closed system is to be used, the reservoir bag, bag mount, corrugated tubing, APL valve, elbow and facepiece are removed from the anaesthetic machine immediately after the operation and placed in a bucket. To this are added other items that have been in contact with the patient, such as the head harness and retaining ring and the airway or endotracheal tube. They

should all be thoroughly washed and then, if possible, autoclaved; failing this, they should be boiled or soaked in a chemical sterilizing solution, such as those mentioned above or mercury biniodide solution. If a closed system is required, a Waters' canister should be used. After use all the metal parts may be autoclaved and the rubber or plastic parts treated in the same way as above. The laryngoscope handle should be swabbed with alcohol or chlorhexidine solution and the blade either autoclaved or soaked in 0.5% chlorhexidine in 70% alcohol solution. The anaesthetic machine and any other surfaces that may have been contaminated should be swabbed down with alcohol or chlorhexidine solution.

The use of bacterial filters such as that shown in Fig. 11.45 may reduce the contamination of breathing attachments and may therefore be deemed desirable in such cases.

Storage of Sterile Objects

Facepieces and other parts of breathing attachments should be hung up to dry and then stored in a dust-free cupboard or drawer. Endotracheal tubes and airways may normally be stored together in a sterile tray and kept covered with a cloth or polythene sheeting. Where the airways or endotracheal tubes are to be used in a patient who has had an operation on the nose, throat or chest, they may be individually packeted before autoclaving. The packet should be either of some transparent material or marked with the size and length of the endotracheal tube and the size and type of airway contained. The individual packaging of endotracheal tubes and airways is becoming increasingly popular. However, the labour costs are increased and there is a tendency for more than one packet to be opened for each case in order to make the selection of an appropriate tube more speedy. A range of tubes and airways of different sizes may be packed in a box for use in emergencies.

Even when the anaesthetist maintains the most strict vigilance, accidents may happen. Monitors, and the warning devices that some of them contain, are described in Chapter 14. Further warning devices and the means of preventing accidents may be incorporated in the anaesthetic apparatus itself. They may be intended to: (a) prevent the selection of the wrong breathing system; (b) prevent the selection of the wrong agent; (c) warn of the failure of the supply of anaesthetic gases, particularly oxygen; and (d) prevent injury to patients, and damage to the apparatus itself, as a result of overpressure.

Wherever possible, safety devices should 'fail safe'. This means that if there is a failure of any sort, the situation remaining should be safe rather than dangerous. For example, on the Walton Five dental anaesthetic machine, should there be a failure of the oxygen supply, not only is the nitrous oxide cut off, but also air is admitted to the breathing system. Similarly a monitor, if it fails due to, say, battery exhaustion, should cease to indicate that all is well, and should show that a fault exists.

The Prevention of the Selection of a Wrong Breathing System or Anaesthetic Agent

There are several devices intended to prevent the use of trichloroethylene (Trilene) in an anaesthetic system containing soda lime. One such device is the Trilene safety interlock (Fig. 6.12b), which mechanically prevents the Trilene vaporizer being turned on if the closed circuit has been selected, and vice versa. Alternatively, a two-way tap may be installed in the back bar to direct the fresh gas flow either to the Magill attachment via the Trilene vaporizer, or to the circle absorber, bypassing it.

The Prevention of the Selection of a Wrong Anaesthetic Agent

The non-interchangeability of cylinders and pipelines has been described in Chapters 3 and 4. Before the pin index system (p. 34) was adopted various accidents (some of them fatal) were reported where, for example, a cylinder of nitrous oxide was con-

18
Hazards and the Psychology of Accidents

nected in place of one of oxygen. Accidents of this sort should now be impossible. However, there have been incidents when, during structural alteration or redecoration, the pipeline installations have been tampered with. In one case several patients were subjected to pure nitrous oxide rather than oxygen following the wrong reconnection of the pipeline system. To prevent this type of 'confusion' the most stringent regulations now apply to the commissioning and structural alterations of piped services.

For many years certain volatile anaesthetic agents have been distinctively coloured. The abandonment of this practice with some of the more modern anaesthetic agents is regrettable. One of the problems has been the small number of distinctively coloured materials available.

The development of temperature-compensated, calibrated vaporizers has resulted in the manufacture of different vaporizers for each of the anaesthetic agents. Those produced by the same manufacturer may closely resemble each other, and there is sometimes no clear indication as to which agent should be used with a particular vaporizer. Since the vaporizer for methoxyflurane (Penthrane), for example, would give a lethally high concentration of halothane if the latter agent were accidentally used, steps have been taken to prevent the charging of a vaporizer with the wrong agent. Cyprane and Fraser Sweatman have developed the Fraser Sweatman pin safety system (Fig. 18.1) for volatile agents. Since anaesthetic agents are sold in different types of bottle, a filler tube for each agent with a cap to fit only the appropriate bottle may be used. This filler

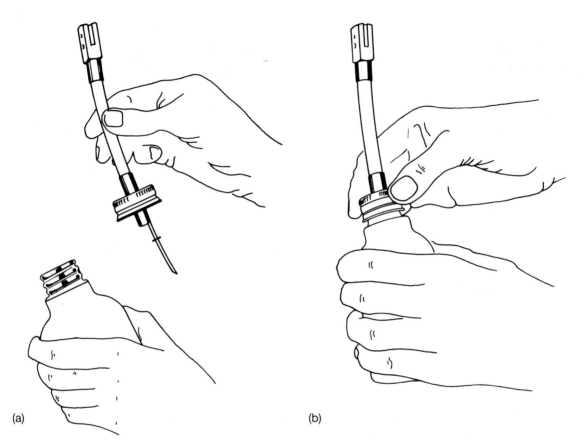

(a)

(b)

tube terminates in a small block that has a slot cut in it in such a way as to be unique to one individual anaesthetic agent. The vaporizer has a filling plug and a draining plug, which accept only the appropriate filling tube block. By inserting the filling tube block in the filling plug the agent may be made to run from the bottle into the vaporizer. When it is desired to drain the vaporizer, the agent may be run back into the bottle via the draining plug.

Warning of Failure of a Cylinder or Piped Gas Supply

Several oxygen failure warning devices have been designed and some of these are obtainable on the market. It is regrettable that the majority of these simply give evidence of the failure of an oxygen supply but do not 'fail safe'.

Figure 18.2 shows the Bosun warning device

produced by BOC. In the event of the failure of the oxygen supply a red light comes on and nitrous oxide blows a whistle. The disadvantage of this device is that if the nitrous oxide is turned off, and this may be done in some models by simply turning off a tap adjacent to it, the audible warning is not given. Similarly, the battery that powers the visible warning may be discharged and in any case it can be switched off.

In most of these devices failure of the oxygen supply does not initiate any remedial measure. Others ensure that should the oxygen fail, the nitrous oxide and any other gases will be turned off or diverted and air admitted to the system. But similarly these devices do nothing to renew the oxygen supply. A warning device has been described that not only gives warning of the exhaustion of the cylinder but also turns on a reserve cylinder in order to continue the oxygen supply (Fig. 18.3). Regrettably no such device is at the moment available, at least on the British market.

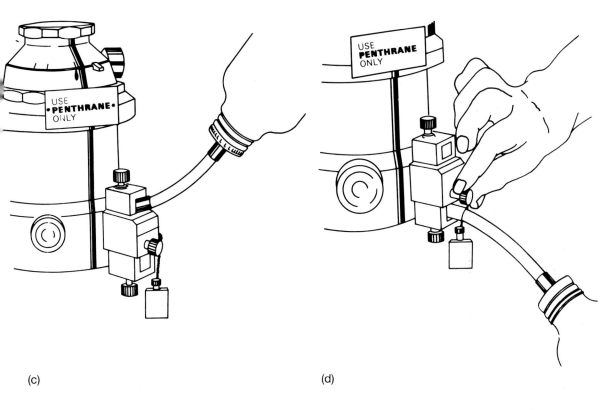

(c)   (d)

Figure 18.1   The Fraser Sweatman pin safety system. (a) The filler tube. (b) The filler tube fits only the bottle for the agent for which it is intended. (c) Filling a vaporizer. (d) Draining a vaporizer.

The problem of fitting a satisfactory oxygen warning device is a complex one. It should be powered by the oxygen remaining in the failing supply, and there should be no question of its being put out of action by the throwing of a switch or the blocking up of an orifice, or whatever. Visible warnings are less useful than those that are audible. The warning sound should be as compelling and characteristic as possible. The fitting of any device that requires structural alteration of the anaesthetic machine and a change of the routine to which the anaesthetist works might in itself present a potential danger. Figure 18.4 shows the Gardner Safety Interlock, which gives both an audible and a visual warning of failure, and Fig. 18.5 shows the latest BOC warning device.

The above warning devices are those that may be fitted to an individual anaesthetic machine. However, warning devices may be installed also in the permanent pipeline system. Not only is there a warning in a central location of the failure of a bank of cylinders on a pipeline manifold, but also it is possible to install a visible or audible warning device in each theatre suite or corridor. This would operate in case of the failure, for any reason, of the piped supply to that section. These are further described in Chapter 4.

Pressure Relief Valves

On an anaesthetic machine with a regulated pressure of 4 bar ($\sim 60\,\text{lb/in}^2$), much damage might be done if the gases were flowing but the outlet obstructed; the whole back bar would be subjected to a pressure of 4 bar. For this reason a pressure relief valve may be fitted to protect the back bar (see Fig. 6.17). Flow restrictors fitted upstream of the flowmeters protect the back bar and patient only from surges of

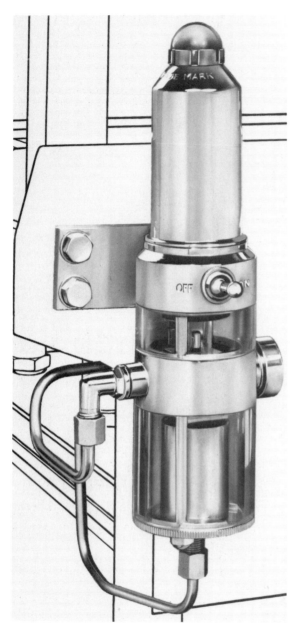

Figure 18.2   The Bosun oxygen failure warning device.

pressure. On pipeline and similar installations, relief valves (safety valves) are fitted to protect the pipeline if the pressure within it were to rise above a set limit owing to a fault.

It should be remembered that safety devices are merely an extra aid to the anaesthetist. He should neither rely upon them nor let them replace his constant vigilance. For this reason some people consider that warning devices may detract from, rather than increase, safety. On the other hand, those with experience know only too well how their attention may be distracted from, say, a cylinder gauge, in the heat of the moment when there are difficulties during an operation or an anaesthetic.

The Removal of Exhaled Gases

There are four reasons for removing a patient's exhaled gases from the atmosphere of the operating theatre or intensive care ward. These are:
1. The risk of airborne cross infection.
2. The possible undesirable effects of prolonged exposure of the personnel to anaesthetic agents.
3. That in a confined space there may be an objection to the odour of anaesthetic agents, which may also cause drowsiness.
4. The removal of inflammable anaesthetic agents where there is a risk of explosion.

The removal of exhaled gases is termed *scavenging* and is discussed in Chapter 15.

Fatal Accidents Associated with Anaesthetic Apparatus

A summary is given below of some of the results of the following three surveys of deaths associated with anaesthesia:
1. Edwards et al. (1955) reported on 1000 cases occurring in Great Britain between 1950 and 1955.
2. Dinnick (1964) investigated 600 cases occurring in Great Britain between 1955 and 1964.

Both these surveys relied on voluntary and confidential reports sent to a specialist committee. There is no doubt that many anaesthetists at whose hands deaths occurred were unaware of the Committee and its request for confidential reports, and so many deaths due to anaesthesia were probably not notified.

3. Holland (1970) investigated 370 cases occurring

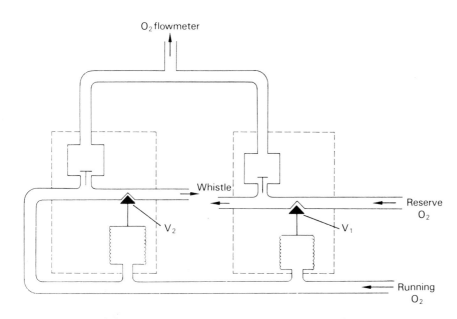

Figure 18.3 A proposed oxygen failure warning device that also turns on a reserve cylinder in order to continue the supply. Failure of 'running' oxygen causes valves V_1 and V_2 to open, thus sounding the whistle. The opening of V_3 also connects the 'reserve' oxygen supply to the flowmeter.

between 1960 and 1968 in New South Wales, where all deaths that occurred within 24 hours of an anaesthetic were reported by hospitals or coroners' offices. It is probable that virtually all anaesthetic deaths were notified.

Both Edwards et al. and Dinnick stressed that theirs were not statistical analyses and that no conclusions of a statistical nature should be drawn from the figures they gave.

Many of the deaths reported in all three series had nothing to do with the anaesthetic and were rather of a surgical or an inevitable nature, and it is likely that in some cases the true cause of death was never discerned. Bearing in mind the limitations of the conclusions that can be drawn, the three surveys will now be examined. Of all the deaths due to anaesthesia, a small number only were due to the failure or misuse of anaesthetic apparatus.

The survey of Edwards et al. (1955)
Of the 1000 cases reported, 589 were considered to be actually associated with anaesthesia, of which the following were due to the apparatus and its use:
(a) *Deaths due to the failure or breakage of anaesthetic apparatus, or to misuse of an excusable nature*
2 cases where an excess of carbon dioxide was unintentionally given.
2 cases where the oxygen flowmeter was leaking.

1 case in which the circle absorber fell off.
1 case in which an explosion occurred due to static electricity.
1 case owing to the confusion of cylinders.
(b) *Malpractice*
3 cases where oxygen was delivered at high pressure during resuscitation.
3 cases in which patients died of anoxia while the anaesthetist failed to achieve intubation.
15 cases where the endotracheal tube was kinked, obstructed by its cuff, in the right main bronchus, or in the oesophagus.
1 case in which the expiratory limb of an Ayres T-piece was obstructed and the patient died of overpressure.
1 case of trauma during intubation.
(c) *Difficulty caused by pre-existing severe disease of the patient*
6 patients died when intubation was impossible owing to conditions such as carcinoma of tongue or larynx.
(d) *Cases of uncertain cause*
9 patients died where the cause was not known but said to be associated with intubation.

Dinnick's survey (1964)
Of the 600 cases reported, 400 were considered to be actually associated with anaesthesia, of which the

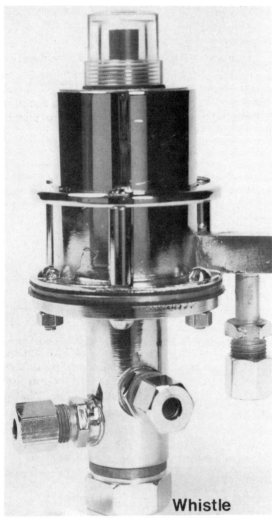

Figure 18.4   The Gardner Safety Interlock oxygen warning device.

Figure 18.5   An oxygen warning device by BOC. A, mixed gases from the back bar; B, regulated pressure oxygen supply; C, to outlet; D, pressure relief valve set at 5 lb/in²; E, restrictor; F, unidirectional air inlet valve; G, magnet; H, spring; I, diaphragm; J, whistle; K, valve seating; L, shut-off valve seating, M, air inlet with whistle. Normally the pressure of oxygen on the left-hand side of the diaphragm is sufficient to keep the spool in the position shown. Failure to maintain this pressure will cause the spool to be attracted by G and so cut off the supply of nitrous oxide at L and allow the ingress of air at M.

following were due to the apparatus and its use:

(a) *Deaths due to the failure or breakage of anaesthetic apparatus, or to misuse of an excusable nature*

1 case where the soda lime canister was not in place.

1 case where an excess of carbon dioxide was accidentally administered.

1 case where the nitrous oxide bypass was turned on instead of the oxygen bypass.

(b) *Malpractice*

1 case where an oxygen catheter was placed in the oesophagus instead of the trachea.

4 cases in which there was obstruction of the endotracheal tube by its own cuff.

2 cases where the endotracheal tube was kinked.

1 case where the endotracheal tube was in the right main bronchus.

1 case where the endotracheal tube was in the oesophagus.

(c) *Difficulty caused by pre-existing severe disease of the patient*

5 cases could not be intubated due to pre-existing disease.

Holland's survey (1970)

Of the 370 cases of death associated with anaesthesia

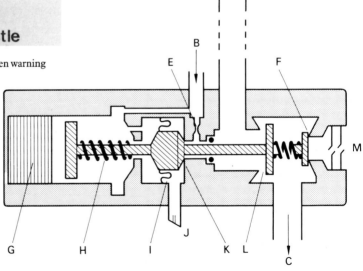

reported, 28 were comparable with those in the surveys above.

(a) *Deaths due to the failure or breakage of anaesthetic apparatus, or to misuse of an excusable nature*

3 cases due to the jamming of a Ruben valve (and in one case there was also overpressure).

2 cases where the vaporizer was set to the wrong concentration.

1 case in which the vaporizer overturned, resulting in liquid halothane entering the breathing attachment and the patient's air passages.

1 case in which the connections in a breathing attachment fell apart.

1 case where a breathing attachment was incorrectly reassembled following cleaning.

(b) *Malpractice*

In connection with endotracheal tubes:

7 cases where the endotracheal tube was kinked or obstructed.

2 cases where the endotracheal tube was in the oesophagus.

2 cases where attempted intubation was unsuccessful.

2 cases of trauma during intubation.

1 case where the endotracheal tube was dislodged.

2 cases in which the expiratory port or valve was omitted from the circuit.

2 cases of oxygen failure.

1 case of incorrect assembly of a breathing attachment.

1 case of confused gas lines.

The changing pattern of accidents associated with anaesthetic apparatus

Owing to the less frequent use of explosive anaesthetic agents, and the institution of precautions to prevent explosions, particularly in connection with static electricity, accidents due to fire and explosion have been virtually eliminated. In recent years, however, deaths from electrocution have been reported, and following the explanation of microshock one is left to wonder how many cases of ventricular fibrillation have been caused in this way.

Other factors that may influence the changing pattern of accidents are as follows:

THE COMPLEXITY OF ANAESTHETIC VENTILATORS

Before the introduction of methods employing controlled ventilation, anaesthetic apparatus was relatively simple, but modern anaesthetic ventilators have become mechanically elaborate. Not only are the breathing systems complicated but also there is a multiplicity of controls that have to be operated to change the mode of operation. For a novice, or an anaesthetist suffering from fatigue, it is a common mistake for only one of the two necessary manipulations of controls to be performed when changing from one anaesthetic technique to another.

Despite the engineering problems involved, it would seem highly desirable that the circuits in an anaesthetic ventilator should be changed by moving one master control knob only. This should be mechanically linked to all those valves, etc. that require to be changed over.

DISPARAGEMENT OF THE MUNDANE

Modern anaesthetic techniques have become so spectacular, and the pharmacology and physiology of anaesthetics so complicated, that the teaching of simple matters such as the functioning of the Boyle's vaporizer have too often been treated with disdain by both teachers and trainees alike. The lack of understanding of the basic tools of his trade can only detract from the safety with which an anaesthetist works.

RELIANCE UPON ASSISTANCE

Theatre technicians have been playing an increasing part in the running of an operating theatre and are particularly of help to the anaesthetist. However, the anaesthetist who has become dependent on the assistance of a theatre technician fares badly in his absence.

PIPED MEDICAL GAS SUPPLY

The installation of a piped medical gas supply to the main operating theatres of the hospital group makes the checking of cylinder contents gauges in those theatres seemingly unnecessary. For this reason the anaesthetist tends to lose the habit of this most necessary safeguard, and may fail to notice the exhaustion of an oxygen cylinder when he is using an anaesthetic machine in one of the remoter hospitals where no pipeline exists.

19

Electrical Hazards and their Prevention

The Mains Electric Supply

Since many items of anaesthetic apparatus and monitors are powered by electricity, it is important to understand some of the principles involved. The 'mains' electric supply is not *direct current*, flowing uninterruptedly in the same direction, as is produced by a battery; it provides an *alternating current*, in which the flow is constantly changing from one direction to the other in a rapid and regular manner. The number of complete cycles of this change of direction, or *frequency*, is 50 per second in Great Britain and 60 per second in some other countries, for example the USA. The two conductors in a cable therefore cannot be said to be *positive* and *negative*, as would be the case with direct current; but since one is at, or at about, the same potential as earth (being connected to earth at the transformer), this is said to be *neutral* or *return*, and the other conductor to be *live*. Because of this earthing of the neutral conductor, any person (or object) who is connected to earth would complete the electric circuit by touching the live conductor, even if no contact were made with the neutral one. Figure 19.1 shows how under certain conditions the circuit may be completed by, say, an earthed diathermy plate, resulting in fatal electrocution. (In most modern diathermy machines the plate is 'earth free'.) Stringent precautions should be taken to ensure that the polarities are correctly identified and connected for all mains electrical apparatus. Furthermore, the interruption of the neutral conductor alone could result in apparatus being at a live potential and yet not operating. Any contact with apparatus in this condition could, if it has not been disconnected from the mains supply, lead to electrocution. It cannot be over-emphasized that if a fault exists, the services of a competent technician should be sought.

The inclusion in an electric supply cable of a third conductor that connects the metal chassis or frame

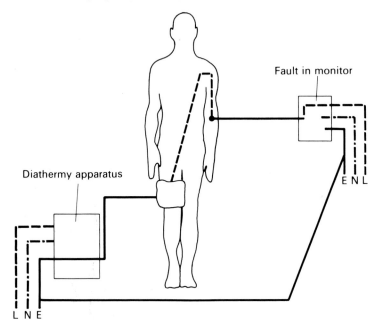

Fault in monitor

Diathermy apparatus

E N L

L N E

Figure 19.1 A fault in a monitor may cause the patient to come into contact with a live wire, the current being returned to earth via a metal object such as diathermy plate (in those types of diathermy machine where the plate is earthed). L = live, N = neutral, and E = earth conductors.

310

of the apparatus to the earthed point of the supply ensures that under faulty conditions, such as an internal short in the equipment, the chassis would not be rendered live. This is said to be the *earth* conductor.

Fuses interrupt the electric supply should the current passing through them exceed a predetermined level that might cause overheating or damage. They may be installed in the mains supply circuit, in the plug-top at the end of the lead to the apparatus, or in the apparatus itself. They usually consist of a fine-gauge wire, which melts if the current passing through it exceeds that against which it is intended to offer protection.

ACCIDENTS ASSOCIATED WITH THE MAINS ELECTRIC SUPPLY

There are three ways in which the mains electric current, or equipment powered by it, may endanger the patient:
1. Electrocution.
2. Burns.
3. Ignition of inflammable materials, leading to fire or explosion.

Electrocution

Until recently the only concept of electrocution was one where two remote parts of the body such as the hands were applied to the two poles of a 240 V mains electric supply.

Figure 19.2a shows how the current may pass through a wide segment of the body so that at any one point within the trunk, the actual 'current density' may be of low order.

The current flowing depends on several factors, including the electrical resistance of the skin at the point of contact. This is particularly influenced by moisture or dryness.

Let us consider the passage of current from one hand to the other, or from one hand to a foot. If the current exceeds 1 mA, a tingling sensation is felt (Fig. 19.2a). If the current is increased, the sensation becomes progressively painful. A current in excess of about 15 mA produces a tonic contraction of the muscles, as a result of which the patient is unable to release his grip upon the electrode: this is known as the 'no let go' threshold (Fig. 19.2b). A current in excess of 75–100 mA can result in ven-

tricular fibrillation (Fig. 19.2c).

A very high current, in excess of 5 A, produces a tonic contraction of the myocardium which could, if irreparable damage has not occurred, be followed, when it ceases, by a normal rhythm. Such a high current is unlikely to be encountered in clinical practice, other than during defibrillation.

Electrocution may cause death relatively slowly by the tonic contraction of the respiratory muscles, leading to asphyxia, or more rapidly by ventricular fibrillation. The onset of ventricular fibrillation may be somewhat delayed, being preceded by ventricular tachycardia, which causes circulatory failure, but which may revert to normal rhythm if stopped in time.

It will be remembered that the neutral pole of the mains electric supply is connected to earth at a point remote from the patient. Since all conductors have some resistance, however low, a loss known as *volts drop* occurs along these conductors, so that the neutral conductor is not *exactly* at earth potential at the patient end of the circuit. This difference in potential can cause 'stray voltage' and may lead to a 'stray current'.

Since earthed electrodes may be attached to more than one part of the patient, and from more than one piece of apparatus supplied by different mains sockets, it is recommended that the earth connections on all the socket outlets in a single clinical area be interconnected by a conductor of low resistance to minimize voltage differences between them. Similarly, all exposed metal objects such as radiators, water pipes, etc. are interconnected to a good earth.

Figure 19.2a, b and c shows the effect of a current passing between the extremities. When it passes across the patient's trunk only a small part of it passes through the heart. However, recent advances in medicine and surgery have led to the placement of electrodes upon or very close to the heart. Under these circumstances a very much smaller current, possibly as low as 100 μA can result in ventricular fibrillation (Fig. 19.2d), since all the current passes through the heart. A very small potential, such as the stray voltage in the mains neutral lead, could be sufficient to produce electrocution in this way. This phenomenon is known as *microshock*.

There are two ways of preventing accidents caused by unwanted currents returning to earth. One is to install an isolating transformer, the output of which is carefully isolated from earth, and the

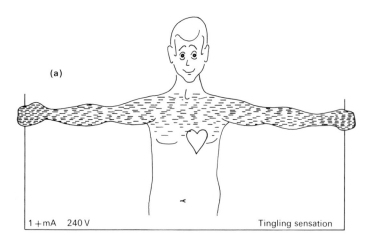

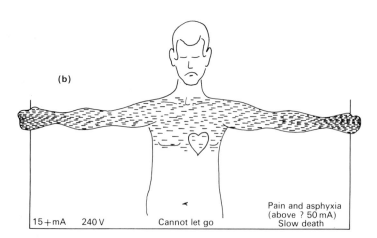

Figure 19.2   (a) A current in excess of 1 mA passing through the body may produce a tingling sensation. (b) If the current exceeds about 15 mA, muscles are held in tonic spasm, the victim cannot let go and will eventually die of asphyxia. (c) Where the current exceeds 100 mA, ventricular fibrillation and rapid death will occur. (d) If one electrode is applied to the right ventricle of the heart itself, a very small current can result in ventricular fibrillation.

second is to detect unwanted currents passing to earth by a device that may then *either* sound a warning *or* automatically switch off the supply. There are advantages and disadvantages of each of these and they will be discussed below.

Such a transformer may supply all the outlets for a whole operating room or theatre suite. This is referred to as *safe patient power* (Fig. 19.3). Apart from the expense, the problems are that if there are several appliances in use, and each of these has a small earth leakage current, harmless in itself, the sum of all these currents may be sufficient to trip the relay and cut off the power to some piece of vital life-support equipment. Similarly, a fault in one piece of equipment may cause the cessation of power to another. If the relay operates a warning device rather than a circuit breaker, it may be observed too late or be unheeded by staff who do not appreciate its importance. Isolating transformers may be used in another and, in the author's opinion, more satisfactory manner. They may be included in the circuitry of each and every item of mains operated electromedical equipment that can be connected to a patient. The patient circuit is earth free and said to

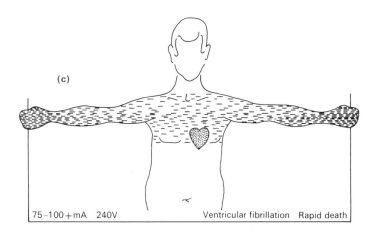

(c)

75–100+mA   240V   Ventricular fibrillation   Rapid death

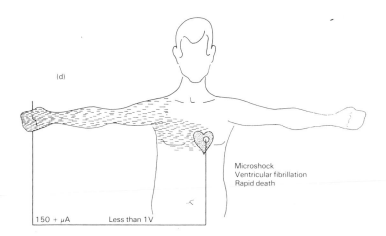

(d)

Microshock
Ventricular fibrillation
Rapid death

150 + μA   Less than 1V

be *fully floating*. The enclosure of the equipment may be earthed, or completely insulated.

The second method of improving safety is to install a current-operated earth-leakage circuit breaker (COELCB, also known as an 'earth trip'; Fig. 19.4). This may be installed in the electric supply to a whole operating room or theatre suite, or may be installed in each item of equipment. The live and neutral conductors each take a couple of turns or so (both exactly the same) around the core of a toroidal transformer. A third winding is connected directly to the coil of the relay which operates the

circuit breaker. If the current in the live and neutral conductors is the same, the magnetic fluxes cancel themselves out. If they differ, there is a resultant field which induces a current in the third winding and this causes the relay to operate and break the circuit. A difference of as little as 30 mA can trip the COELCB in as short a time as 0.03 s. It may be manually reset, and may also have a test button to check its operation.

A similar device may be used instead to merely give a warning of excess earth leakage, or it may perform both functions.

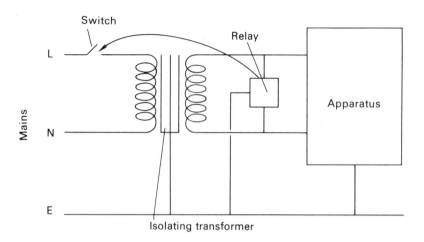

Figure 19.3 Safe patient power. The output of the isolating transformer is free from earth. Should earth leakage above a prearranged level occur, the relay will either disconnect the supply to the input of the transformer or sound a warning device. L = live, N = neutral, and E = earth connectors.

COELCBs may present problems similar to those of isolating transformers, except that they are less expensive. They operate so quickly, and as a result of such a low earth leakage current, that they very greatly reduce the possibility of serious electric shock.

In Great Britain electrical safety in clinical areas is achieved by a high standard of earthing of the fixed wiring, by good earthing of enclosures and by fully floating patient circuits where appropriate. Further safety may be achieved by using battery-operated equipment. In some cases the battery may be recharged between periods of use by 'plugging in' to the mains supply.

Burns

Where an electric current passes through the skin, whether intentionally or not, electrical resistance leads to the generation of heat. Depending on the amount of heat produced, the area over which it is applied and the rate of cooling by the blood circulation, burns may result. This matter is discussed further below, in connection with diathermy.

Fire

Sparks occurring at switches or from the interruption of the supply by the removal of a plug could ignite inflammable vapours. They are prevented in the operating theatre by the installation of spark-proof switches (see Fig. 19.5), and electrical socket outlets that 'capture' the plug, preventing its with-

drawal, whilst the switch is turned on. All electrical apparatus in the operating theatre that does not comply with these precautions is kept outside the 'zone of risk', as described on p. 318. Note that this 'zone of risk' no longer includes the whole operating theatre.

The correct wiring of electrical plugs is essential;

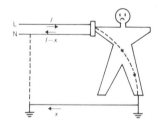

(a)

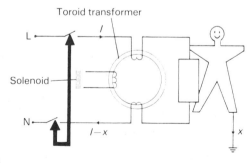

(b)

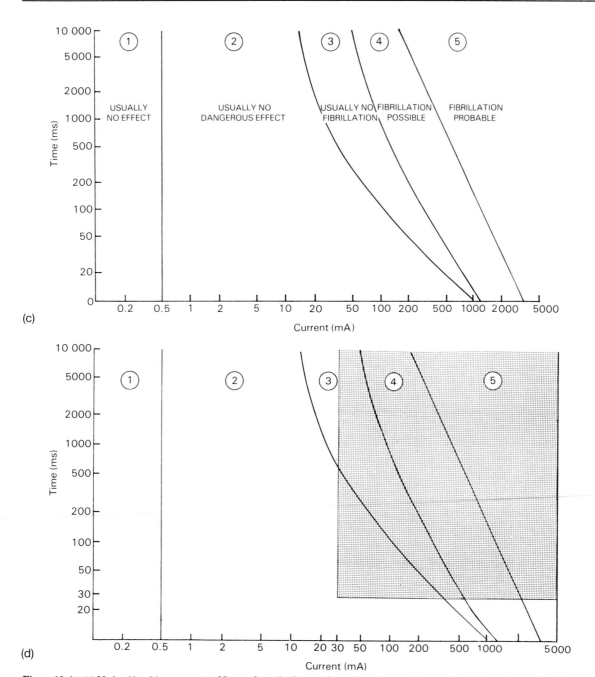

Figure 19.4 (a) If a load is taking a current of I amps from the live conductor L and x amps is returning via the patient and earth, then the current in the neutral conductor N will be $(I - x)$ amps. (b) A current-operated earth-leakage circuit breaker (COELCB). The imbalance between the currents in the live L and neutral N conductors is sufficient to set up a field in the toroid transformer sufficient to induce in the third winding a current that will trip the solenoid and therefore disconnect both the live and neutral supply. (c) The effects of a current passing through the human body (hand to hand or hand to foot). Zone 1, usually no effect; zone 2, usually no dangerous effect; zone 3, usually no danger of ventricular fibrillation; zone 4, ventricular fibrillation possible; and zone 5, ventricular fibrillation probable. (d) The shaded area denotes the protection given by COELCB.

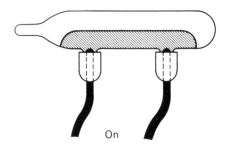

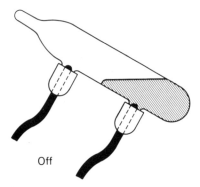

Figure 19.5   The contact of a sparkless mercury tip switch.

this is shown in Fig. 19.6. Fatal mistakes have occurred when the wire intended to be earthed has been connected to the live terminal. Further, when new electrical apparatus is being commissioned, the voltage for which it is intended, and the setting on the voltage control panel (when one is installed), should match that of the mains supply.

Fire and Explosion

For these to occur there are three prerequisites:
1. Combustible material.
2. Oxygen, to support combustion.
3. A source of ignition.

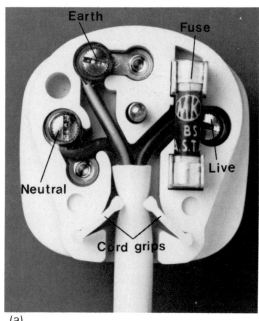

(a)

Figure 19.6   (a) The correct wiring of a ring main 13 A plug top. (b) A cartridge fuse as fitted in portable electric equipment. (c) Colour coding for flexible electric cables.

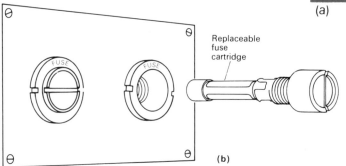

(b)

(c)

	'Old' British	'New' International
Live	Red	Brown
Neutral	Black	Blue
Earth	Green	Green/yellow

The risks arise from two sources:
1. The use of high-pressure oxygen and high concentrations of oxygen at atmospheric pressure.
2. The use of inflammable anaesthetic agents.

Burning consists of the chemical combination of a 'combustible' material with oxygen. The end products of combustion are mainly carbon dioxide and water. Energy is liberated in the form of heat, and if it takes place in a confined space, the pressure may be increased greatly. Rapid liberation of heat and the rise of pressure result in an explosion.

High-pressure oxygen

As stated on p. 14, when there is a rise in the pressure of a gas, heat is generated. If an inflammable material such as oil or grease, in a confined area, is suddenly subjected to oxygen at the pressure of a full cylinder (2000 lb/in^2; ~ 140 bar), the heat liberated is sufficient to ignite it and so cause an explosion. This, incidentally, is the principle of the compression ignition (diesel) engine.

Therefore, oil, grease or other inflammable materials should be kept away from apparatus in which high-pressure oxygen is used.

Under some conditions nitrous oxide may dissociate, producing nitrogen and oxygen, the latter giving rise to the risk of an explosion. Therefore nitrous oxide cylinders should be treated with similar care.

Anaesthetic agents

Cyclopropane, most ethers and ethyl chloride are explosive in anaesthetic concentrations.

Carbon dioxide, halothane (Fluothane), methoxyflurane (Penthrane) and enflurane (Ethrane), are not inflammable, nor is nitrous oxide at atmospheric pressure. Trichloroethylene also is non-inflammable under the conditions in which it is used by the anaesthetist.

Fire or explosion may be caused by the ignition of gases or vapours within the anaesthetic equipment, or escaping from it, or of the vapour of an inflammable substance that has been accidentally spilled or used for purposes such as the cleansing of the patient's skin.

Ignition of inflammable mixtures may be caused by sparks from static electricity, from faulty electrical apparatus, from the cautery and diathermy apparatus, from electric motors, or from an electric plug-top being pulled out of the socket when the switch is turned on and current is flowing. Naked flames are seldom employed in operating theatres now, but they may be encountered in ophthalmic or dental surgery.

Static electricity

Static electrical discharges have probably been responsible for most of the explosions that have occurred.

Today, when nylon and Terylene clothes are so popular, the clicking from sparks as static electricity is discharged is commonplace. Similar static charges are developed on dressing trolleys, operating tables and anaesthetic machines.

Although the quantity of static electricity generated in the operating theatre is relatively small, there is sufficient energy in the spark, when it is rapidly discharged, to ignite inflammable vapours such as cyclopropane and ether. Arrangements should therefore be made not only to prevent the generation of static electricity but also to discharge any that does occur, slowly to earth.

There is therefore an upper and a lower limit to the permissible electrical resistance between any part of the antistatic floor and earth. The resistance between two electrodes set 2 ft (60 cm) apart should nowhere be less than 20 000 ohms or more than 5 000 000 ohms. All mobile equipment in the operating theatre and anaesthetic rooms should make electrical contact with the floor. Trolleys, anaesthetic machines, etc., have wheels, the tyres of which are constructed of antistatic (conducting) rubber. In the absence of such precautions a metal chain, one end of which is attached to the frame of the trolley, is allowed to dangle onto the floor in such a way that at least three links are in contact with the floor. Such chains may become damaged or detached, and are sometimes wound round the frame so that they do not reach the floor. They are therefore a poor substitute for conducting rubber wheels and should be used only where it is necessary to update old equipment.

All footwear worn by the staff should contain conducting material. Tests should be made periodically with an instrument such as a Megger resistance meter to confirm that the electrical conductivity of the above items is still within the prescribed limits.

The most important precaution, however, is the use of antistatic (conducting) rubber or neoprene in the construction of the components of breathing attachments and other flexible parts of anaesthetic machines. As recently as 1982 an explosion occurred with cyclopropane, where a coaxial breathing attachment, the outer tube of which was of a non-conducting material, was damaged. Fortunately it was not in use with a patient at the time. An aerosol spray such as Croxtine (BOC) may be applied at intervals to any part of the breathing system, but particularly to rubber and neoprene, to render them antistatic. This should, however, be considered as an adjunct to, rather than a substitute for the proper materials being used.

Sparks may also be caused by the striking of metal against stone, as occurs when the metal end adaptor of a corrugated hose is dropped on a terrazzo floor.

In 1956 a working party set up in Great Britain by the Ministry of Health reported on the risk and prevention of anaesthetic explosions. This followed a period of seven years during which there had been 36 explosions reported, some of them fatal.

The term *zone of risk* was used to denote the area in which explosive mixtures were deemed to be liable to exist during routine anaesthetic practice.

Within this 'zone of risk' the following precautions were advised:

1. There should be no naked flames.
2. All electric switches should be sparkproof and electric plugs should be 'captive' while the switch is turned on.
3. All parts, especially rubber tubing, etc., of anaesthetic apparatus should be constructed of conductive (antistatic) rubber or other material, and the operating theatre floor should be antistatic. Antistatic rubber, containing carbon, has sufficient conductivity to leach away static electricity, and yet has sufficient resistance to prevent so fast a discharge that a spark occurs.

All trolleys, stools and other mobile equipment should have tyres or feet of a conducting material. These are painted yellow or have a yellow flash or label to indicate that they are antistatic.

The 1956 working party defined the 'zone of risk' as extending from floor level to a height of 4 ft 6 in. ($\sim$ 1.4 m) and 4 ft ($\sim$ 1.2 m) laterally from any anaesthetic apparatus. Because the anaesthetic machine is mobile this included the whole anaesthetic room and operating theatre.

Since 1956 there has been a dramatic decrease in the incidence of explosions. This must be due in part to the advent, a couple of years later, of halothane, which quickly replaced cyclopropane and ether to a very great extent.

In 1968 Vickers enquired into the possibility that the expensive precautions taken were more stringent than was really necessary.

Following investigations described in a paper in 1970, the Association of Anaesthetists of Great Britain and Ireland has recommended that the zone of risk be reduced to 25 cm (10 in.) around any part of the gas pathways of the anaesthetic machine or its breathing attachment.

In Great Britain and other countries this smaller zone of risk has been accepted. It is considered safe to install switches and socket outlets that are not sparkproof in the operating theatre provided that they are permanently attached to the wall. It is also recommended that they be at a height of approximately 15 in. ($\sim$ 40 cm) above the floor. This reduces the risk of damage to flexible cables. All mobile electrical apparatus, and socket outlets on the operating table or floor, should comply with the criteria for sparkproof precautions, since they may be placed within the zone of risk.

The above regulations do not seem to take account of the fact that an anaesthetic machine may be pushed up against a wall at a place where an electric fitting is positioned.

It would seem that the most important precaution for the prevention of explosions where inflammable agents are employed is the use of antistatic materials in the breathing attachments. Certainly explosions are more likely on a cold, winter Monday morning when the air is dry, the water vapour having been precipitated as frost, and the operating list has not been running long enough to generate sufficient steam or water vapour to humidify the air within the operating theatre suite.

The cost of antistatic floors and spark-proof electric switches alone is high. In one operating theatre and its suite of rooms 43 spark-proof switches were counted. It would be pertinent to ask how soon it will be possible to replace all explosive anaesthetic agents with non-inflammable ones and save much expense and trouble. Perhaps the only reason for maintaining the present precautions is that ether, being cheap, simple to use and relatively safe, is still widely used in some parts of the world. Also, a new anaesthetic agent may be discovered that is perfect in all respects except that it is inflammable. The search for the 'ideal anaesthetic' has been pursued since 1846!

Surgical Diathermy

The anaesthetist and his assistants are usually responsible for the correct connection of the diathermy machine. Therefore they should know something of those aspects of the use of diathermy that will concern them.

Surgical diathermy employs the heating effect of an electric current, and may best be explained by the analogy with a domestic electric heater (Fig. 19.7).

Provided that the wiring and plug are in perfect condition and present no electrical resistance, the only part of the circuit offering resistance is the heating element itself, and it is only here that heat is produced.

The amount of heat produced depends on the current (measured in amps) and the resistance (in ohms) of the heating element through which it passes. The power developed is in this case converted to heat and may be expressed as:

$$W = RI^2$$

Where W = power (in watts), R = resistance (in ohms), and I = current (in amps).

If the power is liberated solely as heat, 1 W will give 0.24 calories per second.

In the case of surgical diathermy power in the region of 50–400 W is commonly used.

Returning to the domestic heater, if the prongs of the plug are dirty or a poor fit in the socket, there will be electrical resistance at this point too, and heat will be liberated there as well (Fig. 19.8).

This state of affairs is commonly found to exist when one pulls out the plug to extinguish an electric heater and the plug-top is hot enough almost to burn the hand!

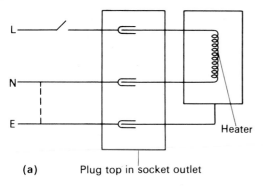

(a)   Plug top in socket outlet

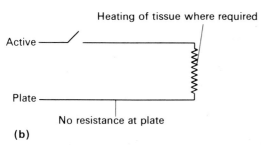

(b)   No resistance at plate

Figure 19.7   Surgical diathermy. (a) An analogy with the circuit of an electric heater. L = live, N = neutral, and E = earth conductors. (b) The circuit of the surgical diathermy.

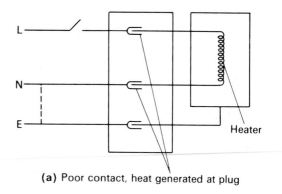

(a) Poor contact, heat generated at plug

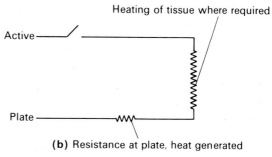

(b) Resistance at plate, heat generated

Figure 19.8   (a) Poor contacts in the socket cause heat to be generated at the plug top. L = live, N = neutral, and E = earth conductors. (b) An anology with resistance at the indifferent plate of the surgical diathermy plate, resulting in the generation of heat and the possibility of a burn.

To complete the analogy, the electric heating element represents the small piece of tissue grasped by the forceps, where it is designed to generate the heat. The plug and socket represent the indifferent electrode (plate) attached to the patient's leg. Should the contact between the plate and the patient present resistance, heat will be generated which may even be sufficient to burn the patient.

Excessive rises in temperature at the site of the plate may be prevented by:

1. Using a large plate so that any heat generated is spread over a wide area. A good contact may be assured if the plate is placed under the patient's buttocks, if this is possible.

2. Applying the plate to an area with good blood circulation, which will help to carry away the heat.

As shown above, if a direct current or an alternating one of mains frequency (50–60 Hz) were passed through a patient, there would be contractions of muscles and even cardiac dysrhythmias or arrest. However, with alternating currents of frequency greater than 10 kHz, these effects do not occur; so high-frequency currents may be passed through the body so that use may be made of their heating effect. A sine waveform is used for cutting, and a damped waveform for coagulation (Fig. 19.9). The sine waveform may be produced by a valve oscillator, while a damped oscillation is best produced by the spark-gap generator. The more recent transistorized diathermy sets produce a satisfactory cutting current, but some users find that the interrupted waveform they produce for coagulation (Fig. 19.10) is not as satisfactory as that of the spark gap.

In practice, the frequencies employed are higher, and though not standardized, are in the region of 0.4 MHz in the spark-gap generator and 1–1.5 MHz in valve oscillators.

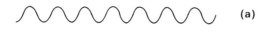

(a)

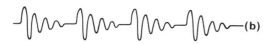

(b)

Figure 19.9 Waveforms for surgical diathermy. (a) A cutting current. (b) A damped waveform for coagulation.

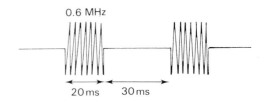

Figure 19.10 Pulsed waveform for coagulation from a transistorized diathermy set.

Modern apparatus is capable of producing modified waveforms that are intended for both cutting and coagulation.

The indifferent lead (i.e. the plate) is at earth potential in many diathermy sets and it is therefore important that it is connected to the correct terminal of the diathermy apparatus. If the plate were accidentally connected to the active terminal, the patient might be burned where his body was in contact with those parts of the operating table at earth potential, when the foot switch was depressed.

The above description is of a unipolar arrangement. However, some diathermy sets are capable of being used with a bipolar system in which the current passes from one blade of a pair of forceps to the other. The circuit is earth-free and the current does not pass through any part of the patient's body other than that grasped by the forceps (Fig. 19.11). The power required is small and it is electrically safer, but it is suitable only for the coagulation of small pieces of tissue or blood vessels. It is particularly suitable for ophthalmic and neurosurgical procedures.

ACCIDENTS DUE TO THE USE OR MISUSE OF THE DIATHERMY APPARATUS

These may be divided into two groups, first where the patient receives electrical burns, and second where fires or explosions are caused by the use of diathermy in the presence of inflammable vapours. The second group of accidents may also be caused by hot wire cautery.

Electrical burns

Electrical burns may be the result of:
1. The accidental depression of the foot switch

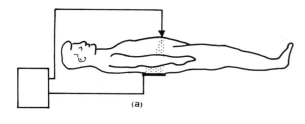

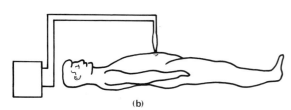

Figure 19.11   (a) Unipolar diathermy. (b) Bipolar diathermy.

when the forceps or cutting electrode is in contact with some part of the patient that it was not intended to burn. This may be prevented by keeping the forceps in an insulated 'quiver' when not in use, and it is also minimized by the installation of a buzzer within the diathermy machine which sounds when the foot switch is depressed. The indicator light on the machine is useful as a confirmation that the apparatus is working, but is not usually heeded as a warning when it is accidentally operated.

2. Poor contact between the plate and the patient, a burn occurring where it actually does touch.

Some diathermy machines give an audible warning if the plate lead is not plugged in, or if the electrical continuity of the lead is broken. However, the fact that the warning is not given is not proof that the plate has been applied to the patient. Some transistorized sets have a fully floating output and the patient is unharmed if the indifferent electrode is neglected.

Where the old-fashioned saline pad is used, it may have dried out, or too dilute a solution of saline may have been used. The plate may have been applied too loosely.

The pad must completely envelop the plate and its terminal, otherwise metal parts might touch the patient's skin and cause burning or mechanical injury.

3. The electrical circuit being completed via the operating table and the floor, or other points through which the patient may be earthed, which may occur if the plate is not applied. It has been known for the tracheal mucous membrane to be severely damaged when the patient was earthed through the damp endotracheal tube and the anaesthetic machine.

Fires and explosions

Fires and explosions may be caused in the presence of any inflammable vapour or liquid. Remember that not only are some anaesthetic agents inflammable, but so are ethyl and isopropyl alcohol, which are often used for cleaning the skin prior to operation. It may be soaked up by and remain in the drapes. This is particularly dangerous, since alcohol flames are barely visible where the part is strongly illuminated by the theatre lamp.

The cause of fire may be a spark at the active electrode itself, or a faulty mains lead, plug or foot switch.

Real safety lies in the abandoning of inflammable vapours and liquids.

The external cases (enclosures) of most diathermy machines are made airtight, i.e. gasproof, but remember that this is difficult to maintain when the machine is to be wheeled about into rooms of varying temperature, so that pressures are developed across the gasproof seal. Also if, owing to over-use or electrical fault, the interior is heated and fumes generated, a dangerous increase of pressure may occur, leading to rupture.

20
Layout and Contents of the Anaesthetic Room

Layout of the Anaesthetic Room

The anaesthetic room, known also as the induction room, is provided in all but the very smallest hospitals in Great Britain. However, in many other countries there is no such room and the patient is taken directly into the operating theatre before induction of anaesthesia. In the latter instance it is common for the operating theatre to be used for one case only rather than for a list of operations, so that adequate cleaning can be carried out after each operation.

It is the author's belief that the anaesthetic room is an essential part of the building, in which not only may the patient experience a tranquil atmosphere, but also the anaesthetist can set about the induction of anaesthesia, possibly the most hazardous part of his work, undisturbed.

Circumstances and temperaments differ, however, and doubtless there are many people who would prefer to induce anaesthesia in the operating theatre and save the problem of wheeling both the patient and the equipment between the anaesthetic room and the theatre after the patient had been induced.

Where work is organized so that the whole list of operations is performed in one operating theatre, during a morning or an afternoon, the presence of an anaesthetic room becomes even more desirable and saves the choice of either having delays between cases or patients waiting in corridors for their turn to be anaesthetized and operated on.

Under these circumstances it is equally important

that there should be a satisfactory recovery area for the immediate postoperative period, up to the stage where the protective reflexes have returned and the patient is awake. Here again there are different practices, but it is the author's preference to have a recovery area immediately adjacent to his theatre and anaesthetic room so that he may, through a suitable window, observe the supervision of patients as they recover from anaesthesia. In other situations one central recovery room may serve several theatres. The only disadvantage that this might have is that more reliance is placed on a large number of skilled staff, since it is impossible for such a recovery room to be close to all theatres in a large suite. Referring to Fig. 20.1, it will be noticed that two recovery areas have been joined together by virtue of removing partitions and made into one relatively large recovery room (5A) accommodating up to six patients. This type of system works satisfactorily, but it will be noted that the area is immediately adjacent to and visible from the neighbouring anaesthetic rooms and theatres.

The size and position of the anaesthetic and recovery rooms are too often dictated by factors outside the control of the anaesthetist. The following points, however, should be borne in mind when the anaesthetist is in a position to influence design.

1. The anaesthetic room, although requiring access to both the operating theatre and the theatre corridor, should not be used as a route for personnel passing between them. The layout should be such that intrusions by surgeons and theatre staff are reduced to a minimum.
2. The floor area should be sufficient to permit both the patient's arms to be abducted and placed on arm boards and there should be sufficient room at each end of the trolley to allow staff to pass from one side to another even with the doors open. The doors should be open in the direction in which the patient trolley passes.
3. In a multiple theatre suite the anaesthetic rooms should be similar, though they may need to mirror-image each other. If the general layout permits, they should be close to each other and to an equipment store or parking area for bulky apparatus such as ventilators. Where each theatre technician is assigned to his own anaesthetic room, small departures from uniformity should be allowed to encourage his initiative and individuality.

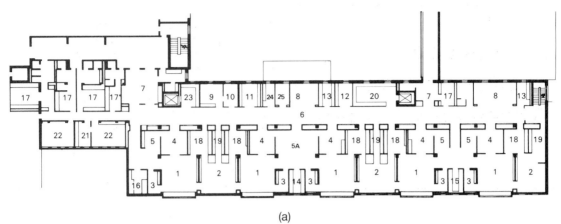

(a)

Figure 20.1 (a) Plan of a multiple operating theatre suite.
1, operating theatre; 2, sterilizing room; 3, scrub room;
4, anaesthetic room; 5, recovery area; 5A, larger recovery area;
6, clean corridor; 7, transfer bay; 8, trolly storage bay; 9 and 10,
offices; 11, ventilator and anesthetic equipment room;
12, Superintendent's office; 13, general store; 14, special store;
15, X-ray dark room; 16, Anaesthetic Department
workshop/store; 17, changing rooms; 18, disposal and
instrument cleaning room; 19, sterile pack store; 20, central
sterile supply department (CSSD) and special instrument room
(with lift direct to main CSSD); 21, kitchen; 22, sitting room;
23, dirty disposal room with decontaminating machine and lift to
incinerator and CSSD dirty receiving room; 24, cleaner's room;
and 25, Sister's office. (b) Detailed plan of a single theatre unit.
1, operating theatre; 2, sterilizing room; 3, scrub room;
4, anaesthetic room; 5, recovery area; 6, main theatre corridor.
Note the direction in which the doors of the anaesthetic room
open.

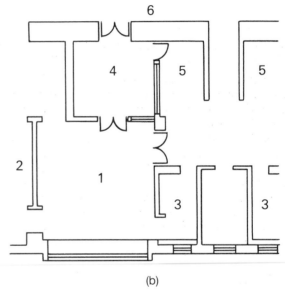

(b)

4. The recovery area should be as close as possible to the operating theatre and anaesthetic room. In large theatre suites consideration should be given to having a separate recovery area adjacent to each anaesthetic room. This arrangement (as shown in Fig. 20.1) is especially suitable where the nursing staff on recovery duty are relatively inexperienced. Windows between the theatre, anaesthetic room and recovery area may be of suitable dimensions to allow the anaesthetist to watch the recovering patient from either of the other two rooms, but not low enough for the patient waiting and awake, in the anaesthetic room, to see anything of the operation in progress or a patient in the recovery area. The window into the theatre should be fitted with a blind operated from the anaesthetic room side! There should be adequate sound proofing between the anaesthetic room and operating theatre and recovery rooms.

5. A cylinder store is required, even if there is a piped medical gas installation. Full cylinders may conveniently be stored on gently sloping shelves, those needed for use being drawn from the bottom of the slope and new ones being added at the top as the stock rolls downhill. This assures that cylinders are used in rotation and none are held in stock for excessive periods of time.

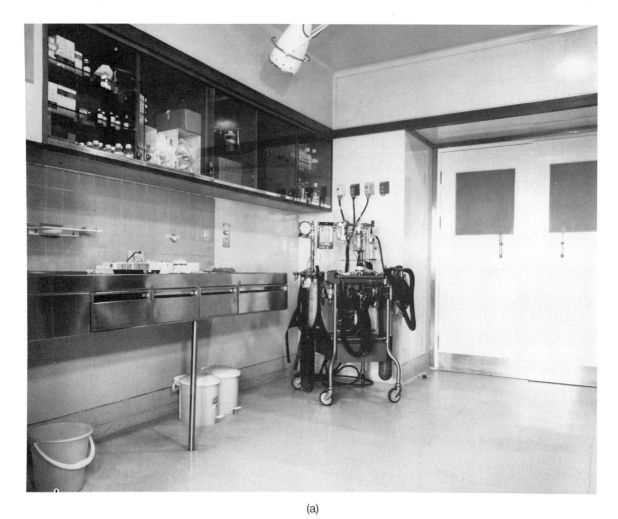

(a)

Figure 20.2   (a) An anaesthetic room. Notice the buckets below the work top, the glass fronted cupboards and the position of the piped medical gas outlets. When this photograph was taken scavenging had not yet been installed. The drug cupboard and sink are to the left (out of the picture). (b) The same anaesthetic room. Note the door and window to the recovery area (on the left), and also the door and window to the operating theatre (on the right).

6. A room should be set aside for storing parts and apparatus that are not intended for everyday or general use. This room should be equipped with a work bench and the necessary tools for day-to-day maintenance (see Schedule 2, p. 342). Where there are many anaesthetic machines to be maintained it is useful to keep one or two spare vaporizers for each agent which may be used to immediately replace those taken out of service for cleaning and recalibrating. In this room it is advisable to keep records in the form of a system such as the 'Cardex', on which details of servicing and alteration to anaesthetic machines and ventilators may be entered. A list of telephone numbers and addresses of the manufacturers and suppliers is also useful.

7. A sterilizing and decontamination room should be provided unless these services are performed elsewhere.

8. A refrigerator should be available for the storage of drugs such as succinylcholine. A separate, special refrigerator is required for the storage of blood.

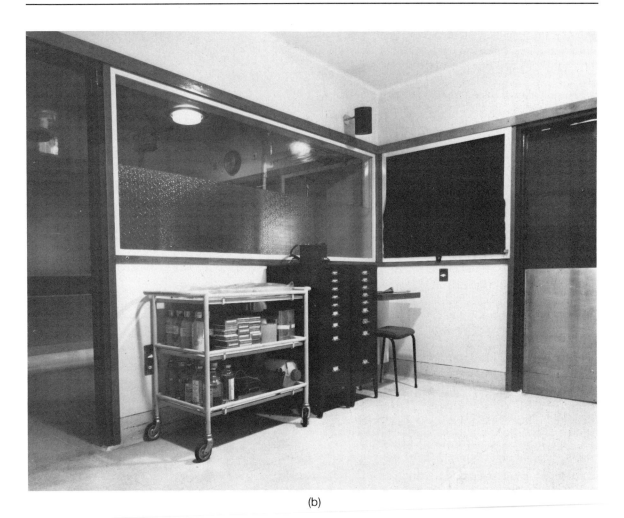

(b)

Contents of the Anaesthetic Room

Furniture

Figure 20.2 shows a typical anaesthetic room.

The cupboard space, which must be ample, should include a proportion of cupboards with glass doors, which may conveniently be at eye level above the worktop. There must be a lock on at least one cupboard for the storage of drugs. Dangerous (controlled) drugs and registers may be kept either in each anaesthetic room or in a central cupboard in the Theatre Superintendent's office.

The worktop should be of generous size, i.e. at least 2.5 m × 0.5 m, and there should be space under it for buckets — plastic, and if possible of different colours. The colours of these buckets should be standard throughout the hospital, for example:

Yellow — two-thirds filled with dilute soap solution, or a suitable detergent such as Neodane, for used tubes, airways, etc. (see Chapter 11).

Blue — for general rubbish.

Green — for broken glass, ampoules, used syringes and needles, etc., which should be handled separately from the general rubbish to avoid injury to those disposing of it.

(Red — for saline solution if 'wet' diathermy plates are still being used. Now outdated!)

Behind the worktop there should be a rack to accommodate prepacked sterile articles such as syringes, needles, etc. Endotracheal tubes and airways may be kept either in this rack or on a trolley which can be wheeled up to the patient during the induction of anaesthesia. Such a trolley may also carry solutions and giving sets for intravenous infusions.

The sink should have a mixer tap, high enough to allow a bucket to be filled, but arranged so that it will not cause splashing on to a surface where sterile articles are laid out.

Each anaesthetic room should have an identical multidrawer cabinet, the contents of each drawer being standardized throughout the hospital (Fig. 20.3). There may also be a second cabinet, with the drawers marked in different coloured labels, containing special equipment for the particular type of work carried out in that theatre. These cabinets should be mounted on castors to enable them to be wheeled out of the room when it is being cleaned, and in the case of the intensive care unit they may be wheeled to the patient's bedside.

There should be a writing surface, where the operation register may be kept and, if desired, a telephone. The clock, with a second hand, should be in a position where the anaesthetist can see it during induction. It has been common practice to provide a heated blanket cupboard, intercommunicating between the anaesthetic and recovery rooms. However, this is not always used, since blankets can more easily be left on the patient's trolley, and most anaesthetists are opposed to their being heated.

The overall lighting intensity should be high but not dazzling to the patient. There may be provision

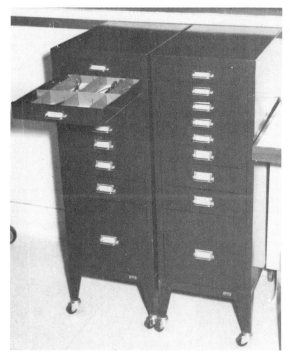

Figure 20.3   Multi-drawer cabinets for instruments and sundries. Note that they are mounted on castors for easy transportation during cleaning.

for an additional spotlight. Especially where infants are anaesthetized, a window or skylight is highly desirable in order to enable the patient's colour to be

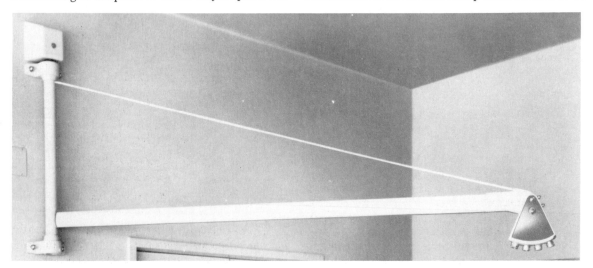

Figure 20.4   A swinging boom for medical piped gases.

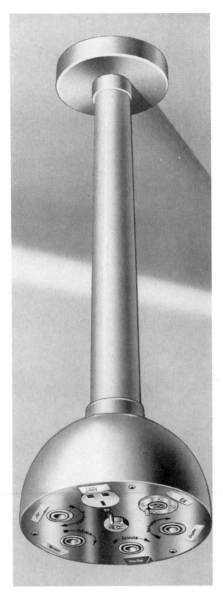

Figure 20.5 A fixed pendant for piped medical gases and electricity supply.

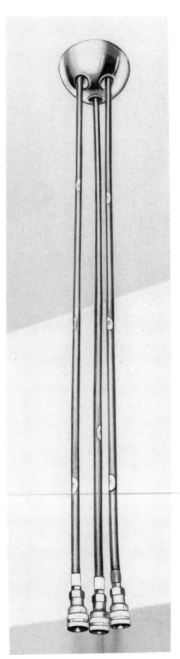

Figure 20.6 Hanging medical gas pipeline hoses.

assessed by daylight. The promises of architects and builders to provide daylight by artificial means are not always fulfilled. Some fluorescent tubes give a close approximation to daylight. The colour rendering (i.e. the colour of the patient when illuminated) given by the Kolorite tube has been found to be the best, and this type should be used in all areas where patients are tended.

The floor should be constructed of an antistatic material. Although the insistence on antistatic precautions has been relaxed, it may well be argued that for floors and instrument trolleys it should be

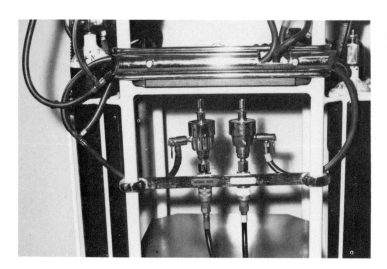

Figure 20.7   The pipeline conversion of an old type 'Basket Boyle's' machine. Note the 5 lb/in^2 pressure regulators.

maintained, since it reduces the static charge on trolleys that attracts dust which may carry infection.

Until recently all electric fittings were required by regulation to be sparkproof; mercury tip switches were usually employed. Recently, however, research has shown that ignition of anaesthetic vapours is not likely at a distance greater than 25 cm from the gaseous pathways of the anaesthetic machine. There has been considerable relaxation of regulations (in Great Britain) with reference to electrical equipment mounted on walls and other situations remote from the anaesthetic machine. There should be at least two socket outlets (for electrical plugs) in the anaesthetic room, and two on each of the walls in the operating theatre. Fire-fighting instructions and apparatus should be placed in a position where they are available to the staff but not where they will frighten the patient.

The whole decor of the anaesthetic room should be reassuring and restful to the patient and possibly include a picture or illustrated calendar and suitable cartoons where the patients are children.

Equipment

When equipping a hospital from the start, it is convenient to make out a list of equipment for a 'standard anaesthetic room'. A copy of this list may then be taken and amended for each anaesthetic room, according to the type of work to be done. A similar list may be made for the recovery area, and

for anaesthetic apparatus required in the theatre. Next, a list can be compiled of equipment intended for general use in the theatre suite as a whole — items such as ventilators, monitors, resuscitation equipment, etc., being specified.

The anaesthetist may be asked also to order equipment for the intensive care and coronary care units, the accident department and for the treatment of cardiac arrests and other emergencies in the hospital.

Typical lists are shown in Schedule 1 (pp. 337–342).

The pipeline outlets may be mounted on the wall, in the floor, in the ceiling or on a swinging boom (Fig. 20.4). Each arrangement has its advantages and drawbacks. It is usually found more convenient to use wall mounting outlets in the anaesthetic and recovery rooms, with a standard position (1.3 m for horizontally engaging probes; 1.6 m for vertically engaging probes) above floor level, and suction units mounted on a special plate screwed on to the wall adjacent to them. In the operating theatre, a fixed pendant (Fig. 20.5) is usually the best arrangement. Although there is the possibility that the height at which it is fixed may be out of the reach of very short anaesthetists, there is less risk of mechanical failure. Flexible tubing of the telescopic type is liable to damage and is not easily accessible for repairs and maintenance. The swinging boom is also liable to mechanical damage or failure, and it is not always possible to prevent its traverse from coinciding with that of the operating light and other objects. A boom may also disperse dust in the operating theatre. Booms and rigid pendants may be fitted with electric outlets, etc.

Piped gases and a vacuum may also be supplied through hanging hoses fitted with non-interchangeable connections (Fig. 20.6). Anaesthetic machines originally designed to be supplied by cylinders may be converted for connection to the pipeline (Fig. 20.7).

21
Management of the Anaesthetic Room

Although the anaesthetic room is connected with both the operating theatre and the outside corridor, no members of staff should be allowed to use it simply as a passage between the two. It should be kept as the private domain of the anaesthetist, in which he is not disturbed during the induction of anaesthesia, and the patient is not molested while still conscious. However, there may be times when minor procedures are best performed in the anaesthetic room rather than the operating theatre. Examples of these are endoscopies, and operations for infected cases such as the simple incision of abscesses, etc., where the contamination and consequent recleaning of an operating theatre can be avoided. The atmosphere should be reassuring and quiet and the walls that the patient can see should not be covered with gloomy hazard notices and the like (Fig. 21.1).

There should be as much standardization as possible between all the anaesthetic rooms in one hospital, though obviously that attached to, say, an ENT theatre will require certain stock items which would not be found in one for orthopaedic surgery. For day-to-day management the care of each anaesthetic room should be assigned to one particular, named, technician who may identify himself with the efficient running of that particular area.

In some establishments drugs are drawn up into syringes by nurses or technicians, in anticipation of the needs of the anaesthetist. This is a dangerous practice and it is the author's opinion that, if allowed at all, it should be limited to the preparation of bulk solutions in vials.

In many hospitals syringes containing anaesthetic drugs are labelled. This would, at first sight, seem to be an admirable practice, but mislabelling or recharging of syringes with a drug other than that for which they have been labelled has occurred and this, of course, defeats the object of the exercise. A much safer practice is to avoid charging syringes with potent drugs earlier than required and certainly to avoid stock-piling a large number of syringes, to be used in successive cases during an operating list. When a drug has been drawn up from an ampoule, that ampoule can be placed over the needle, not only to maintain its sterility, but also to identify it.

Rigid discipline in choosing a particular size of syringe for a particular class of drug can help to prevent accidents. For example, 20 ml syringes for induction agents, 5 ml syringes for non-depolarizing relaxants and suxamethonium for repeated increments, and 2 ml for all other purposes. When an anaesthetist is relieved by a colleague it is wise to avoid, wherever possible, transferring from the care of one to the other, syringes charged with potent drugs.

Care should be taken to avoid the contamination of unused equipment. For example, there should be a clean worktop for the drawing up of drugs, etc., from which all used equipment should be excluded. The anaesthetist should be discouraged from putting down on this surface objects such as syringes and needles which, having been used, are liable to be contaminated with the patient's blood, and laryngoscopes, airways and endotracheal tubes which, being contaminated with the patient's saliva, could well carry infective agents. Discarded syringes and needles should be destroyed or made unusable before being sent to the destructor or rubbish dump, in order to prevent attempts by addicts to obtain them. Broken ampoules and their tops, and other sharp items, should similarly be discarded separately. Used endotracheal tubes, airways and laryngoscopes, which are destined for resterilization, should be kept in a container isolated from items such as syringes, needles and broken ampoules in order to avoid the possibility of fragments getting into these items. For example, there have been cases where an endotracheal tube has been obstructed by the top of an ampoule that had got into it prior to resterilization.

Cleanliness is not only required to avoid the risks of cross-infection, but also to prevent too much contact with drugs, including antibiotics to which an allergy might become established. The career of

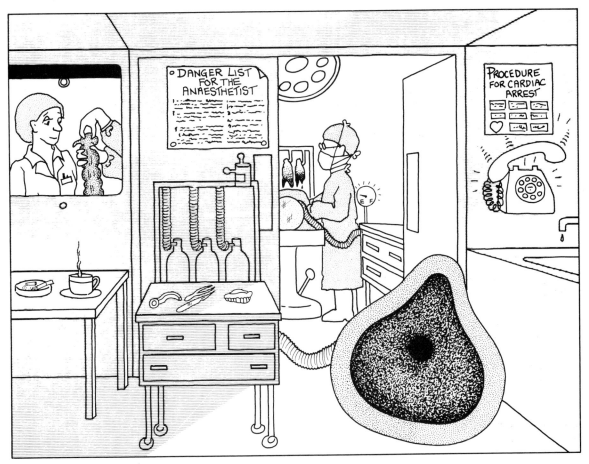

Figure 21.1 How a patient should *not* see an anaesthetic room!

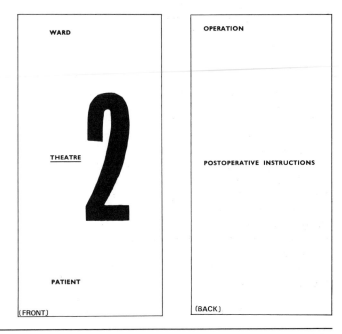

Figure 21.2 The operating theatre card.

331

one member of the nursing profession was jeopardized because she had become allergic to certain antibiotics and had to relinquish her post as ward sister.

It is usually the responsibility of the anaesthetist, or one of his staff, to order the time of the administration of the preoperative medication ('premed') and to send for the next patient at the appropriate time. Where there are several theatres in a suite, a card such as that shown in Fig. 21.2 may conveniently be used. Each theatre may have a different colour and number, and not only does one side of the card identify the patient and the ward from which he has come, but the other side may conveniently carry back to the ward, postoperatively, details of the operation and instructions.

The anaesthetist may also be required to supervise the keeping of a register recording the details of operations and also to keep a record of controlled drugs used.

Nurses, technicians and anaesthetists should be aware of the location of drugs and equipment that may be needed in an emergency, but of which only one is kept in reserve in a whole operating theatre suite.

This chapter is a catalogue of the various instruments and sundries used by the anaesthetist. The number of each that is required must be appraised by those whose concern the department is, but a general guide is laid out in Schedule 1 (pp. 337–342).

22

Instruments and Aids to Anaesthesia

Laryngoscopes

The most commonly used adult laryngoscope is the Macintosh curved folding laryngoscope (Fig. 22.1). There are various sizes of blade, sometimes referred to as 'large adult', 'adult', 'child' and 'infant'. In practice the 'adult' size is suitable for nearly all patients, and although the smaller blade is perhaps rather more convenient for children, it is really not necessary above 1 to 1½ years. Few patients are so large that the 'large adult' is really required. The whole range of blades is detachable and interchangeable and the handle may also be used for other types of blade. The light comes on automatically as the blade is opened to the right-angle position.

The electrical system of the laryngoscope has been greatly improved in recent years, but some points are still worthy of note. The bulb unscrews from the light carrier. On most bulbs the central contact is a 'blob' of solder, but there still remain others in which it is a small wire coil, which may need bending and adjusting so that it will reach the contact in the light carrier but not short circuit on to

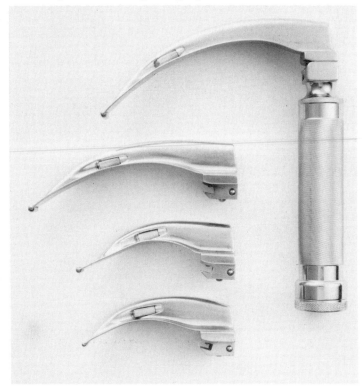

Figure 22.1 The Macintosh laryngoscope with four sizes of blade.

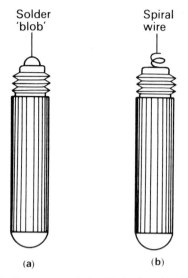

Solder 'blob'   Spiral wire

(a)   (b)

Figure 22.2   Laryngoscope bulbs. Notice the solder 'blob' contact on (a) and the wire spiral on (b).

the side (Fig. 22.2).

The light carriers for different blades are not interchangeable and should be removed and cold sterilized when the blade is autoclaved. The electric contacts between the handle and the mount of the blade may need cleaning from time to time with some fine abrasive material or a smooth file. In some cases the handle may be removed by loosening the retaining screw a couple of turns and then, while pressing the knurled head inwards, slipping the blade off the handle.

When replacing the batteries in the handle, it should be ensured that the spiral spring is still in the base of the battery compartment; leak-proof batteries should be used. (It is most aggravating to find, in an emergency, that not only are the batteries exhausted but they have also corroded within the handle, making replacement impossible.)

The laryngoscope blade may be cleaned between cases with soap and water, applied using a scrubbing brush, followed by spirit or chlorhexidine swabbing, and should be autoclaved, less the light carrier, as often as circumstances permit.

Other laryngoscope blades fitting the same universal handle are shown in Fig. 22.3.

Various child and infant blades, with smaller handles, are shown in Fig. 22.4. Their mode of operation and maintenance is similar to the above.

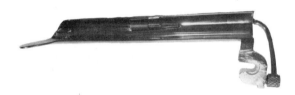

(a)

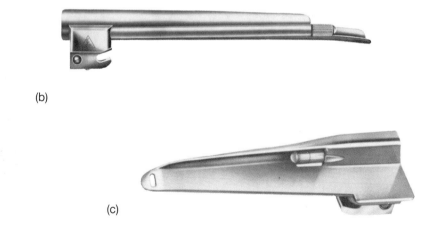

(b)

(c)

Figure 22.3   Various other adult laryngoscope blades. (a) The Magill. (b) The Wis. (c) The Soper. (d) The polio laryngoscope, which is particularly useful for obese patients undergoing caesarian section. (e) A one-piece plastic laryngoscope.

Left-handed laryngoscopes

At least one company (Penlon) manufacture a Macintosh laryngoscope, the blade of which is the mirror image of that to which we are accustomed. The left-handed laryngoscope is not, as sometimes imagined, to be used by an anaesthetist who is left-handed, but for patients in whom the nature of the teeth or maxilla make it undesirable to exert pressure upon a particular area. This may be due to complicated dental restorations, loose or ill positioned teeth, or the presence of cysts or tumours of the maxilla, to which damage could be caused by pressure of the laryngoscope. A left-handed laryngoscope should be carefully marked and kept in an appropriate place. Those with no experience will be amused to find how difficult it is to use it to begin with. It might be considered wise to obtain some practice with it so that when a difficult case does arise the user will be familiar with it.

Fibreoptic laryngoscopes (Fig. 22.5)

Fibreoptic laryngoscopes are currently still under development but are expected to be widely available in the near future. It is the author's view that they will prove to be more reliable than existing models and will soon replace them. (For general information on fibreoptics see pp. 342–345).

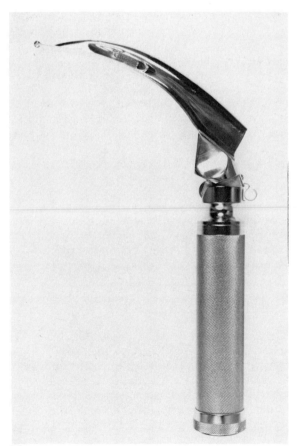

(d)

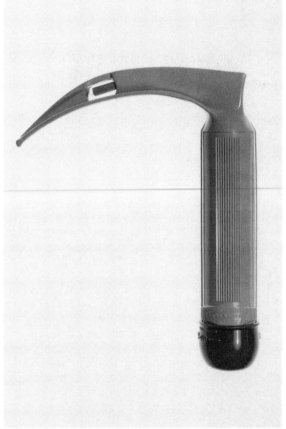

(e)

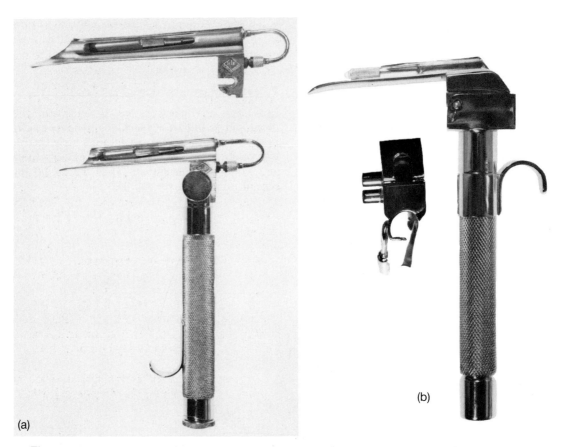

Figure 22.4 Two of the many infant laryngoscopes available. (a) The Anderson. (b) The Whipp's Cross Hospital pattern.

Bronchoscopes

There are simple emergency bronchoscopes which work on the same principles as laryngoscopes. The proportions are different, however, and a smaller bulb is employed.

It is an advantage to obtain blades that fit the same universal handle as the laryngoscope. They are made in various sizes, a set of three, viz. 11 mm, 8.5 mm and 3.5 mm, being convenient.

Figure 22.6 shows three blades for the Magill emergency bronchoscope, which incorporate a side tube through which oxygen may be blown. By occluding the open end with the finger, the patient's lungs may be inflated with what becomes a type of T-piece system. Although this may be less convenient for the operator than a jetting device (see

p. 234), it is pointed out that this is an *emergency* bronchoscope to be used at times when the latter may not be available. Metal suction tubes or plastic suction catheters may be used for aspiration.

Sprays

Nebulizing sprays are used for the topical (surface) application of local analgesic solutions, such as 4% lignocaine, to the larynx and trachea, and sometimes of vasoconstrictors to the nose. The general principle is the same in them all: a jet of air is blown through a venturi and 'sucks up' and nebulizes a solution of the agent to be used. Figures 22.7 and 22.8 show two popular types.

All these sprays tend to block up if they are not

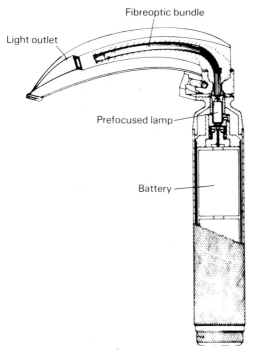

Light outlet

Fibreoptic bundle

Prefocused lamp

Battery

Figure 22.5 The Heine fibreoptic laryngoscope. Note that the lamp is within the handle, thus avoiding unreliable electrical contacts between the handle and the blade.

cleaned shortly after use. This is because the solution remaining at the nozzle dries out, leaving crystals which block the small orifice. This may be avoided by rinsing them out with distilled water or spirit after use.

The spray may be cleaned after use by any cold sterilizing solution, but a scrub with a brush and soapy water followed by a spirit swab is usually considered adequate. In the air inlet to the bulb there is a ball or flap valve. The analgesic solution has a tendency to run back into this and cause corrosion. In the case of the Swerdlow spray (Fig. 22.7) the ball may be removed for cleaning by undoing the knurled nut, care being taken to avoid losing the small retaining spring.

The two other common problems encountered with the Swerdlow spray are that the washer that seals the joint within the container is often damaged by over-tightening, and that the small length of tubing with the sinker often falls off. The tubing may be replaced by a piece cut from the pilot tube of an old red rubber cuffed endotracheal tube.

The maintenance in good working order or otherwise of the sprays may be taken as an index of the efficiency of the theatre technician!

The other instruments used are familiar and no comment is needed with regard to their care and maintenance: they will simply be listed here.

Schedule 1: The Standard Anaesthetic Unit

Boyle's anaesthetic machine, combined with the following:

Rotameter (flowmeter) unit for N_2O, O_2, CO_2 and (if required) C_3H_6

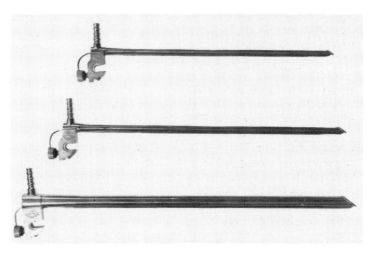

Figure 22.6 Magill emergency bronchoscope blades.

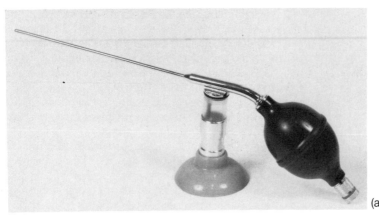

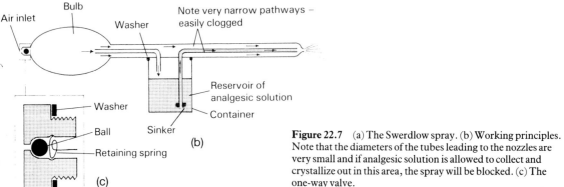

(a)

Bulb

Air inlet

Washer

Note very narrow pathways – easily clogged

Reservoir of analgesic solution

Container

(b)

Washer

Ball

Sinker

Retaining spring

(c)

Magnified diagram of air inlet valve

Figure 22.7   (a) The Swerdlow spray. (b) Working principles. Note that the diameters of the tubes leading to the nozzles are very small and if analgesic solution is allowed to collect and crystallize out in this area, the spray will be blocked. (c) The one-way valve.

Boyle's vaporizing bottle
Temperature-compensated vaporizers
Cardiff swivel outlet
Magill breathing attachment
Circle absorber unit
Emergency oxygen flush control
Provision for CO_2 cylinder
Provision for medical suction
Blood pressure apparatus
Shelves — Formica or glass
Top shelf
Drawer unit
Pipeline attachment
Cylinder labels (Fig. 22.9)
Trilene safety interlock, etc.
Pressure relief valve
Oxygen warning device

Other extras:
Facepieces, various (MIE, BOC, etc.)
Cylinder keys (Fig. 22.10)
Spares: rebreathing bag, corrugated hose,
    expiratory valve, etc.
Airways, various (Fig. 22.11)
    Guedel 1, 1a, 2, 3, etc.
    Phillips 1, 2, 3, 4
Endotracheal connectors
    Magill
    Nosworthy paediatric
    other
Endotracheal tubes
    various adult
    various paediatric
Laryngoscopes, adult and paediatric
Laryngeal sprays
Magill's endotracheal introducing forceps (Fig.
    22.12)

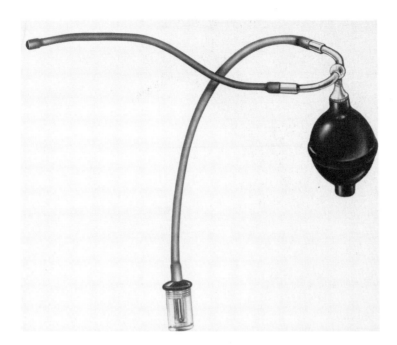

Figure 22.8 The Macintosh spray.

Mitchell's inflater, or syringe for endotracheal cuffs
Spencer Wells' forceps (Fig. 22.13a)
Guy's tongue forceps (Fig. 22.14)
Mayo's tongue and towel forceps (Fig. 22.15) or Thompson's tongue forceps (Fig. 22.16)
Large Kocher's forceps (Fig. 22.13b)
Scissors
Mouth gags (Figs. 22.17–22.19)
Mouth wedge (Fig. 22.20)
Suction end (Yankauer's or other)

Stethoscope
Ayre's T-pieces
Magill emergency bronchoscope, combined with various sized blades
Suction catheters
Kidney dishes and gallipots
Clausen's, Connell's or other head harnesses (Fig. 22.21)
Hudson's head harness (Fig. 22.22)
Catheter mounts (Fig. 7.71)
Plastic buckets

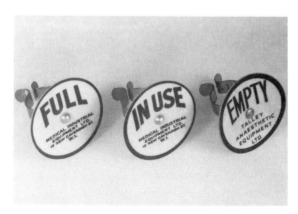
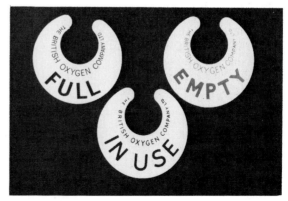

Figure 22.9 Various cylinder labels.

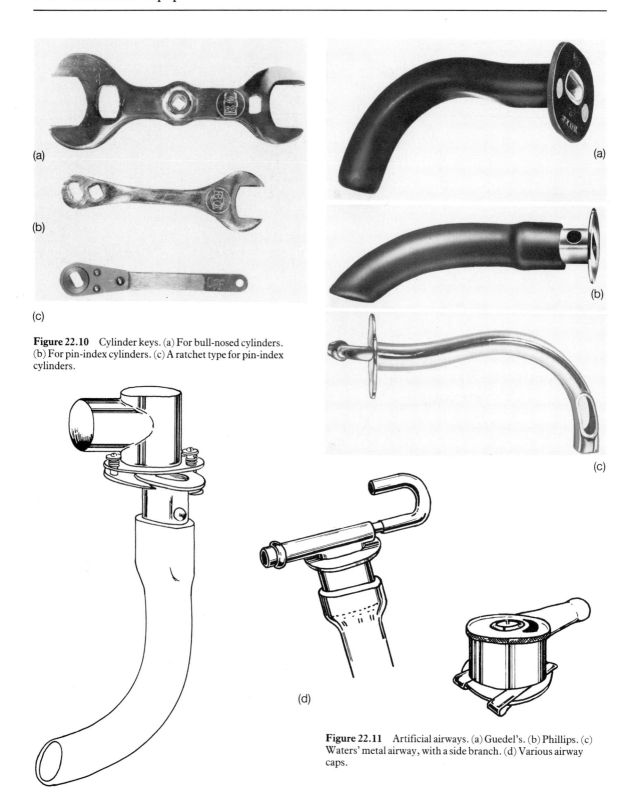

Figure 22.10   Cylinder keys. (a) For bull-nosed cylinders. (b) For pin-index cylinders. (c) A ratchet type for pin-index cylinders.

Figure 22.11   Artificial airways. (a) Guedel's. (b) Phillips. (c) Waters' metal airway, with a side branch. (d) Various airway caps.

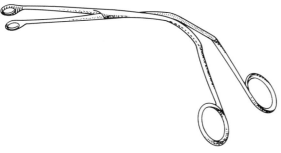

Figure 22.12   Magill's endotracheal introducing forceps.

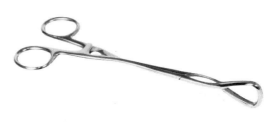

Figure 22.14   Guy's tongue forceps.

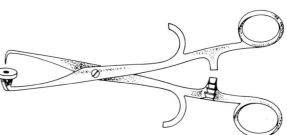

Figure 22.15   Mayo's tongue and towel forceps.

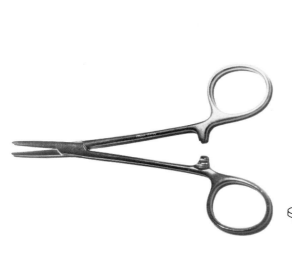

(a)

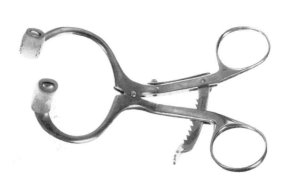

Figure 22.16   Thompson's tongue forceps.

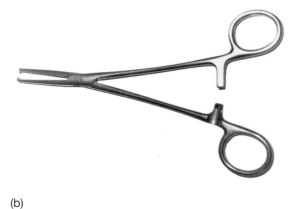

(b)

Figure 22.13   Artery forceps. (a) Spencer Wells'. (b) Kocher's.

Figure 22.17   Sydenham's modification of Doyen's mouth gag.

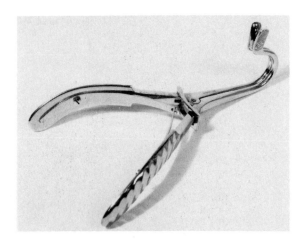

Figure 22.18 Ferguson's mouth gag.

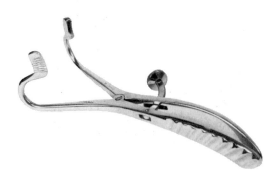

Figure 22.19 Mason's mouth gag.

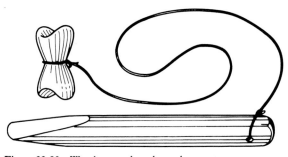

Figure 22.20 Wooden mouth wedge and prop.

Armboards
Ampoule holder block
9 drawer cabinet(s)
Bandages, adhesive plaster, etc.
Analgesic ointment and lubricating jelly
Drip stands
Intravenous infusion equipment

Schedule 2: The Technician's Tool Kit

A set of tools for the technician should include:

Various screwdrivers, including Phillips screwdriver
A set of spanners up to ½ in. Whitworth
Adjustable spanners, one small, one large
Set of hexagonal wrenches (Allan keys), Imperial and metric sizes
Pair of combination pliers
Pair of diagonal cutters
Small hacksaw and spare blades
Set of files
Ball-pein hammer
Wooden mallet
Sharpening stone
Oil can
Vice mounted on the bench
Crimping tool and spare ferrules — *available only to a suitably qualified engineer*
Spare bulbs for laryngoscope and bronchoscope
Spare batteries
Spare washers, including those for cylinder yokes, soda lime canisters, sprays, etc.
Torch
Direct current electric test meter
Grease — Wakefield H. M. Spheerol, and other specified lubricants
Manufacturers' instruction manuals for machines and ventilators
Pressure gauges of various types

Fibreoptics

The object of the fibreoptic system is to transmit light from a powerful external light source through an instrument that, being flexible, can be passed through a series of curvatures, and return to an

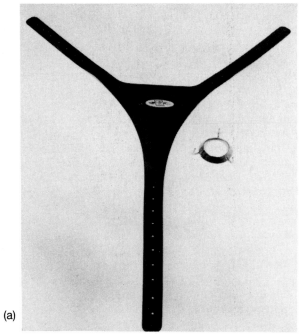

(a)

Figure 22.21 (a) Clausen's head harness and ring. (b) Connell's head harness.

(b)

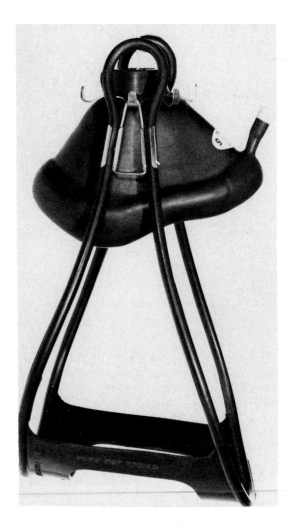

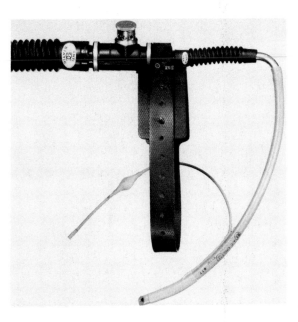

Figure 22.22 Hudson's head harness.

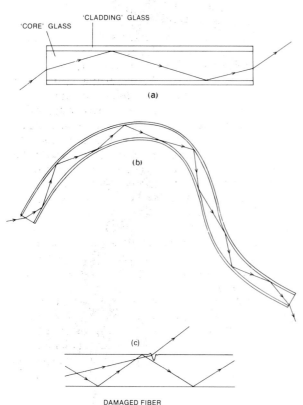

Figure 22.23 (a) A single optic fibre. Note that the light ray is repeatedly internally reflected from the interface between the core and cladding glass. (b) If the fibre is curved, the ray is still internally reflected within it. (c) If the surface of the fibre is damaged, the light may not be totally internally reflected and some may escape from the bundle.

eyepiece or camera an image of the area being illuminated. It may be used for endoscopy by various routes: for example, laryngoscopy, bronchoscopy, oesophagoscopy and colonoscopy. The pathways through which the light and the image pass consist of bundles of thousands of very fine glass fibres. Typically these fibres have a diameter of the order of 20 μm. Each consists of a central glass core surrounded by a thin cladding of another type of glass, having a refractive index different from that of the core. As will be seen in Fig. 22.23, the light ray passing down the fibre is repeatedly internally reflected from the interface between these two elements of the fibre. A bundle of these fibres is called a guide. In the case of a light guide the fibres are arranged in a random fashion,

whereas with the image guide the position of the fibres at each end of the bundle must be precisely located relative to each other. Each fibre carries the light from one small portion of the image in the same way that many small dots make up the printed representation in a book or newspaper of an original photograph. The fibres are so fine that they are easily flexible and they are lubricated so that they can move relative to each other. The whole bundle may therefore be flexed.

The light source of a fibrescope (Fig. 22.24) is usually powered by the mains electric supply and contains a lamp very much brighter than that at the distal end of an endoscope. It provides sufficient illumination not only for visualization, but also for the taking of colour photographs with a suitably adapted camera.

The trunk of the instrument may carry all of the following: an optical bundle (image guide), one or two light guides, a channel for suction or air insufflation, and another channel for the passage of instruments such as a biopsy forceps. At the distal end of the optical bundle there is a suitable lens to focus the image on the ends of the fibres; at the proximal end there is an eyepiece which may be focused. The eyepiece mount also carries a connection for the vacuum/insufflation channel and a valve to make a seal for the instrument channel. A fibreoptic bronchoscope is shown in Fig. 22.25.

The care of the fibrescope and of light cables in general is of great importance. The optical bundles in particular are extremely expensive to manufacture and are easily damaged. Although they can be

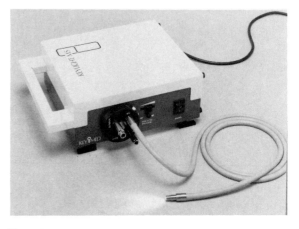

Figure 22.24 A light source and guide.

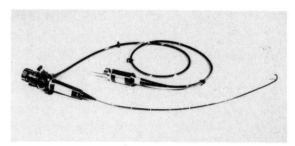

Figure 22.25 A fibreoptic bronchoscope.

flexed into acute angles of relatively small radii, they are easily damaged if they are pinched or knocked, as for example by a towel forceps on the operating table, or by being shut in the lid of the case in which they are transported. The covering over the distal six centimetres or so of the instrument is very delicate, and it is at this point that the greatest flexion takes place. It may well have to be replaced at about yearly intervals; the whole instrument being serviced every six months, according to the maker's instructions.

After use, the instrument may be cleaned by wiping it with a solution of Savlon and then rinsed in water. It can be disinfected between cases with Cidex, but it is essential that the eyepiece and head of the instrument are not immersed in the solution, otherwise water may track down between the fibres and damage the lubricant between them. If the trunk is immersed in the sterilizing solution, it should not be hung vertically, since the pressure at the lower end may be sufficient to drive water inside the cable and damage the lubricant as mentioned above. There are specially designed dishes into which the instrument is laid horizontally, with the head supported well above water level. Disinfectant solution may be sucked through the channels, and there is also a small brush which may be used to clean it. Although the instrument may be better protected by returning it to its carrying case after sterilization, it is, in fact, better to hang it vertically in a cupboard with the eyepiece at the top, so that any moisture contained may evaporate and it may dry out.

For procedures such as laryngoscopy and bronchoscopy the fibrescope is at first very difficult to use, and a prudent manufacturer has suggested that the anaesthetist should practise with it at least forty or fifty times on routine cases before he can expect to benefit from its use in an emergency or difficult situation.

23

Administration, Supplies and Maintenance

training purposes a list of the stock levels of drugs may conveniently be placed on the drug cupboard door, and photographs may be provided of sets of instruments, with details of the equipment that should be available in the anaesthetic room and operating theatre. Photographs of sets of instruments required for procedures such as epidural, subarachnoid and regional blocks are particularly useful. A policy may be laid down specifying the types and manufacturers of items such as endotracheal tubes, to ensure continuity of quality and dimensions. Any special endotracheal tubes, etc. that are not regular stock items should be ordered by the anaesthetist in charge of equipment.

The administration of an Anaesthetic Department requires liaison with the nursing staff, the pharmacist, the engineering staff and the porters.

Daily Care and Management

Arrangements should be made to ensure that all anaesthetic equipment is clean, sterile (where appropriate) and in good working order. This may be done by a theatre technician or nurse, but it is the responsibility of the anaesthetist himself to ensure that everything is in working order, that the appropriate cylinders have been turned on, empty ones replaced, vaporizers replenished and that a test is carried out to ensure that the pipeline hoses are correctly connected. It is good policy to assign the care of each theatre and anaesthetic room to one particular technician or nurse. It should also be the duty of the technician or nurse to check the lists of stock drugs so as to ensure that the drugs have been replenished where necessary. In some establishments he/she is also required to draw up drugs into syringes and to assemble infusion sets, but in the author's opinion this is an unreasonable delegation of a duty that should devolve upon the anaesthetist himself.

Arrangements should also be made to ensure the regular replacement of disposable items and short-lived equipment, such as endotracheal tubes, artificial airways and facepieces. For this purpose it may prove more satisfactory to stipulate stock levels. For

Record Keeping

Daily routine also includes the keeping of a register of operations and anaesthetics, and the identification of the patient. Once a patient has been anaesthetized, and his face perhaps partly obscured by an anaesthetic facepiece, it cannot be deemed the responsibility of the surgeon to identify him.

Within the Anaesthetic Department, or available to it, the following records should be kept:
1. Users' manuals of all equipment.
2. A list of spare parts.
3. Guarantees for the appropriate equipment.
4. A file of hazard notices that have been issued regarding the anaesthetic equipment.
5. The servicing schedules by various companies, including the frequency at which equipment is serviced.
6. Back-up requirements, such as spare batteries and laryngoscope bulbs.
7. Information regarding special equipment not mentioned above.
8. The addresses and telephone numbers of manufacturers and their representatives.

Maintenance

The maintenance of anaesthetic machines falls into three categories:
1. Day-to-day cleaning, replenishment of empty cylinders and vaporizers and general fettling.

2. Planned preventative maintenance (PPM).
3. Breakdown repairs.

In the case of essential apparatus, including life-support systems, the scale of equipment should be such that if any one particular item were to break down, there would be sufficient reserves on which one could call to continue the service.

In a large department it is preferable that there be one named consultant who has a particular interest in, and identifies himself with, the purchase and maintenance of equipment. This consultant may possess the ability to make minor adjustments or repairs himself, but certainly no other unauthorized person should be permitted to tamper with anaesthetic equipment.

Items of anaesthetic equipment that are faulty should *never* be sent to the ordinary hospital engineer ('steam and drains' department), since, although there are in these departments many mechanics who wish to be helpful and are only too pleased to render assistance when asked, they are often ignorant of the principles involved in anaesthetic equipment. Their well-meaning assistance, or interference, has only too often led to accidents resulting from inappropriate repairs or alterations. Their sole function (if any) should be to ensure that the service engineers from the appropriate manufacturing companies have attended and carried out their duties.

The ideal arrangement is to establish an Electronic and Biomedical Engineering Department (EBME), whose members may include both electronic and mechanical engineers. This department could not only carry out the supervisory duties mentioned above but could also make repairs and adjustments to equipment as required. However, the individual engineers must be aware of their own limitations. It is not often that such a department has sufficient expertise to entirely replace the PPM performed by the service engineer of the manufacturer concerned.

PPM should be carried out at regular intervals, usually every three months for anaesthetic machines and every six months for ventilators. Unless there is a comprehensive EBME Department, PPM is best undertaken by manufacturers' engineers. In recent years most of the latter have undertaken PPM and repairs only for their own equipment, whereas previously the engineer from one company would often

service the equipment of others. Records should be kept of the work done by these engineers; their attendance may be supervised by the EBME Department, the hospital engineers, or the supplies department.

With regard to malfunction or apparent breakdown, repairs are better initiated by reporting the incident first to the Consultant Anaesthetist responsible or to the EBME engineer. Either of these may investigate the problem. Very often it is found to be due to maladjustment on the part of the user rather than some fault in the equipment itself. As mentioned above, the ordinary hospital engineer should never be invited to tamper with the equipment; his role should be only to summon the representative of the manufacturer.

Without the preliminary inspection by the Consultant Anaesthetist, or the EBME engineer, there may be many instances when the manufacurer's engineer is called merely to make a minor adjustment. This is not only time consuming but may be very expensive if the travelling time concerned is significant, as this is usually charged for at the same hourly rate as when he is working.

A record of faults occurring in anaesthetic equipment should be kept, so that if there is a particular problem that recurs, the reason may be investigated and if possible eliminated.

The EBME Department should obtain circuit diagrams, etc. of the equipment under its care, and should also keep a stock of spare parts sufficient to deal with most of the common breakdowns. Such spares as reservoir bags, tubing, APL valves and catheter mounts should be kept within the Anaesthetic Department.

Supply of Cylinders of Compressed Gases

These are normally ordered by the pharmacist and stock levels for each gas are agreed between him and the anaesthetists. Some system should be employed to allow regular rotation of the stock of cylinders, so that those longest in store are used first. Labels such as those shown in Fig. 3.6 may be well intended, but in practice are of little use. A full cylinder is identified by the plastic dust cover around the outlet, and an empty one by the letters 'MT' written in chalk upon the body of the cylinder.

The administrative anaesthetist is also responsible for contingency planning for a disaster. This means not only the provision of anaesthetic equipment to take to the scene of, for example, an air crash or industrial calamity within the area, but also the provision of equipment that can be used in the event of the failure of supplies within the hospital. There must, for example, be adequate reserve cylinders to provide a standby service in the event of the failure of the piped medical gas system until all patients being anaesthetized can be returned from the operating theatre with their operations completed.

Purchase of Equipment

Administrative arrangements for the purchase of equipment must obviously vary from one country to another. It is appropriate here only to mention the procedure recommended by the author, variations being appropriate as circumstances demand. Purchases may be divided into three categories.

Category 1. Capital expenditure

This category includes equipment for which the purchase price exceeds a nominal value, say, £400, and which is likely to be used for many years, for example, anaesthetic machines, ventilators, sophisticated monitors and similar equipment. A policy must be agreed between all the anaesthetists as to the type and manufacturer of the anaesthetic equipment to be ordered, so as to maintain a uniformity of standards and the standardization of equipment. This also permits the purchase of adequate spare parts and facilitates the emergency repair of equipment by the EBME Department.

Category 2. Stock orders and disposables

The Hospital Supplies Department should carry stocks of disposable and short-lived items. An agreement should be made with them as to the type and manufacturer selected. For example, if a new manufacturer were to offer endotracheal tubes at a lower price than those already purchased, it would be the responsibility of the Supplies Officer or the CSSD (Central Sterile Supply Department) Manager to confirm with the anaesthetists that they approved of this particular pattern. The range and stock levels (number of each item kept) should also be discussed. Stock orders may be made by theatre technicians or members of the nursing staff.

Category 3. Non-stock orders

Non-stock orders are for items of equipment of low cost, but which are not regularly ordered and therefore not kept in stock. Any item up to a nominal value of, say, £400, may be ordered by the administrative anaesthetist as a 'non-stock' order. The administrative anaesthetist should notify all other anaesthetists of changes in the type or pattern of equipment ordered.

There are certain situations in which it would be difficult or impracticable to provide sophisticated, heavy and bulky anaesthetic equipment on the scale to which we are accustomed in hospitals. Examples are, domiciliary anaesthesia for a single patient and which may be for an emergency or planned minor surgery, and anaesthesia and resuscitation at the site of an accident or disaster. Also, in areas where underdevelopment of transport and other facilities preclude the adequate supply and maintenance of anaesthetic equipment, special arrangements may have to be used.

24
Provision for Anaesthesia in Difficult Situations

Domiciliary Anaesthesia

In a compact country such as the United Kingdom there is seldom any difficulty in providing a portable anaesthetic machine, complete, if necessary, with cylinders for the administration of a single anaesthetic. Minor surgery only would be undertaken. There are several satisfactory portable Boyle's machines, which function in the same manner as their larger counterparts, but very often small cylinders only are carried, and some form of rebreathing system, such as a circle absorber or Waters' canister, is appropriate. These portable anaesthetic machines may, if necessary, be used in conjunction with a manual resuscitator such as the Ambu, the Oxford bellows or merely a reservoir bag to achieve artificial ventilation if relaxants are used. Examples of these are shown in Chapter 11.

In domiciliary practice, care has to be taken if explosive anaesthetic agents are used. In two obstetric cases the author experienced a rather worrying situation. In the first, after the anaesthetic had been completed for the removal of retained placenta, from a patient who had suffered severe haemorrhage, a roaring coal fire was found that had been obscured by a clothes-horse on which various items of laundry were drying. In the second, the coal fire was successfully extinguished with a gallon or two of water, and all seemed to be well until, when leaving, the author was met by the occupants of the flat below. They pointed out the growing soot laden wet patch on their ceiling, immediately under the fire that had been extinguished!

The Major Accident

In this situation there may be many casualties and the incident always occurs unexpectedly. The territory is often unfamiliar to those working, and this can often pose problems to all concerned. Exposure to high temperatures and dehydration in the tropics can be matched in its importance by extremes of cold climate, which may be found even in so-called temperate zones such as the United Kingdom. Low temperatures may not only incapacitate those working and harm the injured, but may also preclude the use of some anaesthetic, agents, such as Entonox. Altitude may also pose problems with the administration of nitrous oxide and the volatile agents.

The lines of communication between the rescue workers and their patients, and the removal of the patients to safety, may be rendered very difficult by local conditions, as, for example, in an underground railway disaster or a mining accident. Darkness, dust and cramped conditions may preclude the carrying of sophisticated equipment. If emergency amputation or disentanglement of patients from wreckage is required, this may well be achieved under intravenous or intramuscular anaesthesia with ketamine, but even so oxygen (bearing in mind inflammability) and Entonox, may be required. The greatest need may be for resuscitation, including endotracheal intubation, and this should be borne in mind when selecting equipment.

Triservice Anaesthetic Apparatus

This compendium of anaesthetic and resuscitation equipment (Fig. 24.1) has been designed by the three British Fighting Forces in order to provide a versatile but standardized system which, with the exception of the oxygen cylinder, is all housed in a box of rugged construction that can be dropped by parachute and weighs no more than 25 kg.

The basis of the compendium is a breathing system which includes a Laerdal folding manual resuscitator and two Oxford Miniature vaporizers (OMVs) (see p. 100 and Fig. 5.29). During spontaneous ventilation the patient draws in air through the OMVs, and if it is desired to enrich it with oxygen the reservoir tubing is added to conserve the oxygen during the expiratory phase. During expiration the exhaled gases are voided to air through a valve mounted adjacent to the facepiece.

The OMVs are a slightly modified version: they have three folding feet which enable them to be stood on a flat surface, and their capacity has been increased to 50 ml. The calibration scale for one agent may be detached and replaced by that for another — halothane or trichloroethylene (Trilene) may be used. Since the wicks in the vaporizing chamber are of metal, and therefore non-absorbent, one agent may be drained out, and after 'rinsing out' the vaporization chamber with a little of the new agent and then discarding it, it may be immediately filled with the new agent. When the control is turned to 'O' (off) the contents will not spill if the vaporizer is accidentally inverted — though during transport it is preferable to empty out the agent. If the control is not turned to 'O', the vaporizer should be maintained still, in the vertical position for a few minutes before use, so that any liquid agent that has entered the bypass or the vapour control mechanism may drain back into the sump. Although the OMV is not temperature compensated, it does contain a heat sink, which helps to keep the output concentration relatively stable. Two OMVs are included in the system so that a quick change can be made from one agent to another, and also so that by using both, in series, for halothane or ether, a high enough concentration of those agents may be obtained for induction (as opposed to maintenance) of anaesthesia.

If the patient is apnoeic for any reason, whether arising from collapse or from the anaesthetic technique, IPPV may be instituted by manual compression of the Resusci bag or by a ventilator, if available.

If a technique employing a muscle relaxant and controlled ventilation is being employed, trichloroethylene may be used as a substitute for nitrous oxide to keep the patient asleep and analgesic.

Situations in Underdeveloped and Distant Countries

In some underdeveloped countries problems may arise not only on account of the apparatus but also due to the experience and training of the anaesthetist. It is not within the scope of this book to discuss the desirability of employing nurse-anaesthetists, but it seems certain that in many countries anaesthetics will have to be given by these 'medical assistants' for many years to come. Furthermore, it may well be argued that a medical assistant who has been well trained may be more efficient at anaesthetizing patients than a doctor who has received little or no training in anaesthesia.

Let us consider the personnel first. In many hospitals there may be one doctor who is helped by several medical assistants. In these cases he may well induce anaesthesia and intubate the patient himself and then hand over to the assistant whilst he performs the operation, returning to the role of anaesthetist at the end. It is quite obvious that the maintenance of a clear airway is one of the paramount duties of the assistant and this will be greatly facilitated if the patient has been intubated. Therefore, under these conditions, endotracheal intubation may be more common than elsewhere, and this should be borne in mind when considering the provision for endotracheal equipment. The anaesthetic apparatus used should be as simple as possible so that there are few controls to operate and the least possible chance of malfunction or maladjustment. A combination of the EMO vaporizer, the OMV ('Oxford Miniature' vaporizer) (equipped and calibrated for both halothane and trichloroethylene (Trilene)) together with a means of inflation such as a manual resuscitator or Oxford bellows, a Ruben or similar valve, and a facepiece or endotracheal connector may well be the most practicable equipment available under these circumstances. The facility for the

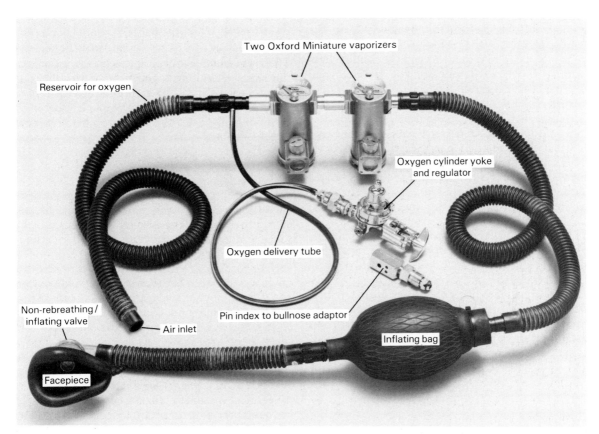

Figure 24.1 The Triservice apparatus. The patient may breathe spontaneously, drawing air through the two Oxford Miniature vaporizers and the inflating bag. There is a valve mounted on the facepiece which prevents rebreathing. The air, which is drawn in through the inlet, may be enriched with oxygen from a cylinder to which is attached the cylinder yoke, with the pin index to bull-nose adaptor if required. During expiration, the oxygen is stored in the reservoir tubing. The two Oxford Miniature vaporizers may be used for a variety of anaesthetic agents, there being interchangeable calibration labels for each. In the case of induction with ether, with spontaneous ventilation, both vaporizers will be required to produce an adequate vapour concentration. However, with spontaneous ventilation, if halothane is employed in the first vaporizer, it may be found convenient to use trichloroethylene in the second in order to make good the deficiency of analgesia caused by the exclusion of nitrous oxide. These vaporizers may be easily cleaned to remove traces of previous anaesthetic agents and in this photograph they are shown without their feet extended.

For controlled or assisted ventilation the inflating bag may be squeezed manually, or it may be replaced by a mechanical ventilator of the bag-squeezing type, the choice being dictated to some extent by the type of power source available. As an alternative to the inflating bag shown, the Laerdal folding silicone bag may be used.

addition of a supply of oxygen would be desirable. The provision of equipment and supplies to these areas is prejudiced by long lines of communication and very often unreliable means of transport. Whilst much equipment can be delivered by air, this is expensive and may be precluded in certain weather conditions, and also it must be remembered that there are problems concerned with the delivery of agents such as ether by air.

Restricted Articles Regulations

The International Air Transport Association publishes regulations concerning the precautions to be taken when transporting by air the following: inflammable gas, oxidizers, corrosives, explosives, poisons, non-flammable compressed gas, inflammable liquids and radioactive material. These regulations are accepted throughout most of the world, and are concerned with the labelling, the general packing requirements and the handling and loading of restricted articles. The labels are all diamond shaped, of different colours, and bear both a word and a symbol to denote the danger.

Agents such as trichloroethylene and chloroform may be carried in both passenger and cargo aircraft, but subject to a restriction in quantity: in both cases 40 *l*. Halothane, unfortunately, is not as yet mentioned. Ether is not accepted at all in passenger aircraft and a maximum of 40 *l* may be carried in cargo aircraft. One litre of ethyl alcohol may be carried in a suitable container in passenger aircraft and up to 40 *l* in cargo aircraft. Up to 70 kg of both nitrous oxide and gaseous oxygen may be carried in passenger aircraft and up to 140 kg in cargo aircraft. Liquid oxygen is not acceptable as cargo in any aircraft, either in a non-pressurized or pressurized package. Cyclopropane is not acceptable in passenger aircraft and up to 140 kg may be carried in cargo aircraft. Up to 70 kg of gaseous or liquefied carbon dioxide may be carried in passenger aircraft and up to 140 kg in cargo aircraft; there is no restriction for solid carbon dioxide.

Maintenance of Equipment

There are some countries in which there are good standards of equipment and work but maintenance may be a problem. The author's experience in an island in the Indian Ocean with a population of less than one million was that the personnel in all categories were well trained. However, problems arose owing to the distance that had to be travelled by service engineers, and so even relatively small matters of maintenance became a problem. It would be difficult to justify the full-time employment of an engineer for just an occasional task, and yet the cost of transporting an engineer by air to perform his work is very expensive. For this reason it is better to avoid complicated and sophisticated equipment such as the larger ventilators, which may need frequent attention and adjustment. Supplies of oxygen and nitrous oxide may be available but very expensive, and consideration should be given to the use of closed, low-flow breathing systems, or oxygen concentrators.

When ordering equipment for these areas, consideration should be given to the provision of adequate spares and it might well be deemed advisable to have one of the anaesthetists trained in some of the less complicated mechanical manipulations required in servicing.

Although SI units have been adopted for scientific purposes, they are not yet universally used in anaesthetic practice. As many pieces of anaesthetic and oxygen therapy apparatus will survive for many years, the older units in which they are calibrated have been retained throughout this book. Conversion tables will be found on the following pages.

The SI units applicable to anaesthesia are as follows:

Appendix 1

SI Units (Système International d'Unités) and Conversion Tables

Function	SI Unit
Mass	kilogram (kg)
Length	metre (m)
Force	newton (N) — accelerates a mass of 1 kg by 1 m/s^2 (1 N = 10^5 dynes)
Pressure	pascal (Pa) = 1 N/m^2 (NB 1 bar = 10^5 Pa)
Energy	joule (J) — force of 1 newton acting through 1 metre (1 J = 10^7 ergs)
Power	watt (W) = 1 J/s
Temperature	kelvin (K) = °C (0 K = −273°C)
Frequency	hertz (Hz) = 1 cycle/s
Capacity	litre (*l*)

LENGTH **AREA**

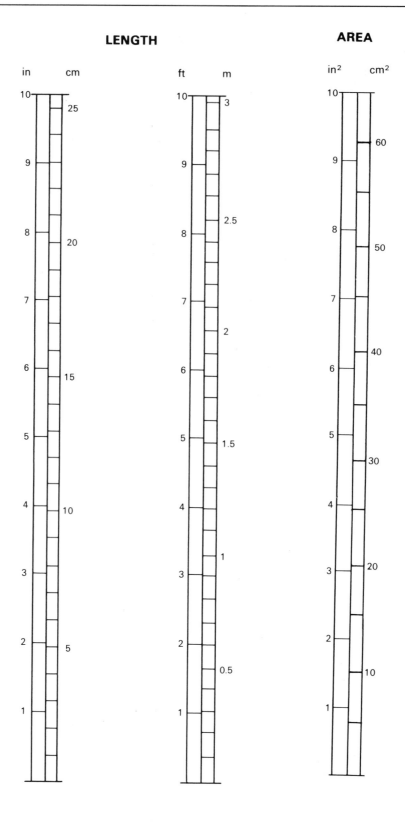

VOLUME

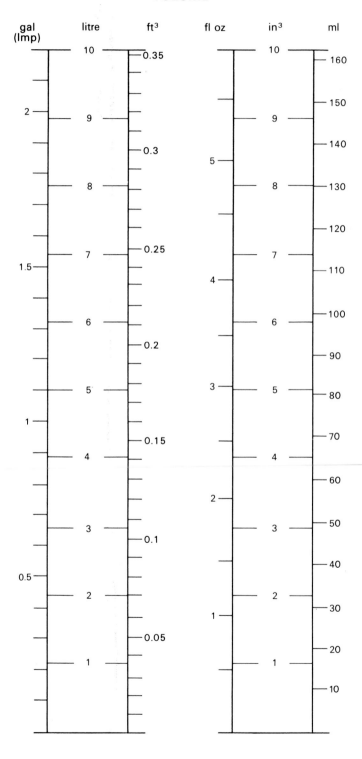

PRESSURE

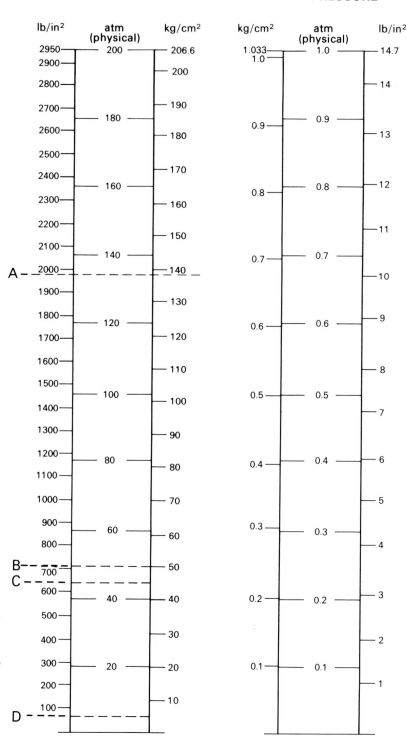

PRESSURE

NB 10^5 Pa = 1 bar = 0.987 atm. (physical)

A   Approximate pressure in full O_2 cylinder/full Entonox cylinder at 15°C (1960 lb/in²).
B   Approximate pressure in full CO_2 cylinder at 15°C (723 lb/in²).
C   Approximate pressure in full N_2O cylinder at 15°C (639 lb/in²).
D   Approximate pressure in full cyclopropane cylinder at 15°C (64 lb/in²).

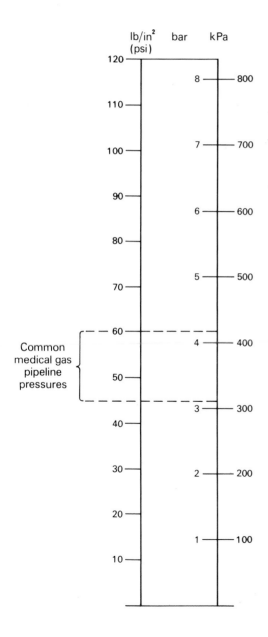

PRESSURE

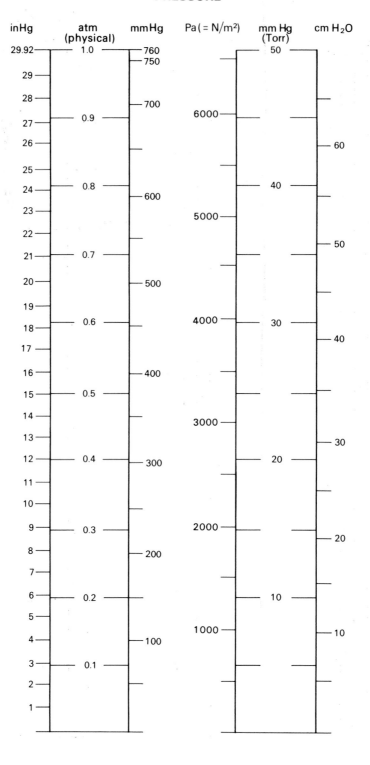

WEIGHT

FLOW RATE
(to estimate duration
of cylinder contents)

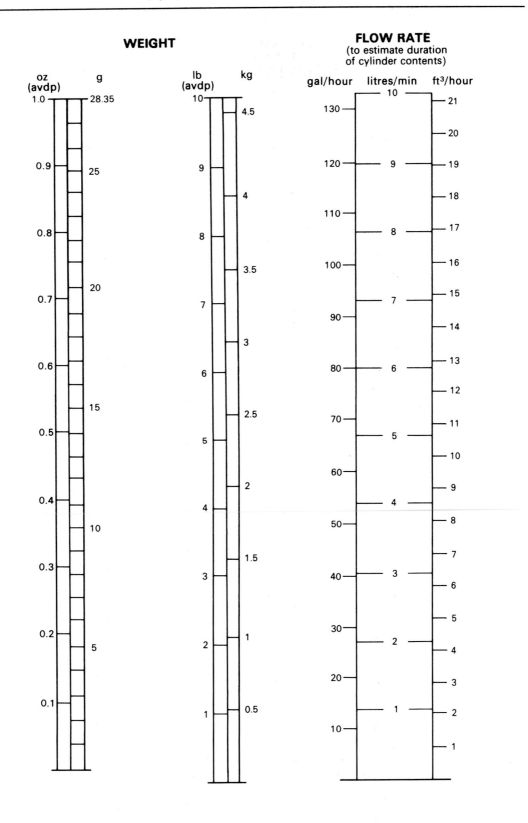

HEAT and TEMPERATURE

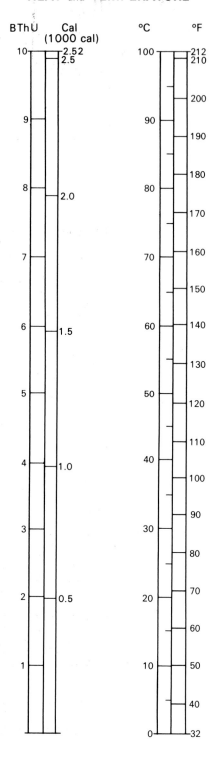

Appendix 2
Equipment Manufacturers

Adsorba. Dutom Meditech Ltd, Ronald Belcher Research Centre, Warwick Street, Birmingham B12 0NH. Tel. no. 021–771 3000. — M

AE. Anaesthetic Equipment Ltd (once part of Cyprane). *See* Ohmeda. — D, W

Ambu International UK Ltd, Charlton Road, Midsomer Norton, Bath BA3 4DR. Tel. no. 0761 416868.
or Ambu International, Marielundvej 32, PO Box 58, DK-2730 Herleu-Copenhagen, Denmark. Tel. no. 02–91 02 22. — E, R, S

AME. Art Medical Equipment (Pty) Ltd, AME House, 93 Bree Street, Newtown, Johannesburg, PO Box 23591, South Africa. Tel. no. 011–834 5741/2/3. — G

Beckman-RIIC Ltd, Norvic House, 7 Hilton Street, Manchester M4 1LP. Tel. no. 061–834 7225. — O

Bedfont Technical Instruments Ltd, PO Box 42, Streatham, London SW16 1JH. Tel. no. 01–769 7518. — A

Bennett. *See* Puritan-Bennett International Corp. — V

Bird Products Corporation, 3101 East Alego Road, PO Box 2007, Palm Springs, California 92263, USA. Tel. no. 619 327 1571.
(In the UK contact MIE.) — V

Blease Medical Ltd, Deansway, Chesham, Bucks. HP5 2NX. Tel. no. 0494 784422. — G, V

BOC. British Oxygen Company. *See* Ohmeda. — C, G, P

British Fluidics and Controls Ltd, Forest Road, Hainault, Ilford, Essex. Tel. no. 01–500 3300. — F

Cape. *See* Penlon Ltd. — V

Childerhouse Developments Ltd, 310A Upper Richmond Road West, East Sheen, London SW14 7JN. Tel. no. 01–876 4078. — G

Cory Bros (Hospital Contracts) Co. Ltd, 4 Dollis Park, London N3 1HG. Tel. no. 01–349 1081. — N, T

Cyprane. *See* Ohmeda. — D, W

Dameca, Islevdalvej 211, DK-2610 Rodovre, Denmark. Tel. no. 02–91 34 80. — A, G, M

Draeger Medical Ltd, Wood Lane, Hemel Hempstead, Herts. HP2 4SU. Tel. no. 0442 3542.
or Dräger, Postfach 1339, Moislinger Allee 53/55, D-2400 Lubeck 1, West Germany. Tel. no. 0451 882 2707. — G, M, V, W

East Health Care, Sandy Lane West, Littlemore, Oxford OX4 5JT. Tel. no. 0865 714242. — G, M, V

Edenvick. Dobromed Ltd, Spring Grove Mills, Manchester Road, Linthwaite, Huddersfield HD7 5QG. Tel. no. 0484 846060. — O

Engström. Gambro Ltd, Lundia House, 124 Station Road, Sidcup, Kent DA15 7AS. Tel. no. 01–309 7800.
or c/o LKB Instruments Ltd, 232 Addington Road, Selsdon, South Croydon, Surrey CR2 8YD. Tel. no. 01–657 8822.
or Gambro Engström AB, Box 20109, S–161 20 Bromma, Sweden. Tel. no. 08–98 82 80. — H, M, V

Eschmann, Peter Road, Lancing, West Sussex BN15 8TJ. Tel. no. 0903 62291. — N, S

Ferraris Development & Engineering Co. Ltd, 26 Lea Valley Trading Estate, Angel Road, Edmonton, London N18 3JD. Tel. no. 01–807 3636. — M

Flomasta. *See* MIE. — V

Frazer Harlake Inc., 145 Mid County Drive, Orchard Park, New York 14127, USA. Tel. no. 716 662 6650.
(In the UK contact Nesor Equipment Co.) — D

Frazer-Sweatman. *See* Frazer Harlake Inc. — D

Gould Medical Ltd, Grovelands House, Longford Road, Exhall, Coventry CV7 9ND. Tel. no. 0203 367676. — A, X

Heine Optotechnik GmbH, Kientalstrasse, 7, D–8036 Herrsching, West Germany. Tel. no. 815 2380. — I, Y

Hoek Loos, Havenstraat 1, PO Box 78, 3100 AB Schiedam, The Netherlands. Tel. no. 010 731122. — G

Hook & Tucker Instruments Ltd, Vulcan Way, Addington, Croydon, Surrey CR0 9UG. Tel. no. 0689 43345. — A

Kay Pneumatics Ltd, London Road, Dunstable, Beds. LU6 3DL. Tel. no. 0582 609292. — F, R. V

Kingston Medical Gases Ltd, 121 Clarendon Street, Hull, W. Yorks. HU3 1AY. Tel. no. 0482 24298. — C, P

Laerdal. Laerdal Medical Ltd, 2 Vincon Close, Orpington, Kent BR6 0EG. Tel. no. 0689 76634.
or Asmund S. Laerdal, PO Box 377, N–4001 Stravanger, Norway. Tel. no. 04–53 40 60. — E, R, S

Leyland Medical International Ltd, PO Box 6, Leyland, Preston, Lancs. PR5 1XR. Tel. no. 0772 431151. — T

Loosco. *See* Hoek Loos. — G

McKesson Equipment Co. Ltd, Tradent House, 110 Park Road, Chesterfield, Derbyshire S40 2JX. Tel. no. 0246 76111. — D

Mallinckrodt (UK) Ltd, Nunn Mills Road, Northampton NN1 5PA. Tel. no. 0604 24853. — N, T

Key

or Mallinckrodt GmbH, Stockstadterstrasse 10, D–8754 Grossostheim, West Germany. Tel. no. 22 47 3020.

Medec Holland. Medical Equipment Development, Postbus 1002, Zaandam, The Netherlands. Tel. no. 075 166412. — U

Medishield. *See* Ohmeda. — C, G

MGI. Medical Gas Installations Ltd, Unit 21, Monmer Close, Stringes Lane, Willenhall, West Midlands WV13 1JR. Tel. no. 0902 631225. — G, J, P

MIE. Medical and Industrial Equipment Ltd, Falcon Road, Sowton Industrial Estate, Exeter, Devon EX2 7NA. Tel. no. 0392 31331. — G

Nesor Equipment Co., Claremont Hall, Pentonville Road, London N1 9HR. Tel. no. 01–278 7401. — D, P

Norgren Enots Ltd, Shipston on Stour, Warks. CV36 4PX. Tel. no. 0608 61676. — F

Ohio. *See* Ohmeda. — G

Ohmeda, Elizabeth Way, Harlow, Essex CM19 5AB. Tel. no. 0279 29692. — C, G, P

Olympus Optical Ltd, San-Ei Building 22–2, Nishi Shinjuku 1–Chome, Shinjuku-ku, Tokyo, Japan. Tel. no. 03–340 2114. — I

Oxylitre Ltd, St Mary's Works, Cambrian Street, Beswick, Manchester M11 3FY. Tel. no. 061–273 1351. — P. Q, S

Pall Biomedical Ltd, Europa House, Havant Street, Portsmouth PO1 3PD. Tel. no. 0705 753545. — B

Penlon Ltd, Radley Road, Abingdon, Oxon OX14 3PH. Tel. no. 0235 24042. — G, U, V, W

Pneupac. *See* Kay Pneumatics Ltd. — R, V

Portex Ltd, Hythe, Kent CT21 6JL. Tel. no. 0303 60551/66863. — N, T

Puritan-Bennett International Corporation, 66 Bognor Road, Chichester, West Sussex PO19 2PH. Tel. no. 0243 787041. *or* Puritan-Bennett Corporation, 9401 Indian Creek Parkway, PO Box 25905, Overland Park, Kansas 66225, USA. Tel. no. 913 661 0444. — P, V

Riken. Weatherall Equipment and Instruments Ltd, PO Box 69, Tring, Herts. HP23 6PL. Tel. no. 024 029 8110. *or* Riken Keiki Fine Instrument Co. Ltd, 2–7–6 Azusawa, Itabashi-ku, Tokyo, Japan. Tel. no. 03–966 1111. — A

Rimer Birlec Ltd, Melingriffith Works, Whitchurch, Cardiff CF4 7XT. Tel. no. 0222 63205. — J

Key

Rotameter. KDG Flowmeters, Rotameter Works, 330 Purley Way, Croydon, Surrey CR9 4PG. Tel. no. 01–688 3816. — Q

Rusch. Willy Rusch, PO Box 1620, D–7050 Waiblingen, West Germany. Tel. no. 07151 405–1/406–0. — N, T

Scott's Electrical. Scott-Western Ltd, Dalling Road, Branksome, Poole, Dorset BH12 1DJ. Tel. no. 0262 766066. — K

Tricomed Ltd, 5–7 Sydenham Road, London SE26 5ET. Tel. no. 01–778 1165. — G, V

Warne Surgical Products Ltd, Walworth Road, Andover, Hants. SP10 5BG. Tel. no. 0264 4261. — N, T

Whitley. Don Whitley Scientific Ltd, Green Lane, Baildon, Shipley, West Yorkshire BD17 5JS. Tel. no. 0274 595728. — L

Key to the principal products of the companies listed

A Analysers (gas and vapour)
B Bacterial filters, etc.
C Cylinders, etc. of medical gases
D Dental anaesthetic equipment
E Educational products
F Fluidic and pneumatic equipment
G General range of anaesthetic equipment
H Humidifiers
I Fibreoptic instruments
J Oxygen concentrators
K Sterilizing equipment
L Leak detectors
M Monitors
N Disposables
O Oxygen analysers
P Medical gas and vacuum pipelines
Q Flowmeters
R Resuscitation equipment
S Suction equipment
T Endotracheal tubes, etc.
U Scavenging equipment
V Ventilators
W Vaporizers
X Pressure transducers
Y Sundry instruments and aids

Further Reading

Adams A.P. & Henville J.D. (1977) A new generation of anaesthetic ventilators. *Anaesthesia*, 32: 34–40.

Aldrete J.A., Lowe H.J. & Virtue R.W. (Eds) (1979) *Low Flow and Closed System Anaesthesia*. London: Academic Press.

Anderson P.K. (1981) Control of carbon dioxide in modified Mapleson A and D (Hafnia) anaesthetic systems. An experimental model. *Acta Anaesthesiologica Scandinavica*, 25: 344–348.

Atkinson R.S., Rushman G.B. & Lee J.A. (1982) *Synopsis of Anaesthesia: General Anaesthesia, Regional Analgesia, Intensive Therapy*, Ninth Edition. Bristol: Wright PSG.

Austin J.C., Shaw R., Crichton R., Cleaton-Jones P.E. & Moyes D. (1978) Comparison of sampling techniques for studies of nitrous oxide pollution. *British Journal of Anaesthesia*, 50: 1109–1112.

Bain J.A. & Spoerel W.E. (1972) A streamlined anaesthetic system. *Canadian Anaesthetist's Society Journal*, 19(4): 426–435.

Boulton T.B. (1966) Anaesthesia in difficult situations, III. *Anaesthesia*, 21(4): 513–545.

Boulton T.B. & Cole P. (1966) Anaesthesia in difficult situations, I. *Anaesthesia*, 21(2): 268–276.

Boulton T.B. & Cole P. (1966) Anaesthesia in difficult situations, II. *Anaesthesia*, 21(3): 379–399.

Brancroft M.E., du Moulin G.C. & Hedley-Whyte J. (1980) The hazards of hospital bulk oxygen delivery systems. *Anaesthesiology*, 52: 504–510.

Campbell D.I. (1976) A new compact, versatile, fluidic controlled ventilator. *Anaesthesia and Intensive Care*, 4(1): 7–15.

Christensen K.N., Thomsen A., Hansen O. & Jorgensen S. (1978) Flow requirements in the Hafnia modifications of the Mapleson circuits during spontaneous respiration. *Acta Anaesthesiologica Scandinavica*, 22: 27–32.

Churchill-Davidson H.C. (Ed) (1984) *Wylie and Churchill-Davidson's Practice of Anaesthesia*, Fifth Edition. London: Lloyd-Luke.

Cohen E.N. (1980) *Anaesthetic Exposure in the Workplace*. Lancaster: MTP Press.

Cooper J.B., Newbower R.S., Long C.D. & McPeek B. (1978) Preventable anaesthesia mishaps. *Anaesthesiology*, 49: 399–406.

DHSS (1982) *Technical Information on Anaesthetic Gas Disposal Systems*. (D265/J01.)

Dinnick O.P. (1964) Deaths associated with anaesthesia. *Anaesthesia*, 19: 536–556.

Dinnick O.P. (1973) Hazards in the operating theatre. *Annals of the Royal College of Surgeons of England*, 52: 349–354.

Dorsch J.A. & Dorsch S.B. (1985) *Understanding Anaesthetic Equipment; Construction, Care and Complications*, Second Edition. Baltimore: Williams & Wilkins.

Duffin J. (1976) *Physics for Anaesthetists*. Springfield, Ill.: C.C Thomas.

Edwards G., Morton H.J.V., Pask E.A. & Wylie W.D. (1955) Deaths associated with anaesthesia. *Anaesthesia*, 11: 194–220.

Grant W.J. (1978) *Medical Gases. Their Properties and Uses*. Aylesbury: HM & M.

Gray T.C., Utting J.E. & Nunn J.F. (1980) *General Anaesthesia*, Fourth Edition (2 vols). London: Butterworths.

Green R.A. & Coplans M.P. (1973) *Anaesthesia and Analgesia in Dentistry*. London: H.K. Lewis.

Harrison G.G. (1978) Death attributable to anaesthesia. *British Journal of Anaesthesia*, 50: 1041–1046.

Helliwell P.J., Laws M.E., Newman T.H. & Williams S.R. (1965) The cleaning, disinfecting and sterilising of anaesthetic equipment at Guy's Hospital. *Anaesthesia*, 20(3): 334–339.

Hill D.W. (1970) *Electronics Measurement Techniques in Anaesthesia and Surgery*. London: Butterworths.

Hill D.W. (1980) *Physics Applied to Anaesthesia*, Fourth Edition. London: Butterworths.

Hoernes G. & Heilwell M.F. (1964) *Introduction to Boolean Algebra and Logic Design*. Maidenhead: McGraw-Hill (UK).

Holland R. (1970) *Safety in Operating Theatres*. Royal Australian College of Surgeons Seminar.

Holland R. (1970) Special committee investigating deaths under anaesthesia. Report on 745 classified cases 1960–8. *Medical Journal of Australia*, 1: 573–594.

Hopkin D.A.B. (1980) *Hazards and Errors in Anaesthesia*. Berlin: Springer-Verlag.

Jackson Rees G. & Cecil Gray T. (1981) *Paediatric Anaesthesia — Trends in Current Practice*. London: Butterworths.

Jenkins J.R.E. & Edgar W.M. (1964) Sterilisation of anaesthetic equipment. *Anaesthesia*, 19(2): 177–190.

Johnson & Johnson (1964) *The Concept of Sterility in Medical Products*. Slough: Johnson & Johnson.

Jones P.L. (1974) Some observations on nitrous oxide cylinders during emptying. *British Journal of Anaesthesia*, 46: 534–538.

Jowitt M.D. (1984) Anaesthesia ashore in the Falklands. *Annals of the Royal College of Surgeons of England*, 66: 197–200.

Kilpatrick A. (1979) *Practical Dental Anaesthesia*. Edinburgh: Churchill Livingstone.

Latham M.J. (n.d.) Bacterial removal efficiency of Pall Ultipor anaesthesia/breathing filter – BB50. *Pall Technical Report BM 20044*. Portsmouth: Pall Biomedical.

Leatherdale R.A.L. (1966) The EMO ether inhaler. *Anaesthesia*, 21(4): 504–512.

Macintosh R, Mushin W.W. & Epstein H.G. (1963) *Physics for the Anaesthetist*, Third Edition. Oxford: Blackwell Scientific.

Mapleson W.W. (1954) The elimination of rebreathing in various semi-closed anaesthetic systems. *British Journal of Anaesthesia*, 26: 323–332.

Mapleson W.W. (1960) The concentration of anaesthetics in closed circuits, with special reference to halothane. *British Journal of Anaesthesia*, 32: 298–309.

Medishield (1980) *General Information: Medical Gas and Cylinders*. Harlow, Essex: Medishield.

Morris L.E. (1974) The circulator concept. *International Anaesthetic Clinics*, 12(3): 181–198.

Mushin W.W., Rendell-Baker L., Thompson P.W. & Mapleson W.W. (1980) *Automatic Ventilation of the Lungs*, Third Edition. Oxford: Blackwell Scientific.

Naimby-Luxmore R.C. (1967) Some hazards of dental gas machines. *Anaesthesia*, 22: 595.

Neff W.B., Burke S.F. & Thompson R. (1968) A Venturi circulator for anaesthetic systems. *Anaesthesiology*, 29(4): 838–841.

Norgren Fluidics (n.d.) *Introduction to Digital Fluidics*. Shipston on Stour, Warks.: Norgren.

Padmore G.R.A. & Nunn J.F. (1974) SI units in relation to anaesthesia. *British Journal of Anaesthesia*, 46: 236–243.

Parbrook G.D., Davis P.D. & Parbrook E.O. (1982) *Basic Physics and Measurement in Anaesthesia*. London: Heinemann Medical.

Penlon (1975) *Instruction Booklet: EMO Outfits and EMO Ether Inhaler*. Abingdon, Oxon.: Penlon.

Portex (n.d.) *The Sterilisation of Plastics*. Hythe, Kent: Portex.

Rees G.J. & Gray T.C. (1981) *Paediatric Anaesthesia: Trends in Current Practice*. London: Butterworths.

Revell D.G. (1959) A circulator to eliminate mechanical dead space in circle absorption systems. *Canadian Anaesthetists' Society Journal*, 6(2): 98–103.

Rosen M. & Hillard E.K. (1960) The use of suction in clinical medicine. *British Journal of Anaesthesia*, 32: 486–503.

Samson H.H. & Moyes D.G. (1980) Valveless anaesthetic circuits incorporating scavenging. *South African Medical Journal*, 57: 955–958.

Schrieber P. (1972) *Anaesthetic Equipment: Performance, Classification and Safety*. Berlin: Springer-Verlag.

Scurr C. & Feldman S. (Eds) (1982) *Scientific Foundations of Anaesthesia*, Third Edition. London: Heinemann Medical.

Stark D.C.C., Green C.A. & Pask E.A. (1962) Anaesthetic machines and cross-infection. *Anaesthesia*, 17(1): 12–20.

Stenqvist O. & Sonander H. (1984) Rebreathing characteristics of the Bain circuit. An equipment and theoretical study. *British Journal of Anaesthesia*, 56: 303–309.

Sykes M.K., Vickers M.D. & Hull C.J. (1981) *Principles of Clinical Measurement*. Oxford: Blackwell Scientific.

Thomas K.B. (1975) The Development of Anaesthetic Equipment. Oxford: Blackwell Scientific.

Thomsen A. & Jorgensen S. (1976) The Hafnia A Circuit. *Acta Anaesthesiologica Scandinavica*, 20: 395–404.

Utting J.E., Gray T.C. & Shelley F.C. (1979) Human misadventure in anaesthesia. *Canadian Anaesthetists' Society Journal*, 26(6): 472–478.

Vickers M.D. (1970) Explosion hazards. *Anaesthesia*, 25: 482.

Vickers M.D. (1971) Explosion hazards. *Anaesthesia*, 26: 155.

Ward C.S. (1968) The prevention of accidents associated with anaesthetic apparatus. *British Journal of Anaesthesia*, 40: 692–701.

Ward C.S. (1968) Oxygen warning device. *British Journal of Anaesthesia*, 40: 907–908.

Ward C.S. (1981) *Electrical Safety in Hospitals*. London: Henry Kimpton.

Wyant G.M. (1978) *Mechanical Misadventure in Anaesthesia*. Toronto: University of Toronto Press.

Wylie W.D. (1975) 'There, but for the grace of God . . .' Eighteenth Joseph Clover lecture. *Annals of the Royal College of Surgeons of England*, 56: 171–180.

Health Technical Memoranda (formerly Hospital Technical Memoranda) of interest to anaesthetists

HTM 1	Anti-static precautions: rubber, plastics and fabrics
HTM 2	Anti-static precautions: flooring in anaesthetising areas
HTM 7	Electrical services: supply and distribution
HTM 8	Safety code for electro-medical apparatus
HTM 11	Emergency electrical services
HTM 22	Piped medical gases, medical compressed air and medical vacuum installations
HTM 22 (Suppl.)	Permit to work system: for piped medical gases, medical compressed air and medical vacuum installations

HTMs are published by HM Stationery Office. A full catalogue of all Department of Health and Social Security documents is available in the form of: *Works Guidance Index*, published yearly by the DHSS, Euston Tower, 286 Euston Road, London NW1 3DN.

Some British and other Standards of interest to anaesthetists

Anaesthetic airways 6153
Anaesthetic breathing bags, rubber 3353
Anaesthetic and analgesic machines, on demand type 4272 (two parts)
Endotracheal tubes 3487
Safety of medical electrical equipment 5724 part 1
Medical gas cylinders 1319
Medical gas pipeline systems 5682
Anti-static flexible products 2050 and 2044
Medical vacuum pipeline services for use in hospitals 4957
Surgical suction apparatus electrically operated (high and low pressure and displacement) 4199 parts 1 and 2
Breathing attachments for anaesthetic apparatus 3849
Bourdon tube pressure and vacuum gauges 1780
Tracheostomy tubes and connections 6149 part 1
A glossary of terms used in anaesthesia 6015

A full list of British Standards may be found in the BSI catalogue published by the British Standards Institution, 197 Pentonville Road, London N1. This catalogue also gives the equivalent ISO standards.

Also of interest
ISO 5358 Continuous flow inhalational anaesthetic apparatus (anaesthetic machines) for use with humans

American National Standard ANSI Z89.8–1979 Minimum performance and safety requirements for components and systems of continuous-flow anaesthetic machines for human use. (This is published by the American National Standards Institute Inc, 1430 Broadway, New York, New York 10018, USA).

Index